T0228020

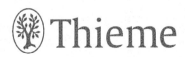

The Wills Eye Handbook of Ocular Genetics

Alex V. Levin, MD, MHSc, FRCSC
Chief
Pediatric Ophthalmology and Ocular Genetics
Robison D. Harley, MD Endowed Chair
Pediatric Ophthalmology and Ocular Genetics
Wills Eye Hospital
Philadelphia, Pennsylvania

Mario Zanolli, MD
Facultad de Medicina Clínica Alemana de Santiago
Universidad del Desarrollo
Santiago, Chile
Former Fellow of Ocular Genetics
Wills Eye Hospital
Philadelphia, Pennsylvania

Jenina E. Capasso, MS, LCGC
Licensed Certified Genetic Counselor
Wills Eye Hospital
Philadelphia, Pennsylvania

Thieme
New York • Stuttgart • Delhi • Rio de Janeiro

Executive Editor: William Lamsback
Managing Editor: Elizabeth Palumbo
Director, Editorial Services: Mary Jo Casey
Assistant Managing Editor: Haley Paskalides
Production Editor: Sean Woznicki
International Production Director: Andreas Schabert
Editorial Director: Sue Hodgson
International Marketing Director: Fiona Henderson
International Sales Director: Louisa Turrell
Director of Institutional Sales: Adam Bernacki
Senior Vice President and Chief Operating Officer:
  Sarah Vanderbilt
President: Brian D. Scanlan

Library of Congress Cataloging-in-Publication Data

Names: Levin, Alex V., 1957- author. | Zanolli, Mario, author.
  | Capasso, Jenina, author. | Wills Eye Hospital
  (Philadelphia, Pa.)
Title: The Wills Eye handbook of ocular genetics / Alex V.
  Levin, Mario Zanolli, Jenina Capasso.
Other titles: Handbook of ocular genetics
Description: New York : Thieme, [2018] | Includes
  bibliographical references.
  Identifiers: LCCN 2017035629 (print) | LCCN 2017037367
  (ebook) | ISBN 9781626232945 (e-book) |
  ISBN 9781626232938 (print)
Subjects: | MESH: Eye Diseases, Hereditary–genetics |
  Eye Diseases, Hereditary–therapy
  Classification: LCC RE48 (ebook) | LCC RE48 (print) |
  NLM WW 140 | DDC
  617.7/042–dc23
LC record available at https://lccn.loc.gov/2017035629

© 2018 Thieme Medical Publishers, Inc.

Thieme Publishers New York
333 Seventh Avenue, New York, NY 10001 USA
+1 800 782 3488, customerservice@thieme.com

Thieme Publishers Stuttgart
Rüdigerstrasse 14, 70469 Stuttgart, Germany
+49 [0]711 8931 421, customerservice@thieme.de

Thieme Publishers Delhi
A-12, Second Floor, Sector-2, Noida-201301
Uttar Pradesh, India
+91 120 45 566 00, customerservice@thieme.in

Thieme Revinter Publicações Ltda.
Rua do Matoso, 170
Rio de Janeiro, RJ, CEP 20270-135, Brasil
+55 21 2563 9700

Cover design: Thieme Publishing Group
Typesetting by Thomson Digital, India

Printed in the United States by King Printing   5 4 3 2 1

ISBN 978-1-62623-293-8

Also available as an e-book:
eISBN 978-1-62623-294-5

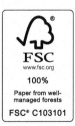

We offer our deepest thanks to the families who allowed us the privilege of participating in their ocular genetic care, as well as our own families who accompanied us in the writing of this book, which we hope will better the care of patients with ocular genetic disorders. We thank our spouses and children for the borrowed time that was used to write this book. At the end of the day, it is about patients and families, all of them.

Contents

Preface

Ocular genetics is an emerging subspecialty of ophthalmology. At the time of this writing, it is estimated that there are only 70 to 80 ocular geneticists in the world. Yet, the world of genetics continues to evolve at a rapid pace. Virtually every issue of every journal in ophthalmology contains articles with genetic relevance. Genetic eye disease is one of the leading causes of blindness worldwide. Genetic factors also have influence on ocular infection, inflammation, wound healing, and disorders such as retinopathy of prematurity or other acquired disorders. This leaves every ophthalmologist with the task and burden of obtaining some mastery within the realm of ocular genetics.

Ocular genetics sometimes may seem like a confusing realm, difficult to understand and connect to our common clinical practice. With an explosion of information and technology in almost every facet of ophthalmology, learning genetics can be daunting. The Wills Eye Handbook of Ocular Genetics was written to assist ophthalmic practitioners at every level and from every specialty on this path. Our goal was to provide a basic, yet detailed, reference for a variety of ocular genetic conditions that would serve to increase the reader's fund of knowledge while also giving the reader a practical approach to diagnosis and differential diagnosis. Each chapter offers background information on ocular genetic disease, which is then linked to modern genetic concepts relevant to the disease with pathways to attain the correct diagnosis while considering pitfalls and pearls along the way. Each topic then concludes with questions and answers to allow the reader to test their knowledge in real-life practical scenarios that they may face in clinical practice. This leaves the reader with a basic knowledge of genetics that they can then apply to a wide variety of ocular genetic disorders while assisting their patients attain diagnosis and receive appropriate genetic counseling.

We need more ocular geneticists in the world. This book is not intended to replace the few fellowship training opportunities that currently exist. The services of an ocular geneticist and genetic counselor will remain essential. Rather, this book is designed to help the nonocular geneticists to navigate the complicated world of ocular genetics in a fashion that will allow them to provide practical basic understanding and care to their patients with ocular genetic disease. Likewise, clinical geneticists will also continue to play a critical role in the management of patients with genetic disorders, especially those systemic disorders with ocular manifestations (such as neurofibromatosis) that are largely excluded from this textbook due mainly to the vast amount of information that would need to be covered. Ophthalmologists and other nongenetic professionals must continue to use consultation with ocular geneticists, clinical geneticists, and genetic counselors to provide advanced-level sophisticated genetic care to their patients. This book will allow the nongeneticists to have some mutual understanding to enhance and optimize these collaborations.

Ocular genetics is about patients and their families. Although the diseases are fascinating, so much more than information is part of the world of affected individuals. Counseling must address the issues such as reproduction, emotions surrounding a genetic diagnosis, prognosis, and future options. Care inevitably extends beyond the probands into their families where there may be individuals affected genetically or emotionally by the probands' disorder. As we are getting closer to a time when gene therapy or cell therapy will become a reality, patients want and need to know what possibilities there may be to prevent vision loss due to ocular genetic disease. Getting there will require the bringing together of patients with these rare disorders for research investigation as well as for mutual support. As ophthalmic practitioners become familiar with ocular genetic disease, they can better recognize these disorders and thus facilitate these efforts.

Contributors

Jenina E. Capasso, MS, LCGC
Licensed Certified Genetic Counselor
Wills Eye Hospital
Philadelphia, Pennsylvania

Christian R. Diaz, MD
Facultad De Medinina
Clnica Alemana De Santiago
Universidad De Desarrollo
Santiago, Chile

Vikas Khetan, MD
Senior Consultant
Department of Vitreoretina and Ocular Oncology
Chennai, India

Yu-Hung Lai, MD
Attending Physician
Department of Ophthalmology
Kaohsiung Medical University Hospital
Kaohsiung City, Taiwan
Assistant Professor
Department of Ophthalmology
School of Medicine
College of Medicine
Kaohsiung Medical University
Kaohsiung City, Taiwan

Alex V. Levin, MD, MHSc, FRCSC
Chief
Pediatric Ophthalmology and Ocular Genetics
Robison D. Harley, MD Endowed Chair
Pediatric Ophthalmology and Ocular Genetics
Wills Eye Hospital
Philadelphia, Pennsylvania

Michelle D. Lingao, MD Ophthalmologist
Asian Eye Institute
Department of Ophthalmology and Visual Science
University of the Philippines College of Medicine
Philippine General Hospital
Makati City, The Phillipines
Sentro Oftalmologicio Jose Rizal
PGH Compound
Manila, the Philippines

Juan P. López, MD
Department of Opthalmolgy
Universidad de Chile
Las Condes, Santiago, Chile

Jagadeesan Madhavan, MBBS, DO
Consultant
Dualhelix Genetic Diagnostics Private Ltd
Chennai, India

René Moya, MD
Assistant Professor
Opthalmology
Universidad de Chile. Department of
    Ophthalmology.
Centro de la Visión (CEV)
Santiago. Chile

Diego Ossandon Villaseca, MD
Clinica Alemanda De Santiago
Santiago, Chile

Pablo Romero, MD
Associate Professor
University of Chile-Clínica Alemana de Santiago
Vitacura, Santiago, Chile

Carol L. Shields, MD
Director
Ocular Oncology Service
Wills Eye Hospital
Thomas Jefferson University
Philadelphia, Pennsylvania

Mario Zanolli, MD
Facultad de Medicina Clínica Alemana de Santiago
Universidad del Desarrollo
Santiago, Chile
Former Fellow of Ocular Genetics
Wills Eye Hospital
Philadelphia, Pennsylvania

1 Basic Genetics

Abstract

Understanding the underlying mechanisms related to deoxyribonucleic acid (DNA) structure and function allows us to use and interpret genetic testing, which in turn helps diagnose and treat human genetic diseases. Genes serve to create proteins, whereas other DNA sequences are transcribed into RNA (ribonucleic acid), which itself may have a regulatory function. Molecular genetic testing has become an important tool in clinical medicine.

Keywords: deoxyribonucleic acid, gene, ribonucleic acid, protein, mutation, pathogenic variant, polymorphism

Key Points

- A gene is a region of DNA, composed of nucleotides, that is structured to serve the special function of making RNA, which may then be translated into protein.
- When a change in the nucleotide sequence leads to a structural or functional disruption of a gene, an associated clinical abnormality, it is called a mutation. Non–disease-causing variations in our gene sequences are called polymorphisms.

1.1 What is DNA?

Deoxyribonucleic acid (DNA) is the basic blueprint for the creation and functioning of an organism. DNA is made up of the nucleotides adenine (A), guanine (G), cytosine (C), and thymidine (T). These nucleotides are lined up in such a way that reading three nucleotides at a time creates a genetic code. Each triplet, also known as a codon, encodes a specific amino acid for the resultant protein. Some triplets are known as stop codons, in that they instruct the body to stop reading the DNA at that point and thus end the process of making the protein. For example, "GAGAAACGGCACTAG" would be read in triplets, where GAG codes for glutamine, AAA for lysine, CGG for arginine, CAC for histidine, and TAG is a stop codon, thus stopping protein formation. DNA exists to make proteins. Proteins may be structural (e.g., collagen, fibrillin), enzymes for metabolic processes, or proteins that regulate other genes. Just as you are reading the words on this page from left to right, a molecule of DNA is said to be oriented from its 5 prime (5') to 3' end and is read in that direction.

Some DNA sequences do not encode for proteins. In the past, these areas of the genome were referred to as "junk DNA," but today it is well established that many of these sequences have important functions, including sequences for ribonucleic acid (RNA) molecules that play a role in transcription, translation, and post-translational protein modification.

1.2 What is a Gene?

A gene is a region of DNA that is structured to serve the special function of making RNA and then, usually, a protein. Humans each have approximately 20,000 to 25,000 genes distributed throughout 23 pairs of chromosomes. Chromosomes are identified by number: from largest (1) to smallest (22) with two additional sex chromosomes, X and Y. The first 22 chromosomes are known as autosomes. We have two copies of each autosome. Additionally, females have two X chromosomes, and males have one X and one Y chromosome. Each copy of a pair is called an allele. Each chromosome contains thousands of genes. Each chromosome pair has the same genes although the sequence of each copy of the gene may be different. Each cell in our body, no matter what tissue we are speaking of, has the same chromosomes and the same genes. The difference is that different genes are expressed, or activated, in different tissues. For example, a phototransduction protein is turned off in the lateral rectus but turned on in cells of the retina. Some genes are used in multiple tissues (e.g., the gene that encodes the protein fibrillin), whereas others are more specific to a single tissue.

1.3 What is RNA: Transcription and Translation?

DNA is *transcribed* into messenger RNA (mRNA), a single chain made up of the same nucleotides, with the exception of thymidine, which is replaced by uracil (U). The enzyme RNA polymerase catalyzes synthesis of RNA from DNA. Enzymes may modify RNA after it is transcribed from DNA. Each mRNA sequence is created by reading the DNA 3' to 5' strand of the double helix and assembling corresponding complement RNA nucleotides. Given that the 3' to 5' strand is transcribed, the mRNA strand should directly correspond to the sequence of the 5' to 3' DNA strand.

mRNA is converted to protein by the process of *translation*. Like DNA, the nucleotides of mRNA are read in triplets, each of which codes for one amino acid. As there are 22 possible amino acid choices and a greater number of triplet possibilities (considering the permutations of the four nucleotides), there is redundancy such that more than one triplet can code for the same amino acid. mRNA is decoded by ribosomes, which are made up of ribosomal RNA (rRNA), to produce a specific amino acid chain that will fold into an active protein. Transfer RNA (tRNA) delivers amino acids to the ribosome where they are linked together to form the protein as the mRNA is being read.

Some RNA molecules are not translated into protein. These are called noncoding RNAs. Examples include tRNA and rRNA. Micro-RNAs (miRNAs) and short interfering RNA (siRNA) are other noncoding RNAs that are involved in regulation of gene expression.

1.4 Introns and Exons

Genes have a characteristic structure. *Exons* are the parts of the gene transcribed into the mRNA product of that gene, and then subsequently translated into protein. A gene can have just a few exons or dozens. *Introns* are noncoding nucleotide sequences that occur between exons of a single gene. They are transcribed but not translated. Although they do not code for the final gene product, introns are involved with ensuring the proper processing of mRNA, which results in the joining together of transcribed exons on either side of the intron. This process is called splicing. The exon–intron junctions are known as the donor site (5' end) and acceptor site (3' end), representing the end of one exon and the beginning of the next exon, respectively. Alternative splicing can generate multiple different functional proteins from a single gene, referred to as isoforms.

A promoter is an area of DNA, usually upstream (5') from a gene, which is transcribed to produce RNA, and potentially a protein, that initiates and/or regulates RNA transcription of that gene. Promoters are usually 100 to 1,000 nucleotides long.

1.5 Protein Functions: Building Blocks versus Enzymes versus Transcription Factors

Genes that code for proteins have different functions. Some proteins have structural functions, such as myosin, fibrillin, and the many collagens. Other proteins are enzymes that catalyze biochemical reactions such as rhodopsin in phototransduction or rhodopsin kinase. Other genes, sometimes referred to as developmental genes (their expression is necessary in embryonic development), encode proteins that act as transcription factors, which regulate the expression of other genes. Structural genes and genes that encode enzymes are like the instruments in an orchestra. They require a conductor to function in harmony, being expressed at the right time in the right places. Genes that encode transcription factors serve as the conductor by turning on and off other genes in the appropriate places at the correct times.

Every gene is present in every cell of the body, but only certain genes are being used (expressed) in certain cells, thus allowing for unique cell identity. Genes that are used to make a photoreceptor may not be used in the liver and vice versa. Some genes are used in more than one tissue. For example, genes that are involved with the maintenance and function of cilia are expressed in the retina and may also be used in adipose cells, brain cells, and tissues involving hair cells in the ears. When mutated, the resulting disorder may have features involving all of these tissues as seen in Bardet–Biedl syndrome: retinitis pigmentosa, obesity, developmental delay, hearing loss, and other findings. The expression in multiple tissues may be necessary because the structural protein is used in each tissue (e.g., fibrillin in the lens zonules and the aorta) or because a transcription factor regulates different genes in different cells.

1.6 Types of Mutations

A change in the nucleotide sequence that leads to a structural or functional disruption of a gene product is called a mutation if there is an associated clinical abnormality. A mutation may involve only one nucleotide (point mutations) or more than one. A missense mutation occurs when the change in a nucleotide results in a different amino acid in the protein primary structure. A nonsense mutation occurs when a nucleotide change causes a codon to change from one that codes for an amino acid to one that indicates protein production to stop, known as a stop codon, thus truncating the protein. There can also be nucleotide insertions or deletions, which cause the reading frame to be shifted (frameshift mutation), resulting in an entire change in amino acids for a whole segment of the protein thereafter until it eventually comes to a stop. Having such a jumbled protein is usually deleterious. Mutations can also be an alteration in chromosomal structure, thus affecting the ability of one or more nearby genes to function normally. One example is the increase in the number of repetitive sequences known as triplet repeats (e.g., CAGCAGCAG) that may normally be present in a gene. This repeat expansion can cause the gene to malfunction, depending on the size of the expansion.

A somatic mutation is one that occurs in a somatic cell, any cell after the fertilized egg (zygote) begins to divide into progeny cells. All descendants of the cell carrying the new mutation will also harbor that mutation. The earlier in development the mutation occurs, the larger the number of cells that are affected. When a person has a mutation confined to a population of cells that derived from a cell that experienced a somatic mutation, the individual has somatic mosaicism: one population of cells with the

3

mutation and the remainder without. A germline mutation originates in a gamete (sperm or egg) so that it is present in the zygote and therefore in all cells in the body. Germline mosaicism may also occur, in which case only some of the egg or sperm population of the transmitting parent has the mutation. Germline mutation is required to transmit a mutated gene to offspring. Somatic mutations are usually not heritable. However, it is possible an individual exhibiting somatic mosaicism in multiple tissues may have mosaicism for their mutation in their gonadal tissue as well and would therefore have a risk of transmitting their mutation to their offspring.

1.7 Mutation versus Polymorphism

Despite all of the variations between us, it has been estimated that the difference between the DNA sequences of individuals is only 0.1%. This is equivalent to 30 million nucleotides. These differences in our gene sequences do not cause disease but result in normal human variation such as iris, skin and hair color, height, and variable facial features. Such non–disease-causing variations in our gene sequences are called polymorphisms. By definition, genetic polymorphism is a variant that occurs with a minimum frequency of 1% in a given population.

1.8 Genetic Heterogeneity, Phenotypic heterogeneity, Expressivity, and Penetrance

Genetic heterogeneity means that a single phenotype (e.g., retinitis pigmentosa) may be caused by a number of different genes. Conversely, phenotypic heterogeneity means that different mutations in the same gene may be associated with multiple diseases. For example, mutations in *ABCA4* can result in phenotypes such as Stargardt disease, retinitis pigmentosa, cone–rod dystrophy.

Variable expression refers to a difference in severity of the same disorder due to the same gene mutation between individuals. For example, in the same family we might see a patient severely affected with neurofibromatosis, while another is more mildly affected. This is presumably due to polymorphisms in other genes that cause the gene mutation to "act differently" in different people. Expressivity should not be confused with penetrance, which refers to the presence or absence of a particular clinical phenotype associated with a particular gene mutation. A person who has the gene mutation but shows no phenotype is termed "nonpenetrant."

1.9 Nomenclature

DNA variations are reported with specific notation. A deeper insight can be found at the Human Gene Mutation Database (HGMD) website (http://www.hgmd.cf.ac.uk/docs/mut_nom.html; last accessed July 2016). Changes in genes, which code for proteins, are designated with a "c" followed by the position number of the affected nucleotide in the gene and then the change at that position: c.192C>A, indicates that a cytosine is replaced by an adenine at the 192nd nucleotide position within this coding gene. If a nucleotide change occurs in exon–intron boundaries, a "+" (splice donor) or "–" (splice acceptor) notation can be seen. For example, 123+1C>T means substitution of thymidine for cytosine one nucleotide beyond the splice donor site, which starts at nucleotide 123 from the 3' end of the coding sequence of the gene. Likewise, 247–2A>G means substitution of guanine for adenine two nucleotides upstream from the splice acceptor, which ends at nucleotide number 247. In other words, the next exon begins at nucleotide position 247.

Protein variations are annotated with a "p" that stands for "protein" followed by the amino acid change and position of the change in the protein: p.Arg650Cys indicates that the amino acid arginine at position 650 in the protein is replaced by the amino acid cysteine. This is a missense mutation. The nomenclature proposed in the HGMD reports the same change using the single letter, which is designated for the amino acid: R650C indicating the change from arginine (R) to cysteine (C).

Nonsense mutations are annotated by the nucleotide change in the coding DNA, but the resultant truncation of the protein is indicated by using "X," "*," or "ter" for the result of the change. For example, c.374 C > G indicates that a cytosine is changed to a guanine at nucleotide 374 of the gene. If this was the last nucleotide in the codon TAC, which encodes for tyrosine, it would now be TAG, which is a stop codon. The resulting change in the protein would be denoted as Y109X, p.Tyr109*, or p.Tyr109ter, indicating that the tyrosine is no longer added to the protein at this position. Rather, the protein is truncated at this point in the amino acid chain (▶ Fig. 1.1). When there is an insertion of one or more nucleotides to DNA, the inserted nucleotides are indicated in the nomenclature. This can produce a change that may lead to a mutation. An insertion can also occur at the chromosome level, but instead of nucleotides, large pieces of chromosomes are inserted. On the other hand, a *deletion* is when a sequence of DNA or a piece of chromosome is missing, leading to an imbalance that may express as a mutation or absence of protein expressed by the genes that were deleted.

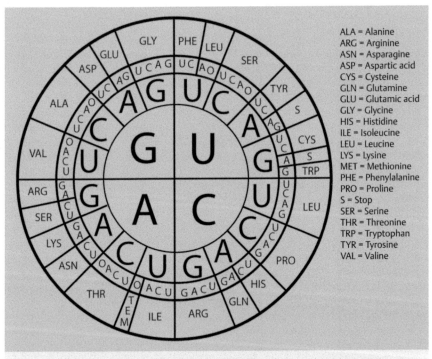

ALA = Alanine
ARG = Arginine
ASN = Asparagine
ASP = Aspartic acid
CYS = Cysteine
GLN = Glutamine
GLU = Glutamic acid
GLY = Glycine
HIS = Histidine
ILE = Isoleucine
LEU = Leucine
LYS = Lysine
MET = Methionine
PHE = Phenylalanine
PRO = Proline
S = Stop
SER = Serine
THR = Threonine
TRP = Tryptophan
TYR = Tyrosine
VAL = Valine

Fig. 1.1 Codon wheel, showing the combination of nucleotides to form different amino acids.

1.9.1 Frameshift Mutation

Frameshift mutation is a mutation caused by insertion or deletion of a number of nucleotides in a DNA sequence that cannot be divided by 3. This changes the reading frame, resulting in a different protein translation. The earlier the frameshift mutation, the more the protein is altered. It is also called a framing error or a reading frameshift. Frameshifts are designated by "fs" after the amino acid affected by the change. It can be "fs" only (short description) or "fs*#" (long description); the latter should include the change occurring at the site of the frame shift. The "*#" indicates at which codon position the new reading frame ends in a stop codon (*). The position of the stop codon in the new reading frame is found by starting at the first amino acid that is changed by the frameshift and following the new sequence to the first stop codon (*#). For example, p.Pro97Argfs*23 denotes a frameshift change with proline at amino acid location 97 as the first affected amino acid, changing into an arginine, and the new reading frame ends in a stop codon 23 codons after the beginning of the new reading frame.

When a gene has more than one mutation, the variants can be in *trans* or *cis*. Mutations in *trans* are present on separate alleles. Mutations in *cis* are present on the same allele. This becomes particularly important when considering the origin of the mutations. Mutations in *cis* are usually present on the allele inherited from one parent, whereas mutations in *trans* are usually inherited one from each parent. Knowledge of the inheritance pattern of a disorder and the position of the mutations identified in an individual is important in interpreting the significance of a person's gene test result.

1.10 Is There Gene Therapy for my Patient?

Gene therapy refers to any therapy based on repairing gene function, replacing gene products, manipulating genetic pathways, replacing genes, or otherwise treating the patient in a fashion that directly addresses the genetic defect. Alternatives to gene therapy may include symptomatic interventions (e.g., cataract surgery), stem cell delivery, or implantable electronic devices.

Ocular gene therapy includes intraocular delivery of DNA or other genetic material, repair mechanisms, or pathway manipulations. Genetic material is most often delivered using viral or nonviral mechanisms, which can carry genes or other molecules that interact with genes (e.g., transcription factors, siRNA). Viral vectors can transfect living cells to deliver the desired material, for example, DNA, which then incorporates into the host cell DNA or replicates using the viral systems. The desired effect could be blocking a dysfunctional gene, inserting a new functional gene, or repairing the malfunctioning gene.

The eye has many advantages for gene therapy: well-defined anatomy, immune privilege, easy accessibility of target cells (e.g., topical, intravitreal injection, subretinal injection), the ability to easily view and test the treated tissue effect directly, and the ability to use an untreated fellow eye as a comparative control. If the delivery is efficient, long-term gene expression is achieved, complications such as inflammation or infection are limited, and tissue function is improved, then gene therapy can be defined as a success.

In genetic disorders characterized by a loss of cells (e.g., photoreceptor death), there are few cells to act as target for gene therapy. In such cases, stem cell treatment or tissue transplantation may allow for cell replacement. Alternatively, artificial devices, such as implantable retinal chips, are beginning to show promise, although it does require inner retinal preservation.

As research advances and new trials and techniques become available, clinicians may find it difficult to keep up to date and knowledgeable in a way that patients may request in their search for therapies. A database of clinical studies can be found at www.clinicaltrials.gov. This web-based resource provides information for patients, families, health care professionals, and researchers. Clinicians can discuss with patients the basic concepts of enrolling in research trials. Clinical trials are conducted in a series of phases. Each is designed to answer a different research question. In Phase I studies, researchers test an intervention in a small group of people for the first time to evaluate its safety, determine a safe dosage and identify side effects. In Phase II, the treatment is given to a larger group of people to see if it is effective and to further evaluate its safety. Phase III studies confirm treatment effectiveness, monitor side effects, compare to commonly used treatments, and collect information that will allow the drug or treatment to hopefully proceed to clinical use. Finally, Phase IV studies are carried out after the drug or treatment has been marketed to gather information on the effect in various populations and any side effects associated with long-term use. In ophthalmology, experimental trials usually start with adults and eyes with very low vision. It is important that physicians use appropriate language in discussing the possibility of research options with families. Even the term "gene therapy" suggests a therapeutic intervention rather than research. Patients must know the implications and uncertainties of research.

We live in a time of exciting advances in the therapies for genetic disorders. Gene therapy, retinal chips, anti-VEGF (vascular endothelial growth factor) injection and other possibilities are becoming active therapeutic options. For young patients with retinal dystrophies, treatment will certainly occur within their lifetimes. A better understanding of the disease mechanisms that cause visual defects combined with the rapid advances in technology will be crucial to the development of effective treatments. Promising results for the treatment of Leber congenital amaurosis (LCA) due to *RPE65* mutations or choroideremia have been encouraging, although long-term follow-up shows a weakening of the improvement over time. In patients with LCA2 treated with recombinant adeno-associated virus 2/2 (rAAV2/2) vector carrying the *RPE65* complementary DNA, 3 years after therapy, improvement in vision was maintained, but the rate of loss of photoreceptors in the treated retina was the same as that in the untreated retina. Topographic maps of visual sensitivity in treated regions 6 years after therapy for two of the patients and 4.5 years after therapy for the third patient suggest progressive diminution in the areas of improved vision. Progress is so rapid that we do not include specific interventions for each disease covered in this book as it is likely that therapeutic options will occur so rapidly that the world will have changed significantly by the time the book is published. Clinicians are encouraged to consult online resources and consult with ocular geneticists to offer their patients the most current options.

1.11 Problems

1.11.1 Case 1

A 4-year-old male presents with high myopia, cleft palate, micrognathia, hearing deficiency, and a flat midface (▶ Fig. 1.2). He has had retinal detachment surgery of one eye. Slit-lamp examination of the anterior vitreous shows membranous and optically empty vitreous. The clinical features suggest a diagnosis of Stickler syndrome. Which of the following mechanisms best explains the pathophysiology of this disease?

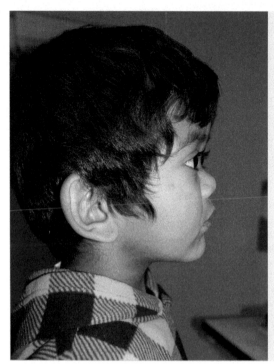

Fig. 1.2 Profile of a 4-year-old male patient with Stickler syndrome. Note the micrognathia and flat midface.

a) A change from a cytosine to an adenine at nucleotide 192 (c.192C > A) in the *COL2A1* gene results in a change from a cysteine to a tyrosine at amino acid position 57 (Cys57Tyr) in the collagen 2A1 protein, which renders the protein dysfunctional.

b) A change to uracil instead of thymine in the RNA made by the *COL2A1* gene causes the protein to be translated incorrectly.

c) The RNA sequence is created reading the 3' to 5' direction of DNA instead of the 5' to 3' direction, causing the protein to be jumbled and thus dysfunctional.

d) A nucleotide change in the intron of the *COL2A1* gene is incorrect, thus leading to a different amino acid in the collagen 2A1 protein.

Correct answer is a.

Stickler syndrome is a connective tissue disorder that can include ocular findings of myopia, cortical wedge-shaped cataracts, vitreous abnormalities, and retinal detachment. Systemic features include hearing loss, midfacial underdevelopment, cleft palate and/or bifid uvula, and joint abnormalities. It is caused by mutations in at least six different genes (*COL2A1*, *COL9A1*, *COL9A2*, *COL9A3*, *COL11A1*, and *COL11A2*).

a) **Correct.** This nucleotide change in a codon of an exon in *COL2A1* results in a change of the amino acid coded for by the triplet, which renders the protein dysfunctional.

b) **Incorrect.** Uracil is always used in RNA instead of thymine.

c) **Incorrect.** In mRNA transcription, DNA is always read in the 3' to 5' direction to create an mRNA 5' to 3' sequence.

d) **Incorrect.** Introns are transcribed but not translated as they are removed from mRNA before translation. Although mutations in introns can cause disease, they do so by altering mRNA splicing, which *indirectly* alters the protein that is subsequently made.

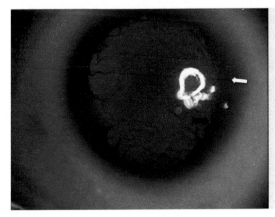

Fig. 1.3 Aniridia. White arrow indicates iris stub. Black arrow indicates lens edge. Note the multiple vessels of a persistent tunica vasculosa lentis that is sometimes seen in this condition.

1.11.2 Case 2

An 8-month-old patient is referred to you with regard to corneal haze in both eyes. You find corneal epithelial edema, enlarged corneal diameters, high intraocular pressure, no iris except for a tiny peripheral iris stub, macular hypoplasia, and nystagmus. Regarding the diagnosis of aniridia (▶ Fig. 1.3), which of the following mechanisms are likely to be the primary cause?

a) A structural protein that is used in different parts of the eye is not being produced properly, causing the anatomic eye abnormalities.

b) A mutation in a developmental gene impacts the expression of other genes in different parts of the eye during embryonal development.

c) A mutation in the *PAX6* gene, which codes for a critical enzyme for eye metabolism, results in abnormalities in multiple parts of the eye.

d) A gene is mutated that produces an abnormal protein that stops the cell cycle.

Correct answer is b.

Aniridia is usually due to a mutation in the *PAX6* gene. The *PAX6* gene belongs to a family of genes, called homeobox genes, which are transcription factors that play a critical role in the formation of tissues and organs during embryonic development. When *PAX6* is mutated, the expression of multiple other ocular genes is affected, resulting in an eye with multiple problems such as glaucoma, corneal disease, cataract, and macular hypoplasia in addition to the characteristic near absence of iris.

a) **Incorrect.** Aniridia is not the result of an abnormality in a specific structural protein, although multiple structural proteins may be abnormal as a result of the effect of the mutated *PAX6* gene on genes that encode for structural proteins.

b) **Correct.** Aniridia is usually caused by mutation in *PAX6*, a developmental gene, which affects the expression of many other genes in various parts of the eye during critical periods of embryonal development.

c) **Incorrect.** Aniridia is not the result of an abnormality in a specific enzyme, although multiple enzymes may be abnormal as a result of the effect of the mutated *PAX6* gene on genes that encode for enzymes.

d) **Incorrect.** *PAX6* does not exert its primary effect by arresting the cell cycle.

1.11.3 Case 3

A 5-year-old boy presented with ectopia lentis in both eyes. He has normal fingers, toes, and sternum without any signs of systemic disease and specifically no other manifestations of Marfan syndrome. Family history was positive for ectopia lentis in multiple family members on his mother's side, but not the patient's mother who is clinically normal. Eye examination of the mother was normal. Genetic testing revealed an *FBN1* mutation (c.1948 C > T, p.Arg650Cys). The mother was found to have the same mutation. How can one explain the unaffected mother?
a) Phenotypic heterogeneity.
b) Incomplete penetrance.
c) Genotypic heterogeneity.
d) Variable expression.

Correct answer is b.

Incomplete penetrance is a phenomenon where an individual with no signs of the disease has the gene mutation known to otherwise cause a phenotype. Nonpenetrance may also be a sign of age. For example, the mother may yet still develop ectopia lentis or aortic root dilatation at which point she would be penetrant.

a) **Incorrect.** Phenotypic heterogeneity refers to many different diseases being caused by mutations in the same gene. For example, a mutation in the *PAX6* gene may cause aniridia or autosomal dominant keratitis with a normal iris. *ABCA4* mutation can produce a wide range of disorders including Stargardt disease, retinitis pigmentosa, and cone–rod dystrophy.

b) **Correct.** As we can see in this pedigree, though the mother has the mutation, she does not exhibit the disease.

c) **Incorrect.** Genotypic heterogeneity refers to multiple possible genetic causes for a similar phenotype. Retinitis pigmentosa can be caused by mutations in many different genes. Likewise, features of Marfan syndrome can be seen as a result of mutation in either *FBN1* or *TGFβR2*.

d) **Incorrect.** Expression refers to the extent to which a genotype shows its phenotypic expression. In the same family, different individuals with Marfan syndrome may show varying severity of the aortic, skeletal, and ocular involvement as well as other manifestations, but some detectable clinical feature is always present.

1.11.4 Case 4

A 30-year-old male with night blindness is diagnosed with retinitis pigmentosa. Family history reveals that one brother, one sister, his father, and paternal grandmother are also affected. Genetic testing reveals a mutation in the *RHO* gene, which encodes for the protein rhodopsin (c.68C > A; p.Pro23His). Which of the following best corresponds to the mutation type?
a) Missense.
b) Deletion.
c) Nonsense.
d) It is not a mutation. It is a polymorphism.

Correct answer is a.

The DNA variation involves the substitution of a cytosine for an adenine at nucleotide number 68 in the *RHO* gene. This results in a proline being replaced by a histidine at the protein level. When a nucleotide change results in a disease-causing change in an amino acid in the protein, it is a missense mutation.

a) **Correct.** This is a missense mutation.

b) **Incorrect.** Frameshift mutations occur from insertions or deletions, resulting in a DNA read that is out of frame causing an entire change in the amino acids translated thereafter.

c) **Incorrect.** A nonsense mutation occurs when a nucleotide change causes a codon to change from one that encodes an amino acid to that of a stop codon.

d) **Incorrect.** This change has been well described in the literature as the most frequent mutation in the *RHO* gene that results in autosomal dominant retinitis pigmentosa.

1.11.5 Case 5

A 40-year-old female from Spain with night blindness, photophobia, and altered peripheral vision is diagnosed with retinitis pigmentosa. Family history reveals that her father is also affected. Genetic testing reveals a sequence change in the *CRB1* gene, reported as a variant of unknown significance that has not been reported previously (c.98C > A). Further testing reveals that her affected father does not have the change, but her mother, who is not affected (normal clinical examination and normal electro-retinography), has the same variation. The sequence change results in an isoleucine being replaced by a leucine at the protein level, which is predicted to be benign. Further testing revealed a known *RP1* gene mutation. The patient's affected father had the same mutation. Which of the following best describes the interpretation of the *CRB1* sequence change?

a) Mutation causing the disease.

b) Dysfunctional CRB1 protein.

c) Retinopathy due to abnormal transcription of the *CRB1* gene.

d) Polymorphism.

Correct answer is d.

In this case, the DNA variation involves the change of a cytosine for an adenine at nucleotide number 98 in the *CRB1* gene. The key finding is that this variation does not segregate with the disease: it is seen in both affected and unaffected individuals. Therefore, it cannot be the cause of the disease.

a) **Incorrect.** Although this is a missense change that results in a change of an amino acid in the protein, it does not segregate with the phenotype and thus is likely not related to the disease and more likely is a benign variant.

b) **Incorrect.** Although the protein now has one different amino acid, it is neither dysfunctional nor disease causing.

c) **Incorrect.** Transcription is not affected by this change. Transcription will proceed without dysfunction and the new mRNA will be corresponding to the new DNA sequence. As the sequence change does not segregate with the disease, it is not causing the retinopathy.

d) **Correct.** The most likely explanation is that this is a non–disease-causing polymorphism.

1.11.6 Case 6

A 35-year-old man comes to your office complaining of blurry vision in his left eye. You find that he has a retinal detachment. Family history reveals that his father had Wagner syndrome, which is a vitreoretinopathy due to abnormalities in the *VCAN* gene, which encodes the protein versican. In your patient's right eye you find moderate myopia, dotlike cortical cataract, perivascular pigmentation, and chorioretinal thinning, all of which are concordant with the diagnosis. Mutations in *VCAN*, which result in Wagner syndrome, are typically found in the splice acceptor or splice donor site. Which of the following is true?
a) Mutations that cause Wagner syndrome are typically located in intronic regions.
b) An intron is a section of the gene that codes for important parts of the final protein.
c) Splicing is the process that divides exons to help assemble the final protein.
d) Introns are located at the beginning and end of genes.

Correct answer is a.
   Wagner syndrome is characterized by optically empty vitreous and vitreous strands and veils, mild to severe myopia, cataract, and progressive chorioretinal atrophy. There is a high rate of retinal detachment. It is an autosomal dominant disorder. Mutations in *VCAN* that result in Wagner syndrome are typically found in the splice acceptor or splice donor site of introns 7 and 8 resulting in abnormal splicing of the exon products and a dysfunctional versican protein.
a) **Correct.** Mutations related to Wagner syndrome are typically found in the splice acceptor or splice donor site, which are found in introns.
b) **Incorrect.** Introns are nucleotide sequences that occur between exons within genes and are not translated into protein.
c) **Incorrect.** Splicing is the process that describes how introns are removed from the mature mRNA so that mRNA transcribed from intact exons is linked together.
d) **Incorrect.** Introns can be located between exons within a gene.

1.11.7 Case 7

Slit-lamp examination of a 55-year-old man shows keratoconus. He also has an anterior cortical cataract. Topography confirms keratoconus. Blood testing reveals a heterozygous substitution mutation in the gene *MIR184* at position number where there is an adenine instead of a guanine (+3A>G). *MIR184* is a gene located at 15q25.1, which encodes for a noncoding miRNA. Which of the following is correct?
a) The RNA created by all genes is translated into protein.
b) The mutation causes the gene to be transcribed correctly, but it is the tRNA that does not work well.
c) The mutation in this gene will lead to a different amino acid and thus abnormal protein function.
d) miRNA is not translated into protein but still affects the function of other genes.

Correct answer is d.
   The mutation described in this patient is associated with keratoconus and EDICT syndrome, an autosomal dominant syndrome characterized by **E**ndothelial **D**ystrophy, **I**ris hypoplasia, anterior polar **C**ataract, and **T**hinning of the corneal stroma.
a) **Incorrect.** Not every RNA is translated into protein.

b) **Incorrect**. A DNA gene mutation results in abnormal transcription to mRNA. tRNA is only involved if the mRNA is being translated into protein.

c) **Incorrect**. This is a gene that gets transcribed to mRNA, but that mRNA is never translated into amino acids as part of a protein.

d) **Correct.** Some RNA is not translated into protein but still has a positive or negative regulatory function on other genes. The mutation in this patient causes abnormal noncoding miRNA to be formed, which adversely affects the function of other genes, thus resulting in the phenotype.

1.12 Summary

Understanding the underlying mechanisms related to DNA structure and function allows us to use and interpret genetic testing, which in turn helps diagnose and treat human genetic diseases. Genes serve to create proteins, whereas other DNA sequences are transcribed into RNA, which itself has a regulatory function. Molecular genetic testing has become an important tool in clinical medicine.

Suggested Reading

[1] McAlinden A, Majava M, Bishop PN, et al. Missense and nonsense mutations in the alternatively-spliced exon 2 of COL2A1 cause the ocular variant of Stickler syndrome. Hum Mutat. 2008; 29(1):83–90

[2] Mukhopadhyay A, Nikopoulos K, Maugeri A, et al. Erosive vitreoretinopathy and Wagner disease are caused by intronic mutations in CSPG2/Versican that result in an imbalance of splice variants. Invest Ophthalmol Vis Sci. 2006; 47(8):3565–3572

[3] Lechner J, Bae HA, Guduric-Fuchs J, et al. Mutational analysis of MIR184 in sporadic keratoconus and myopia. Invest Ophthalmol Vis Sci. 2013; 54(8):5266–5272

[4] Iliff BW, Riazuddin SA, Gottsch JD. A single-base substitution in the seed region of miR-184 causes EDICT syndrome. Invest Ophthalmol Vis Sci. 2012; 53(1):348–353

[5] Bainbridge JW, Mehat MS, Sundaram V, et al. Long-term effect of gene therapy on Leber's congenital amaurosis. N Engl J Med. 2015; 372(20):1887–1897

[6] Jacobson SG, Cideciyan AV, Roman AJ, et al. Improvement and decline in vision with gene therapy in childhood blindness. N Engl J Med. 2015; 372(20):1920–1926

2 Inheritance Patterns

Abstract

Inheritance patterns describe the transmission of phenotypes within families. They are crucial for genetic counseling and diagnosis. Inheritance patterns reflect on the genetic basis for the disease and may involve one or more autosomal chromosomes, sex chromosomes, and/or the mitochondrial genome. Inheritance patterns include autosomal recessive, autosomal dominant, X-linked recessive, X-linked dominant, mitochondrial inheritance, and other infrequent patterns.

Keywords: inheritance pattern, pedigree, autosomal recessive, autosomal dominant, X-linked recessive, X-linked dominant, mitochondrial inheritance

Key Points

- Inheritance patterns describe patterns of transmission of specific phenotypes within families.
- Inheritance patterns include autosomal recessive, autosomal dominant, X-linked recessive, X-linked dominant, mitochondrial inheritance, and other less frequent patterns.

2.1 Introduction

Inheritance patterns show the transmission of determined phenotypes or diseases to offspring. The inheritance patterns will depend on whether the allele is found on an autosomal chromosome (chromosomes 1–22) or a sex chromosome (X or Y) and whether one or both alleles need to be mutated to result in a disease phenotype. Mutations in the mitochondrial genome have their own inheritance pattern.

2.2 Autosomal Recessive Inheritance

If a phenotype is only manifest when both copies of an autosomal gene are abnormal, then the condition is called autosomal recessive. Females and males are affected equally. When only one copy of the gene is affected (heterozygote), an individual is considered to be a carrier, and does not develop the disease, although they may have detectable signs of the carrier state such as reduction of an enzyme level in the blood (e.g., hexosaminidase A in Tay–Sachs disease), mild physical findings (e.g., mild iris transillumination in carriers of oculocutaneous albinism), or changes detectable only by other testing (e.g., mild electroretinogram (ERG) changes in carriers of autosomal recessive retinitis pigmentosa [RP]). The phenotype of the affected patient may depend on the nature of the mutation. If the mutation on each allele is identical, then the patient is homozygous. If the mutation on each allele is different, then the patient is a compound heterozygote.

The chance for parents that are both carriers of having an affected child is 25% for each pregnancy. There is a 50% chance with each pregnancy of having an asymptomatic carrier and 25% for a noncarrier. A carrier and an affected individual both have to mate with another carrier to have an affected child. Constricted populations in which couples are knowingly or unknowingly consanguineous or members of a constricted gene pool increase the possibility of autosomal recessive conditions. Although autosomal recessive pedigrees usually show more than one affected member in the same generation (e.g., siblings), in multiply consanguineous families, the likelihood that an affected individual will mate with a carrier is higher, thus leading to the transmission from one generation to the next, a pattern called "pseudo-dominant." Another characteristic of autosomal recessive disease in nonconsanguineous families is the wide separation of affected individuals often by many generations, as the chances of a carrier mating with another carrier is low. In nonconstricted gene pools, this chance is estimated to be less than 3%.

2.3 Autosomal Dominant Inheritance

If a condition is manifest in individuals that are heterozygotes for an autosomal gene abnormality, then the condition is autosomal dominant. Females and males are affected equally. The phenotype often appears in multiple generations, as each affected patient has a 50% risk with each pregnancy to have an affected child. Exceptions may be de novo mutations or cases in which the condition is not expressed (nonpenetrant) or is mildly expressed (variable expression) and therefore unknown. Clinically normal family members may have subclinical findings (e.g., peripheral ischemia seen only on fluorescein angiogram of autosomal dominant familial exudative vitreoretinopathy) and still transmit the full phenotype to their children. For example, neurofibromatosis type 1 is caused by heterozygous mutation in the gene *NF1* on chromosome 17. An intellectually normal parent may simply have Lisch's nodules of the iris and café au lait birthmarks of the skin, while their affected child might have these findings as well as severe developmental delay.

2.3.1 Dominant Negative Mutations

A mutation that leads to a mutant protein that disrupts the activity of the normal protein is a dominant negative mutation. This mechanism has been described in tumor suppressor genes.

2.4 X-Linked Recessive Inheritance

X-linked recessive phenotypes are not clinically manifest when there is a normal copy of the gene on one allele. In males, X-linked recessive disorders are clinically manifested because they have only a single copy of the X chromosome, and thus no normal copy of the mutated gene. Females are usually not affected by X-linked recessive conditions as they do have a normal copy of the mutated gene. It also may occur that a carrier has subtle or subclinical findings, such as electroretinogram mild scotopic alterations in a female carrier of X-linked recessive RP. If both copies of the gene are mutated, as seen in conditions where the population frequency of mutated genes is high (e.g., red–green color vision deficiency) or if there is skewed inactivation of the normal X chromosome, then a female may show a clinical phenotype.

In X-linked recessive disorders, there is no male-to-male transmission. All daughters born to an affected father will be carriers (heterozygous). A carrier female must conceive with an affected male to have an affected child. X-linked recessive disorders may also occur in males due to a de novo mutation. The pedigrees of families of X-linked recessive disease usually show unaffected heterozygous females as transmitting individuals with affected fathers and/or sons with only rare affected females.

2.5 X-Linked Dominant Inheritance

In X-linked dominant disorders, such as incontinentia pigmenti, only one copy of the mutated gene is needed to cause the disease. Therefore, heterozygous females and hemizygous males who have a single mutated gene on the X chromosome are affected. Males tend to be much more severely affected than the females and often die pre- or postnatally from the disease, as in incontinentia pigmenti. Males who survive may have XXY or other genotypes that provided them with a normal copy of the gene in addition to the mutated copy.

Each male and female offspring of affected females have a 50% risk of inheriting the condition. Like X-linked recessive, the pedigree is also characterized by not only the absence of male-to-male transmission, but also a preponderance of affected females and often a higher frequency of male fetus miscarriage.

2.6 Mitochondrial Disease

Mitochondria are organelles found in the cytoplasm of all cells. Mitochondria possess multiple copies of a circular deoxyribonucleic acid (DNA) strand that is different than nuclear DNA and encodes some of the transfer ribonucleic acid (tRNA) and proteins necessary for mitochondrial function. The primary function of mitochondria is the creation of energy for cellular metabolism. Thus, many diseases transmitted by mitochondrial inheritance affect multiple organs, especially those characterized with high-energy use such as the skeletal muscle, heart, or the eyes. Disorders of mitochondrial function may result from mutations in nuclear genes that encode proteins that are transported into the mitochondria. In this case, the inheritance pattern follows those patterns mentioned earlier. If the mutation is in a gene within the mitochondrial genome, then the typical maternal transmission pattern of mitochondrial inheritance applies. Some disorders, such as chronic progressive external ophthalmoplegia, may be inherited in more than one way.

Homoplasmy describes a cell whose copies of mitochondrial DNA (mtDNA) are all identical. Most mitochondrial mutations are heteroplasmic, meaning they only occur in some copies of mtDNA. The degree of heteroplasmy in specific tissues determines the phenotype. Only females can transmit a mitochondrial condition to offspring, because mitochondria are transmitted only from the egg. Male and female offspring are affected equally (with the unexplained exception of Leber hereditary optic neuropathy, which for unknown reasons affects males more than females). All children of females homoplasmic for a mutation will inherit the mutation. There is no male-to-male transmission. Females who are heteroplasmic for mitochondrial genome mutations will also pass them on to all of their children. However, the proportion of mutant mitochondria in the offspring, and therefore the expression and severity of disease, can vary considerably.

2.7 Other Patterns of Inheritance

2.7.1 Digenic

Monogenic inheritance refers to genetic expression of a phenotype by a single gene resulting in the patterns discussed earlier. Less frequently, the interaction of two genes is required for expression of a phenotype, which is known as digenic inheritance. In this situation, mutations in at least one copy of each gene are required for the expression of a phenotype. If the patient only has a mutation in one of the two genes, then they will be clinically normal. In RP, individuals with heterozygous ROM1 or PRPH2 mutations may be normal, but individuals who are heterozygous for both a ROM1 and a PRPH2 mutation have RP. Another example is Bardet–Biedl syndrome which may also occur as a result of digenic mutations (e.g., BBS2 and BBS6) or even triallelic mutations in which two mutations are found in one gene (compound heterozygote) and a third in a different gene.

Sometimes, one gene acts as a modifier of the other. In families with autosomal dominant primary glaucoma with both adult and juvenile onset, segregation of both MYOC and CYP1B1 mutations may be observed. All affected who carry the MYOC mutation have the adult onset form, and those with both MYOC and CYP1B1 mutations have the more severe juvenile presentation. Individuals carrying only a heterozygous CYP1B1 mutation are not clinically affected.

2.7.2 Polygenic

A polygenic phenotype is one that is influenced by more than one gene. Typical examples include height or skin color, which displays a continuous distribution. Many polygenic traits are also affected by the environment and are called multifactorial.

2.7.3 Multifactorial or Complex Inheritance Patterns

Many diseases and other phenotypes have multifactorial inheritance patterns. Examples include Alzheimer's disease, heart disease, obesity, diabetes, age-related macular degeneration, or even intelligence level. These conditions are not caused by a single gene mutation, but rather are a result of interaction between genetic and environmental factors. A mutation may predispose an individual to a disease, but does not directly cause the condition. Other factors contribute to whether or not the disease develops.

Because of this complexity, multifactorial conditions are more difficult to trace through pedigrees although they do have a higher prevalence in a given family. Diseases with complex inheritance often demonstrate familial segregation because relatives of a patient are more likely to have disease-predisposing alleles in common. However, relatives may still be discordant for phenotype. An example is the lack of identical phenotypes in monozygotic twins.

The underlying mechanisms by which genetic and environment factors interact are still largely unknown and may involve direct effects on DNA by external factors or effect on noncoding RNA. Thus, counseling is based on empirical estimates of recurrence risks. The recurrence risk is higher for first-degree relatives of affected family members than for more distant relatives. In general, the recurrence risk is also increased by the presence of more than one affected patient in a family, a severe form, or an early onset of the disorder.

2.7.4 Loss of Heterozygosity

If a patient has mutation in one copy of a gene that by itself does not cause disease, and then acquires a mutation of the remaining copy of that gene, the patient is said to have loss of heterozygosity (LOH) and becomes affected with the disease. This process is particularly common in tumors. Individuals with retinoblastoma who are heterozygous for an RB1 gene mutation only develop retinoblastoma when the second RB1 gene becomes abnormal in a retinal cell. LOH represents the "second hit" of the remaining allele. LOH may occur by interstitial deletion, mitotic recombination or nondisjunction. The tumors of neurofibromatosis and tuberous sclerosis are also examples of this phenomenon.

The initial abnormal gene is only transmitted to offspring if it is found in the sperm or eggs (germ line mutation) of the affected individual. The offspring would still need to acquire their own "second hits" to develop tumors. Therefore, the inheritance pattern is autosomal dominant although within the tumors, there is not a normal functioning copy of the gene.

2.7.5 Isoparental/Uniparental Disomy

This phenomenon occurs when a patient inherits both copies of all or part of a chromosome from only one parent with no contribution for that region from the other parent. Prader–Willi syndrome can result from paternal deletion or maternal uniparental disomy (UPD) of 15q11-q13, due to lack of allele inherited from the father. This region of the chromosome is imprinted (methylated) such that we only use the paternal allele. If there is no paternal allele, the disorder becomes manifest. Similarly, Angelman syndrome can happen from maternal deletion or paternal UPD of 15q11-q13, due to lack of allele inherited from the mother. Angelman locus within that region is imprinted such that we only use the maternal allele. UPD should be considered (1) in an autosomal recessive disorder with only one carrier parent (assuming correct paternity), (2) in a known syndrome with uncommon features to the disorder, (3) if the parent and patient have an autosomal recessive condition in the absence of consanguinity, and (4) in male-to-male transmission of an X-linked recessive disorder.

2.7.6 Mosaicism

When a patient has a chromosome abnormality, the abnormality is usually present in all of the cells of the body. However, if the chromosome aberration, or single gene mutation, occurs after fertilization in the developing embryo, only the cells that descend from the first abnormal cell will have the same karyotype. The individual thus has two (or more) different genetic complements. Only tissues with the aberration show signs of the clinical abnormality. This is called mosaicism. The earlier the mutation occurs in embryonic development, the more cells and tissues that will be affected. For example, although Sturge–Weber syndrome represents a somatic mosaic mutation in the GNAQ gene, which may occur late in development and thus only affect unilateral periocular skin (port wine birthmark) and the globe (glaucoma, choroidal hemangioma), if the mutation occurs early in embryogenesis, the child may have severe bilateral disease with extensive port wine birthmarks, severe developmental delays, seizures, and glaucoma. Mosaicism is confirmed by sampling more than one tissue for analysis (e.g., skin and blood).

A mosaic abnormality can only be passed to offspring if the aberration or mutation is also found in germ cells. Germ cells may also be mosaic for the change (germ line mosaicism). Although theoretically one could test sperm for the change, it is impractical to do so and eggs are inaccessible. Therefore, germ line mosaicism is implied through the pedigree. For example, if a mother has two children with a genetic disorder, by different unaffected fathers, but her blood tests negative for the mutation found in her two children, then we can presume that the mutation is in her eggs.

2.7.7 Trinucleotide Repeat Expansion

These conditions are defined by an expansion within the affected gene of a segment of DNA consisting of repeating units of three nucleotides in tandem. For example, the repeat unit often consists of a run of CCGs (CCGCCGCCGCCG). The number of repeats can increase from generation to generation, until the normal range is exceeded, causing a disruption of gene function. Examples are Huntington's disease, Fragile X syndrome, spinocerebellar ataxia with retinal dystrophy, and Fuchs' endothelial corneal dystrophy. Although the disorders are inherited in an autosomal dominant fashion, families may show anticipation, wherein the disease appears to be increasingly severe with each successive generation.

2.8 Problems

2.8.1 Case 1

A 15-year-old male with neurofibromatosis comes for genetic counseling. Clinical examination confirms the diagnosis. Family history reveals no history of consanguinity. According to the pedigree (▶ Fig. 2.1), which inheritance pattern is most likely?
a) Autosomal recessive.
b) Autosomal dominant.
c) X-linked recessive.
d) Mitochondrial.

Correct answer is b.

This pattern shows two affected generations, male-to-male transmission and individuals of both genders affected, which is compatible with autosomal dominant. The father seems to have a de novo mutation in *NF1* because his parents and their parents are unaffected.

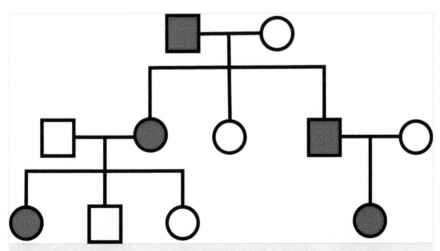

Fig. 2.1 A 15-year-old male with neurofibromatosis comes for genetic counseling. Clinical examination confirms the diagnosis. Family history reveals no history of consanguinity. According to the pedigree, which inheritance pattern is most likely?

a) **Incorrect.** Although the grandparents could be carriers, the father would need to conceive with a carrier to pass the condition, which is unlikely in the absence of a constricted gene pool (no consanguinity or common ancestry). In addition, the clinical diagnosis is neurofibromatosis, which is always an autosomal dominant disorder.

b) **Correct.**

c) **Incorrect.** Male-to-male transmission rules out X-linked inheritance.

d) **Incorrect.** Male-to-male transmission rules out mitochondrial inheritance.

2.8.2 Case 2

A 52-year-old female patient comes for genetic evaluation for a retinal condition. In this inheritance pattern (▸ Fig. 2.2), which mechanism best explains the proband's status?

a) Incomplete penetrance.

b) Variable expressivity.

c) Anticipation.

d) Mosaicism.

Correct answer is a.

Three generations with both genders affected raise the possibility of an autosomal dominant pattern of inheritance. The proband's mother does show clinical signs of the condition, as does the proband's son. Therefore, incomplete penetrance is suspected. Penetrance refers to individuals who are obligate carriers, or known by molecular testing, to harbor the mutation that causes the disease but do not develop any features of the disorder.

a) **Correct.**

b) **Incorrect.** The proband is asymptomatic. Variable expressivity refers to the range of signs and symptoms that *do* occur in different people with the same genetic disease.

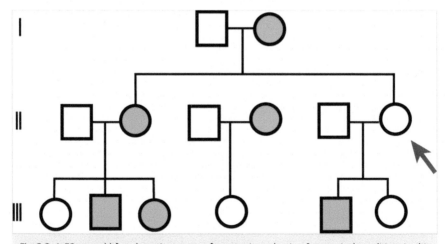

Fig. 2.2 A 52-year-old female patient comes for genetic evaluation for a retinal condition. In this inheritance pattern, which mechanism best explains the proband's status?

c) **Incorrect.** This is not the case. Anticipation is a phenomenon seen in conditions that develop from trinucleotide repeat expansion, where the disease appears to be increasingly severe with each successive generation. One would therefore expect the proband to be affected worse than her affected mother.

d) **Incorrect.** A patient with mosaicism will present with some phenotype in the tissues that have the mutation and often do not transmit as the mutation is not in their germ cells.

2.8.3 Case 3

Based on this pedigree (▶ Fig. 2.3) of a family affected by red–green color blindness, how is it that the proband is affected?

a) Consanguinity in an X-linked dominant condition.
b) Autosomal dominant with complete penetrance.
c) Autosomal recessive in a constricted gene pool.
d) Consanguinity in an X-linked recessive condition.

Correct answer is d.

This pedigree shows consanguinity in a family with an X-linked recessive condition, such as red–green color blindness. As a result, the affected female is homozygous for the mutation (both alleles are affected) having inherited one copy from her affected father and the other from her carrier mother.

a) **Incorrect.** In X-linked dominant disorders, males usually die or are very severely affected. Nonpenetrance in an obligate carrier, such as the paternal grandmother of the proband, is highly unusual.

b) **Incorrect.** Although the pedigree could support an autosomal dominant pattern of inheritance, the paternal grandmother of the proband would be nonpenetrant. We also know that red–green color deficiency is always X-linked recessive.

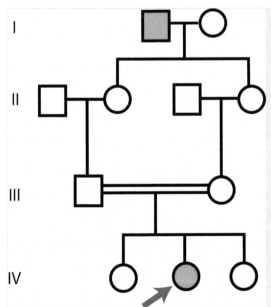

Fig. 2.3 Based on this pedigree of a family affected by red–green color blindness, how is it that the proband is affected?

c) **Incorrect.** Although this pedigree may represent an AR condition, the paternal grandfather would have to be a carrier. Without known consanguinity or a constricted gene pool, this would be highly unlikely. In addition, red–green gene color deficiency is always an X-linked recessive disorder.

d) **Correct.**

2.8.4 Case 4

A 36-year-old man comes for genetic consultation. His two children present a condition that is typically autosomal dominant (▶ Fig. 2.4), confirmed by DNA testing, but clinical and genetic testing was negative. What is the best explanation for this finding?

a) Mitochondrial.

b) Variable expressivity.

c) Anticipation.

d) Mosaicism.

Correct answer is d.

This pedigree shows affected siblings from different mothers with a clinically and genetically normal father. A probable explanation is mosaicism such that the mutations are only present in the father's germline tissues (sperm).

a) **Incorrect.** Males cannot transmit mitochondrial disorders to their children.

b) **Incorrect.** The father is asymptomatic and thus not expressing. If he had the mutation, he would be referred to as nonpenetrant. The terms expression and penetrant only refer to individuals who have the mutation in their blood.

c) **Incorrect.** Anticipation requires successive generations affected to increasing extents. In this pedigree, only one generation is affected.

d) **Correct.**

2.8.5 Case 5

In this family (▶ Fig. 2.5) with optic neuropathy, which inheritance pattern best describes the condition?

a) Autosomal dominant.

b) Mitochondrial.

c) Autosomal recessive.

d) X-linked dominant.

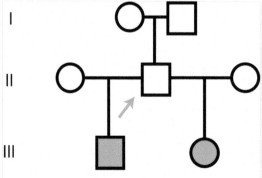

Fig. 2.4 A 36-year-old man comes for genetic consultation. His two children present a condition that is typically autosomal dominant confirmed by DNA (deoxyribonucleic acid) testing, but clinical and genetic testing was negative. What is the best explanation for this finding?

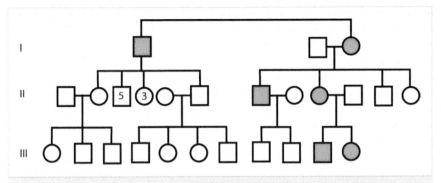

Fig. 2.5 In this family with optic neuropathy, which inheritance pattern best describes the condition?

Correct answer is b.

This pedigree shows that this condition is inherited through maternal lineage. No affected male transmits the disease, increasing the chances of mitochondrial disease.

a) **Incorrect.** Autosomal dominant inheritance has 50% chance of transmission with each pregnancy, yet the affected male in generation I had 10 children with none affected. The chance for this $(0.5)^{10}$.

b) **Correct.**

c) **Incorrect.** The affected woman in generation I as well as her affected daughter would have to conceive with carriers to have affected children. This is highly unlikely in the absence of consanguinity or a constricted gene pool.

d) **Incorrect.** Many affected males rule out X-linked dominant disease, which is usually lethal in males. In addition, the daughters of affected males would all be affected.

3 Genetic Testing

Abstract

Molecular genetic testing is a powerful tool for the care of patients with genetic ocular conditions. Benefits include confirmation or ruling out of an underlying genetic disorder and determining the risk of inheriting or transmitting a genetic disease. Before testing, considerations include the target and goal of testing, cost, availability, possible unintended outcomes, risks, limitations, and benefits. There are many forms of genetic testing and the choice of a specific test must be based on knowledge of the likely target finding. Result analysis and disclosure is a complex process that often requires an experienced genetics team.

Keywords: molecular genetic testing, karyotype, microarray, gene sequencing, deletion/duplication analysis, whole exome sequencing, whole genome sequencing

> **Key Points**
>
> - There are many forms of genetic testing. The choice of test must be based on knowledge of the likely target finding.
> - Test selection is based on a complete phenotype characterization and consideration of cost-effectiveness.
> - Result analysis and disclosure is a complex process that requires an experienced genetics team.

3.1 Introduction

Molecular genetic testing is one of the cornerstones for the care of patients with genetic ocular disease and their families. The results of these tests provide many benefits, including confirmation or ruling out of an underlying genetic disorder or helping to determine the risk of inheriting a genetic disease. With many options for studying the genetic etiology of a disorder, one should consider the target and goal of testing, cost, availability, possible unintended outcomes, risks, limitations, and benefits.

Molecular tests can range from the search for a specific mutation in a single gene to sequencing of the entire genome. Chromosomal tests analyze whole chromosomes or specific lengths of deoxyribonucleic acid (DNA) to identify deletions, duplications, or rearrangements of chromosomal material. Biochemical tests study the quantity or functional level of proteins, which can suggest causative DNA changes that result in a specific disorder.

Genetic testing is voluntary. Because these tests have benefits as well as risks, patients should always be well informed prior to the initiation of testing. A clinical/ ocular geneticist or genetic counselor can provide valuable information about the limitations, advantages and disadvantages of a particular test, risks (e.g., discovery of unreported nonpaternity, identification of a health risk unrelated to the indication for testing), and the potential social, insurance, and emotional implications of genetic testing. Counseling should also include information on the nature, inheritance, and implications of the genetic disorder for which testing is being ordered. Similar counseling should be performed after the results of the test become available.

3.1.1 Karyotype

Karyotype is a test performed with a light microscope, and describes the number and appearance of chromosomes in the nucleus of a eukaryotic cell (▶ Fig. 3.1). Chromosomes are removed from the nucleus at a specified stage of the cell cycle to allow for a desired length of chromosome and then stained with a variety of chemicals to create a characteristic banding pattern, which allows for identification of specific regions on each chromosome. Variables analyzed include large gains or losses of chromosomal material, chromosome number, alteration in chromosomal position or configuration, and the presence of satellite/marker material. To identify possible mosaicism, more than one cell is analyzed. A karyotype is requested when there is no specific recognizable single gene syndrome and more than two involved organ systems, when there is a phenotype that is specific for a chromosomal aberration (e.g., trisomy 21), or the family history suggests a chromosomal basis (e.g., multiple miscarriages due to unbalanced translocation).

3.1.2 Chromosomal Microarray

Chromosomal microarray (CMA) should be considered when a karyotype is normal, but the clinical picture is still highly suggestive of a chromosomal aberration. CMA is a microchip-based testing platform that allows high-volume, automated analysis of many segments of DNA at once. The entire nuclear genome can be screened for

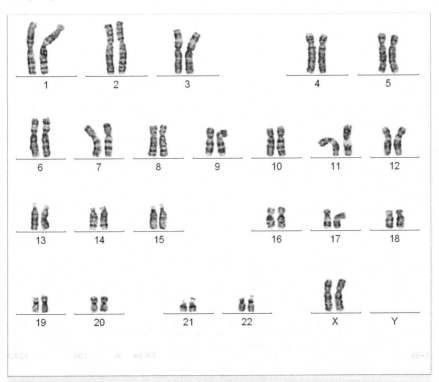

Fig. 3.1 Human female karyotype. (This image is provided courtesy of Silvia Castillo, MD.)

submicroscopic copy number variations (CNV): deletions or duplications. These changes are too small to be seen under a light microscope, but may contain multiple genes, and therefore lead to a disease phenotype. Internet databases allow the coordinates of an identified CNV to be entered and affected genes in the particular region are displayed (see section "Mutation and Copy Number Variation Databases"). Associated known phenotypes are also available in the medical literature. The physician then correlates these findings with the phenotype of an affected individual. Genes within the CNV may not be clearly related to the patient's condition, thus requiring further investigation. CMA may also detect regions of homozygosity, which may be suggestive of risk for recessive disease or imprinting disorders. CMA does not detect balanced translocations, sequence variations within a single gene, or low-level mosaicism (usually below 20%). There may also be intragenic deletions or duplications that are smaller than the resolution of CMA. Deletion/duplication analysis (del/dup) for intragenic changes too small for detection by CMA may be found using probe amplification methods. Deletion and duplication analysis should be considered when sequencing is negative but the clinical picture is very suggestive of a particular syndrome caused by mutations in that gene or when a mutation is found on only one allele for a presumed autosomal recessive disease.

3.1.3 Mutation and Copy Number Variation Databases (Accessed June 2016)

- LOVD: Leiden Open Variation Database:
  - http://www.lovd.nl/3.0/home.
- RetNet:
  - https://sph.uth.edu/retnet/.
- CentoMD:
  - https://info.centomd.com/.
- Retina International Mutation Database:
  - http://www.retina-international.org/sci-news/databases/mutation-database/.
- RetinoGenetics:
  - http://www.retinogenetics.org.
- Keio Mutation Databases: KmeyeDB:
  - http://mutview.dmb.med.keio.ac.jp/MutationView/jsp/index.jsp.
- University of California, Santa Cruz (UCSC) Genome Bioinformatics:
  - https://genome.ucsc.edu/.
- DECIPHER:
  - http://decipher.sanger.ac.uk.

3.1.4 Fluorescein In Situ Hybridization

Fluorescein in situ hybridization (FISH) involves the labeling of metaphase chromosomes with fluorescent probes that bind to specific target regions and thus identify if these regions are deleted or duplicated. The selection of FISH requires a known target region for examination as seen for conditions such as Prader–Willi/Angelman syndrome (del15q11-q13), 22q11 deletion syndrome (del22q11.2), Cri-du-chat syndrome (del5pter), retinoblastoma with systemic malformations (del13q14.1), or Wilms tumor, Anirida, Genitourinary anomalies, Retardation of growth and development, del(11)(p13) (WAGR) syndrome (del11p13). FISH has the advantage of being able to find abnormal cells more easily than standard cytogenetic methods, not requiring living cells and its ability to be quantified automatically. However, a trained technologist is required to distinguish subtle abnormalities.

3.1.5 Gene Sequencing

Gene sequencing is the test of choice when monogenic disease is suspected. Sequencing is the process of defining the precise order of nucleotides within the gene DNA. Sanger sequencing has been the "gold standard" method for many years. It is based on the selective incorporation of chain-terminating dideoxynucleotides by DNA polymerase during in vitro DNA replication. More recently, next-generation sequencing (NGS) methods have allowed for large-scale, automated gene studies including multigene panels where numerous genes can be sequenced in parallel. The Sanger method is still widely used for validation of next-generation results.

3.1.6 Whole Exome Sequencing

Whole exome sequencing (WES) is a technique for simultaneous sequencing of all known coding genes in the nuclear genome, using the NGS technology. This test could render a molecular diagnosis in the setting of a nonspecific phenotype or when standard diagnostic testing has been exhausted. It may also be cost efficient as compared to multiple specific tests. WES is only able to identify those mutations found in coding regions (although some protocols will involve some exon–intron boundaries or deeper intronic sequencing). Approximately 99% of the human genome is not covered using WES.

With WES and whole genome sequencing (WGS; see section "Whole Genome Sequencing"), there is potential for the recognition of incidental findings unrelated to the indication of the test, but which may or may not be valuable for the patient. The American College of Medical Genetics (ACMG) published a policy statement on clinical WES that emphasizes the importance of disclosing the possibility of such results in pretest patient counseling. A gene list of "medically actionable" genes requiring mandatory disclosure if mutated is provided (because of the potential for important preventative interventions). WES has the potential to uncover changes in many other genes as well, which may be unrelated to the patient's phenotype and not actionable. Therefore, most testing laboratories conduct a "filter" of the generated data such that results given to the patient, which are not on the ACMG mandatory disclosure list, are only for those genes felt to be potentially relevant to the phenotype. Another option offered by some laboratories for managing the risk of excessive and unwanted information is to create customized panels using exome testing that restrict result reporting to specific genes, a process very similar to the next-generation array sequencing panels.

3.1.7 Mitochondrial Genome Sequencing

Mitochondrial diseases are a heterogeneous group of disorders that arise as a result of dysfunction of the mitochondrial respiratory chain. They are associated with mutations of genes encoded by either nuclear DNA or mitochondrial DNA (mtDNA). There are different options for studying mitochondrial DNA, including specific panels (e.g., targeted sequencing for Leber hereditary optic neuropathy [LHON]), sequencing of the entire mtDNA, or whole mitome sequencing, which includes all mtDNA and nuclear genes that encode mitochondrial proteins.

3.1.8 Whole Genome Sequencing

WGS assesses the complete DNA sequence, including the noncoding regions. This is the most comprehensive test to analyze the genome. Dropping sequencing costs and large-scale data management makes WGS an emerging technology. In the future, WGS will likely guide "personalized medicine" wherein diagnostic services, therapeutic interventions, disease susceptibility, and drug response may all become available.

3.1.9 X Chromosome Inactivation

X chromosome inactivation studies are indicated when a female is suspected of manifesting clinical signs of an X-linked recessive disorder. The test assesses whether there may be unfavorable skewing of X chromosome inactivation such that a disproportionate number of cells are using the mutated X chromosome.

3.1.10 Methylation Studies

Methylation studies can reveal significant gene expression changes. This is particularly useful when considering uniparental disomy (isodisomy and heterodisomy), a condition in which an individual receives two copies of a chromosome (or part of a chromosome), from one parent and no copy from the other. This may lead to the expression of imprinting disorders including some cancers, Prader–Willi/Angelman syndromes, or rare autosomal recessive disorders.

3.1.11 Genome-Wide Association Study

In the field of genetic epidemiology, a genome-wide association study (GWAS) is an examination of frequent genetic variants in different individuals to see if there is an association with a trait. This approach reveals susceptibility loci for complex diseases, such as glaucoma or diabetes mellitus, and can provide insight into the allelic architecture of multifactorial traits.

3.1.12 Linkage Studies

Although linkage studies are uncommonly used today, this method uses blood from multiple family members, both affected and unaffected, to isolate an inherited segment of DNA, on a particular chromosome that is "linked" to the phenotype and thus presumably contains the causative mutated gene. Using statistical tests, such as the log of odds (LOD) score, one can assess the probability that the identified DNA locus is indeed the correct associated locus. The test is time-consuming and involves multiple family members, making it somewhat impractical in these days of high throughput sequencing, but it is a useful tool to help discover an otherwise unidentified gene that is mutated.

3.2 Interpreting Test Results by Michelle D. Lingao

The interpretation of genetic test results is complex. A "negative" result does not necessarily invalidate the clinical diagnosis. A "positive" result may actually be inconsequential and unrelated to the clinical diagnosis. One may also encounter "uncertain" results that require further investigation. When selecting and ordering a genetic test, we recommend a four-step approach, which includes a complete phenotype characterization, test selection, analysis of the test result, and report of the findings.

1. **Phenotype characterization**. Careful documentation of the ocular and possible systemic findings is the foundation for genetic testing. This process begins with a thorough history and multigenerational pedigree along with a complete review of systems. Diagnostic testing such as IVFA (intravenous fluorescein angiography), OCT (optical coherence tomography), mf ERG (multifocal electroretinography), ff ERG (full-field electroretinography), visual fields, FAF (fundus autofluorescence), color vision testing, and ocular ultrasound may be requested as indicated. Systemic testing may also be needed such as abdominal ultrasound, neuroimaging, or echocardiography. Where indicated, blood tests to assess possible manifestations of mitochondrial or metabolic disease may be needed. Precise characterization of the phenotype indicates the most likely clinical diagnosis, which in turn creates a pathway to identify the most appropriate genetic test.

2. **Test selection**. If the phenotype aligns well with a known genetic disorder for which there is a specific test (e.g., Down syndrome suspected then order karyotype, Marfan syndrome to order *FBN1* sequencing), then that test would be the test of choice. It is recommended by the AAO (American Academy of Ophthalmology) Task Force report on genetic testing to avoid unnecessary parallel testing when a more specific test can be performed. If the phenotype suggests a disorder for which there is genetic heterogeneity (e.g., retinitis pigmentosa), then gene array panel testing may be appropriate. If the phenotype does not identify a specific disorder, but more than one organ system is involved, a search for CNV by karyotype or CMA may be selected as the first choice. If the phenotype does not identify a specific disorder, but there is another disorder that has overlap features, then testing for that disorder may reveal phenotypic heterogeneity. Some pedigrees may suggest a nontraditional pattern of inheritance for which translocation is a possible explanation, in which case karyotype may be the best test. When testing for the suspected disorder fails to reveal the genetic etiology or the phenotype does not suggest a genetic testing pathway, then WES may be most appropriate. Selection of a genetic test will also depend on cost, availability, reliability, insurance coverage, and methodology.

3. **Analysis of the result**. Test results can be positive, negative, or inconclusive. A positive test is a test that shows pathogenic genetic variants that correlate with a particular phenotype. This may be deduced on the basis of prior reports indicating pathogenicity. The abnormality should also segregate with the disease in the family and be either previously reported as disease causing or have a clear molecular level effect that would be expected to be pathogenic. For example, if the test reveals a novel frameshift, but a downstream frameshift was previously reported as pathogenic, then the likelihood is strong that the upstream frameshift is also pathogenic. The reported abnormality should also be consistent with the inheritance pattern observed in the family. A "negative" test does not necessarily rule out the suspected phenotypic diagnosis. Alternatively, the phenotypic diagnosis may be incorrect. A test may also be negative because the test resolution was not adequate (e.g., a karyotype cannot detect submicroscopic deletions), the entire gene may not have been examined (e.g., promoter region, deep intronic areas), the gene that is being sequenced may be deleted in part or completely, the sequence of the gene may be normal but all or part of the gene is duplicated, or it may be the wrong gene or test for the disease. Other possibilities could be the specimen may have been mislabeled or there was a technical error in the testing laboratory.

Some tests may reveal a variation that is not immediately apparent to be disease causing or not. This is called a variant of unknown significance (VOUS). It may be a variant never reported before in the medical literature and thus called a novel change. Sometimes it is the function of the gene or its relationship to the phenotype that is unknown. The current standard terminology describes five categories ("pathogenic," "likely pathogenic," "uncertain significance," "likely benign," and "benign") to describe variants identified in Mendelian disorders. Moreover, the classification of variants should be based on criteria using subtypes of variant evidence (e.g., population data, computational data, functional data, segregation data, etc.). Some laboratories will provide a prediction of pathogenicity based on a variety of computer-based algorithms that estimate the predicted pathogenicity of the change (e.g., PolyPhen-2). One group has developed an estimate of pathogenic probability (EPP) score for which 0 is very unlikely to 3 is probably disease causing. Interpretation of a variant's significance may also require testing and phenotyping of family members (segregation analysis) and literature review to ascertain the possible biologic significance of the change. Finding the proband's VOUS in their normal parents reduces, but does not entirely eliminate, the chance that the variant is responsible for the child's findings as variable expression or nonpenetrance may also explain the finding. Knowledge of these concepts in context of the disease in question may assist with interpretation as well. Testing of additional family members may be helpful as nonpenetrance is rare. The interpretation of a VOUS may also change over time as more evidence emerges. A detected sequence variation change should also be consistent with the suspected pattern of inheritance if it is to be considered as pathogenic and related to the patient's phenotype. Access to appropriate databases becomes essential to search for similar reported changes (e.g., in the same codon or exon) that may give insight into the variant's pathogenicity.

3.3 Problems

3.3.1 Case 1

An 18-month-old boy comes with retinoblastoma. He also has developmental delay and dysmorphic facies. His karyotype is normal. Family history is unremarkable. Which test from the following is the most appropriate to order?
a) *RB1* sequencing.
b) Methylation tests.
c) WES.
d) CMA.

Correct answer is d.

This patient presents with retinoblastoma and other features that affect other systems but has a normal karyotype. The phenotype strongly suggests 13q deletion syndrome. CMA can detect microdeletions or microduplications that are submicroscopic and therefore not seen on the karyotype.
a) **Less appropriate.** Sequencing cannot detect a fully deleted gene, which is suspected based on the phenotype.
b) **Incorrect.** Although some retinoblastoma is due to methylation abnormalities, it is a less common cause and these tests are considered when sequencing is negative.

c) **Incorrect.** WES should be used after targeted testing for a recognized phenotype is found to be negative. In addition, WES cannot detect the suspected microdeletion in this case.

d) **Correct.**

3.3.2 Case 2

A 1-year-old boy comes for genetic counseling. He was diagnosed with Leber congenital amaurosis (LCA) because of congenital blindness associated with isoelectric ff ERG. An LCA gene panel revealed heterozygous variants in *IQCB1* (previously reported mutation c.1090C > T and a novel variation, c.1549A > T, predicted to be probably damaging by PolyPhen-2 with a score of 0.995 out of 1.0). The mutations are in *trans*, and the parents were asymptomatic heterozygotes. Which from the following would *not* support pathogenicity of the *IQCB1* variant?

a) An abnormal renal ultrasound and impaired renal function.
b) PolyPhen-2 score above 0.85.
c) Unaffected sibling with the same two variations as proband.
d) Both variants were *in cis*.

Correct answer is c.

Nonpenetrance rarely occurs for autosomal recessive disease. If the unaffected sibling was compound heterozygous for the same changes seen in the proband, then one cannot likely attribute the phenotype to these changes.

a) **Incorrect.** Knowledge of the phenotype helps assess if the genotype is responsible. LCA due to *IQCB1* mutations is associated with renal medullary cysts or nephronophthisis (Senior–Løken syndrome).

b) **Incorrect.** PolyPhen-2 over 0.85 is considered to be probably damaging. Variants below 0.15 are predicted to be benign and between 0.15 and 0.85 are possibly damaging.

c) **Correct.**

d) **Incorrect.** Unaffected parents who are each heterozygous for one of the sequence variations seen in the proband are consistent with the autosomal recessive pattern of inheritance. The parents are carriers.

3.3.3 Case 3

A 16-year-old girl was diagnosed with Stargardt disease. Her sister is also reported to be affected. No other family members are affected. After your examination, you confirm the clinical diagnosis and select *ABCA4* testing by a laboratory that does sequencing of the coding exons and deletion/duplication analysis. Two mutations in *cis* (c.5882G > A and c.5929G > A) are found and revealed to be inherited from the child's father. Which from the following is the most appropriate next step?

a) Disclose the results as pathogenic mutations causing the child's disease.
b) Perform a retinal dystrophy panel looking for another mutated gene.
c) Repeat exonic *ABCA4* testing with a different laboratory.
d) Intron sequencing of *ABCA4*.

Correct answer is d.

This disease is usually autosomal recessive. One would expect a sequence variation on the other allele of the proband. *ABCA4* intronic pathogenic variants are considered more frequent than previously thought. In this case, a mutation was found (c.302 + 68C > T) in the maternal allele.

a) **Incorrect.** The exonic mutations were in *cis*, meaning that both came from one parent. This is inconsistent with an autosomal pattern of inheritance as suggested by the pedigree.

b) **Incorrect.** It is considered that up to 30% of patients with one *ABCA4* mutation will have intronic pathogenic variants in the other allele. Digenic disease has not, to our knowledge, been reported as a cause of the typical Stargardt phenotype.

c) **Incorrect.** If a laboratory is CLIA (Clinical Laboratory Improvement Amendments) certified, reputable, and uses standard techniques, the chance of lab error is remote.

d) **Correct.**

3.3.4 Case 4

Two sisters have ocular coloboma along with other congenital malformations. CMA reveals a 519-kb duplication involving chromosome 12q in both girls. The unaffected mother has the same CNV. Research using UCSC Genome Browser revealed that the affected region contains a gene that is expressed in the lens of the eye. Which from the following statements is correct?

a) The unaffected mother has the same CNV. Therefore, it is likely not causative, though careful ocular examination of the mother should be documented.

b) Since there is an ocular gene in the region, the CNV is likely causative.

c) CNV cannot explain multiple congenital malformations involving different systems.

d) The sisters may be exhibiting variable expression of the CNV.

Correct answer is a.

As the mother is completely healthy and has the same CNV, we can conclude that the duplication is not likely related to the abnormalities seen in these girls. Although there are well-documented microdeletion and duplication syndromes in which the CNV is present in some asymptomatic parents, when a CNV does not have a documented association with phenotype and the parent is normal, the CNV is likely not related to the proband's phenotype.

a) **Correct.**

b) **Incorrect.** Not necessarily. If the gene in the affected region does not match the phenotype or inheritance pattern, then it may be unrelated. For example, in this case, a lens gene is expressed in surface ectoderm derivatives, whereas a gene involved with coloboma is more likely the one confined to neuroectodermal derivatives.

c) **Incorrect.** CNV does indeed usually cause involvement of multiple systems because more than one gene is often located in the affected region.

d) **Less appropriate.** The absence of a phenotype in the mother, who has the same CNV, strongly argues against its pathogenicity. Nonpenetrance would be highly unusual for a CNV that is pathogenic, though not impossible.

Suggested Reading

[1] Stone EM, Aldave AJ, Drack AV, et al. Recommendations for genetic testing of inherited eye diseases: report of the American Academy of Ophthalmology task force on genetic testing. Ophthalmology. 2012; 119(11): 2408–2410

[2] Koenekoop RK, Lopez I, den Hollander AI, Allikmets R, Cremers FP. Genetic testing for retinal dystrophies and dysfunctions: benefits, dilemmas and solutions. Clin Experiment Ophthalmol. 2007; 35(5):473–485

[3] Nishiguchi KM, Tearle RG, Liu YP, et al. Whole genome sequencing in patients with retinitis pigmentosa reveals pathogenic DNA structural changes and NEK2 as a new disease gene. Proc Natl Acad Sci U S A. 2013; 110(40):16139–16144

[4] Zanolli MT, Khetan V, Dotan G, Pizzi L, Levin AV. Should patients with ocular genetic disorders have genetic testing? Curr Opin Ophthalmol. 2014; 25(5):359–365

[5] Brandt DS, Shinkunas L, Hillis SL, et al. A closer look at the recommended criteria for disclosing genetic results: perspectives of medical genetic specialists, genomic researchers, and institutional review board chairs. J Genet Couns. 2013; 22(4):544–553

[6] Richards CS, Bale S, Bellissimo DB, et al. Molecular Subcommittee of the ACMG Laboratory Quality Assurance Committee. ACMG recommendations for standards for interpretation and reporting of sequence variations: revisions 2007. Genet Med. 2008; 10(4):294–300

[7] Ellingford JM, Barton S, Bhaskar S, et al. Whole genome sequencing increases molecular diagnostic yield compared with current diagnostic testing for inherited retinal disease. Ophthalmology. 2016; 123(5): 1143–1150

[8] Nussbaum RL, McInnes RR, Willard HF. Thompson & Thompson genetics in medicine. Philadelphia, PA: Elsevier Health Sciences; 2015

[9] Hu H, Xiao X, Li S, Jia X, Guo X, Zhang Q. KIF11 mutations are a common cause of autosomal dominant familial exudative vitreoretinopathy. Br J Ophthalmol. 2016; 100(2):278–283

[10] Small KW, DeLuca AP, Whitmore SS, et al. North Carolina Macular Dystrophy Is Caused by Dysregulation of the Retinal Transcription Factor PRDM13. Ophthalmology. 2016; 123(1):9–18

[11] Weisschuh N, Mayer AK, Strom TM, et al. Mutation detection in patients with retinal dystrophies using targeted next generation sequencing. PLoS One. 2016; 11(1):e0145951

[12] Sun W, Huang L, Xu Y, et al. Exome sequencing on 298 probands with early-onset high myopia: approximately one-fourth show potential pathogenic mutations in RetNet genes. Invest Ophthalmol Vis Sci. 2015; 56(13):8365–8372

[13] Green RC, Berg JS, Grody WW, et al. American College of Medical Genetics and Genomics. ACMG recommendations for reporting of incidental findings in clinical exome and genome sequencing. Genet Med. 2013; 15(7):565–574

[14] Richards S, Aziz N, Bale S, et al. ACMG Laboratory Quality Assurance Committee. Standards and guidelines for the interpretation of sequence variants: a joint consensus recommendation of the American College of Medical Genetics and Genomics and the Association for Molecular Pathology. Genet Med. 2015; 17(5): 405–424

4 Ethical Issues

Abstract

Complex ethical problems may require consideration of multiple principles that have simultaneous bearing on a given situation. Ethics reflects many individual perspectives, which are based on past experience, upbringing, values, religion, political beliefs, and culture. Ocular genetics ethical challenges include prenatal diagnosis, presymptomatic testing or screening, and confidentiality. Genetic tests can reveal crucial information that patients may not want to know or can also lead to stigmatization. Other issues include interactions with medical industry, innovative therapies, informed consent, truth telling, and research ethics. Genetic counseling must consider that individuals have different values regarding choices with regard to electing to have children or alter the course of a pregnancy based on genetic information.

Keywords: ethics, prenatal diagnosis, presymptomatic testing, genetic screening, confidentiality, incidental findings

> **Key Points**
>
> - Complex ethical problems may require consideration of multiple principles that have simultaneous bearing on a given situation.
> - Ethical issues include prenatal diagnosis, presymptomatic testing or screening, confidentiality, information disclosure of incidental findings, and stigmatization.
> - Genetic counseling is essential to properly address the complexity of ethical problems associated with ocular genetic diseases.

4.1 Overview

Ethics is a plural word reflecting the many perspectives individuals may have, based on past experience, upbringing, values, religion, political beliefs, and culture. Basic principles of ethics include autonomy (patient's right to make decisions and have knowledge about their medical condition), beneficence (acting in the best interest of the patient), nonmaleficence ("do no harm"), and justice (fairness). Complex ethical problems may require consideration of multiple principles that have simultaneous bearing on a given situation.

Ethically challenging areas of genetics include prenatal diagnosis, presymptomatic testing or screening (especially when one is testing for genotypes that predispose to late-onset or adult-onset untreatable conditions), and confidentiality (in particular where genetic knowledge may impact insurance coverage). Genetic tests can reveal information that patients may not want to know (e.g., nonpaternity or previously unknown incest). Genetic information can lead to stigmatization or feeling of guilt and shame. More traditional bioethics issues also appear in the field of genetics: interactions with medical industry, innovative therapies, informed consent, truth telling, research ethics, and involvement of trainees.

Genetic counseling presents a unique set of ethical issues in that each individual may have different values regarding choices with regard to electing to have children or alter the course of a pregnancy based on genetic information. Whereas one family may regard a recurrence risk of 25% for a blinding autosomal recessive (AR) disease as too high for them to elect pregnancy, another couple may consider this a relatively low risk. It is for this reason that genetic counseling must be nondirective, offering options rather than a specific action. Counseling for ocular disorders may raise specific concerns. For example, should prenatal testing for an untreatable disorder that only affects a child's vision be made available? Should prenatal screening be done for untreatable ocular disorders the genotype–phenotype correlation for which may be difficult to predict (e.g., *ABCA4* mutations)? Should a child have predictive testing for a currently untreatable adult-onset cause of vision loss such as retinitis pigmentosa (RP)? To what extent should medical professionals be the "gatekeepers" to such testing or should access be freely available and each individual decide for themselves? Although some societies have issued policy statements around such issues, specific recommendations or medical literature regarding ocular genetic literature are sparse.

Presymptomatic testing, also known as predictive testing, is becoming an increasing issue of concern in ocular genetics as the genotype for more patients becomes available. Much of what has been learned about the ethical challenges in this come from experience with Huntington's disease, an adult-onset, highly penetrant and untreatable fatal neurological disease. Individuals may be asymptomatic for many years before they develop signs of this progressive illness. Depression or even suicide can occur following a positive or negative predictive test, and the same has occurred for patients with RP. Patients may be adversely affected not only by knowledge that they will likely develop the disease, but also because their expectation of getting the disease, and perhaps altering their lifestyle (e.g., quitting work and traveling), is not fulfilled. They may feel guilty or feel like an "outsider" in the family by being unaffected. Benefits of presymptomatic testing may include the capability of making decisions about reproduction, career choice, or preparing for later life with vision disability. A negative result may bring relief. The decision to undergo testing is highly personal and should be made only after counseling with a genetics professional. Patients should make an informed decision using all available information concerning the risk versus benefits, in particular their own perceptions of risk versus benefit that could result from testing, in the context of the severity, penetrance, and progression of the condition.

If the individual of concern is a child, bioethics principles must be adapted to consider the vulnerability of this population and the inability of the child to express their own voice and autonomy. Testing children for a disease predisposition when the condition can be treated or morbidity significantly reduced (e.g., homocystinuria) is certainly indicated. Testing of children also has the risk of psychological sequelae, stigmatization, and discrimination. Children's autonomy must be balanced with the desire of parents to obtain genetic information. It is usually accepted that unless there is a clear benefit to the care of the child, genetic testing of asymptomatic children for adult-onset disease should be performed only when the patient is mature enough to decide for himself or herself whether to accept such testing.

Individuals have the right to keep their medical information confidential. This is part of a patient's autonomy: everyone has the right to make their own decisions about how their medical information is used and communicated to others. Nevertheless, in genetics, another important factor is the family. An individual's desire for privacy may collide with the desire of other family members to know about their risk for a particular condition. If one family member refuses consent to share information, then the provider is usually obligated to uphold their privacy, perhaps not even disclosing whether that individual is affected or whether they have even been evaluated. One difficult exception may be when there is a serious threat to another family member's health or safety, for example, the risk of retinoblastoma. Recommendations are not unanimous in this area. Under the U.S. Health Insurance Portability and Accountability Act (HIPAA), a physician can disclose a patient's protected health information to another patient without the patient's authorization only if he/she believes that disclosure can prevent or diminish a serious and imminent threat to a person or the public.

The principle of justice becomes particularly important when considering the availability of genetic testing. Some individuals or societies may not have access to genetic testing on the basis of either technology or cost. If we assume that all individuals deserve equal access to care, it becomes challenging to provide the same opportunities in certain environments. As the breadth of available genetic testing increases, even though the cost of specific tests may be decreasing, this issue, as well as the parallel issue of underserved geographic areas, becomes increasingly concerning.

4.2 Problems

4.2.1 Case 1

A mother comes with her 2-year-old boy with a concern about his risk for RP. The pedigree shows that she is an obligate carrier as she is the daughter of an affected male. Previous testing in the family has revealed a mutation in *RPGR*. The child is asymptomatic. The mother would like her child to have deoxyribonucleic acid (DNA) testing for the family mutation. How should you proceed?

a) Test the boy for the mutation without discussion of the risks of presymptomatic testing.

b) Discuss the risks and benefits of presymptomatic testing and proceed only if the mother wishes to do the test after being fully informed.

c) Perform an electroretinogram (ERG) under general anesthesia.

d) Do not offer testing of the boy.

Correct answer is b.

Although for some diseases presymptomatic testing may allow for preventive therapy before damage occurs, there is no current effective treatment for RP. Adverse consequences of both positive and negative tests results include significant psychosocial alterations. Yet some research shows that some patients may benefit from testing. Therefore, the risks and benefits of testing should be discussed with the patient/family to allow an informed decision about whether or not to proceed with testing.

a) **Incorrect.** Parents should be informed of the risks and benefits before presymptomatic testing.

b) **Correct.**

c) **Incorrect.** ERG may or may not determine whether an individual is affected. Perhaps the ERG at this young age would be normal but later become abnormal. Especially in AR disease, an abnormal ERG may simply indicate that the patient is a carrier. In autosomal dominant (AD) disease, an abnormal ERG does not predict severity of later expression. DNA testing is a more definitive way of determining the extent to which the individual is affected.

d) **Incorrect.** Family should always be counseled regarding options before determining the plan.

4.2.2 Case 2

A 30-year-old man with decreasing central vision comes for ophthalmic evaluation of a condition that his mother had. Clinical and laboratory examinations reveal that he has a pattern dystrophy due to a *PRPH2* mutation. Two months later, his 25-year-old sister comes with similar vision complaints and history. She asks about your findings on her brother. Should this information be disclosed?
a) Yes, always as it is relevant to her.
b) Yes, but first ethics committee should be involved.
c) Information must not be disclosed without consent of her brother.
d) Depending on the laboratory results performed on her. If testing shows the same condition, we can disclose his medical information.

Correct answer is c.
Pattern dystrophy due to *PRPH2* mutation is an AD condition that is not associated with any serious systemic condition and is currently untreatable. Patients have a right to confidentiality the abrogation of which may only be considered in emergent or vision-/life-threatening treatable situations or when the law otherwise dictates (e.g., reporting of child abuse). Therefore, in the absence of such considerations here, the brother's confidentiality must be respected and information shared (including even the fact that he was examined) withheld from the sister until he gives informed consent to share.
a) **Incorrect.** Although the information may be relevant, it may not be shared without consent.
b) **Incorrect.** There is no need to involve an ethics committee as the principles and policies in this matter are quite clear and fairly universal. Use of the committee should be reserved for particularly challenging or emergent issues.
c) **Correct.**
d) **Incorrect.** Knowing her molecular diagnosis does not induce the right to violate her brother's confidentiality.

4.2.3 Case 3

A 45-year-old woman presents with a clinical disorder compatible with Best disease and is found to carry a mutation in the *BEST1* gene. Her father, from whom she is estranged, was known to have reduced vision. She is planning to discuss the results with her teenage son but insists that her father and younger adult half-siblings from her father's second marriage not be informed that they may be at risk and that testing is available. What is your next step?
a) You are obligated to respect her right to privacy.
b) Relatives have to be informed because of the risk of vision loss.
c) You must inform her father but not her siblings.
d) Admonish her for her insensitivity and convince her to disclose the information herself to her father and siblings.

Correct answer is a.
Physicians should only consider overriding such requests from patients when there may be preventable risks of death or blindness to family members. Many cases of Best disease are not severe and do not develop legal blindness. It is untreatable except for

the uncommon possibility of subretinal neovascularization. These factors do not likely rise to a level of concern, which obligates the physician to disclose without authorization. In addition, asymptomatic family members may choose not to know their risk.

a) **Correct.**

b) **Incorrect.**

c) **Incorrect.**

d) **Incorrect.** Although one can discuss the risk and benefits of disclosing such information to her family, we cannot admonish a patient for their choices and our counseling should remain nondirective.

Suggested Reading

[1] Nussbaum RL, McInnes RR, Willard HF. Thompson & Thompson Genetics in Medicine. Philadelphia, PA: Elsevier Health Sciences; 2015

[2] Godard B, Hurlimann T, Letendre M, Egalité N, INHERIT BRCAs. Guidelines for disclosing genetic information to family members: from development to use. Fam Cancer. 2006; 5(1):103–116

[3] Greely HT. Banning genetic discrimination. N Engl J Med. 2005; 353(9):865–867

[4] Harper PS. Genetic testing, life insurance, and adverse selection. Philos Trans R Soc Lond B Biol Sci. 1997; 352 (1357):1063–1066

[5] Lapham EV, Kozma C, Weiss JO. Genetic discrimination: perspectives of consumers. Science. 1996; 274 (5287):621–624

[6] Nowlan W. Human genetics. A rational view of insurance and genetic discrimination. Science. 2002; 297 (5579):195–196

[7] Offit K, Groeger E, Turner S, Wadsworth EA, Weiser MA. The "duty to warn" a patient's family members about hereditary disease risks. JAMA. 2004; 292(12):1469–1473

[8] Ossa DF, Towse A. Genetic screening, health care and the insurance industry. Should genetic information be made available to insurers? Eur J Health Econ. 2004; 5(2):116–121

[9] Golden-Grant K, Merritt JL, II, Scott CR. Ethical considerations of population screening for late-onset genetic disease. Clin Genet. 2015; 88(6):589–592

[10] Mezer E, Babul-Hirji R, Wise R, et al. Attitudes regarding predictive testing for retinitis pigmentosa. Ophthalmic Genet. 2007; 28(1):9–15

[11] Dheensa S, Fenwick A, Shkedi-Rafid S, Crawford G, Lucassen A. Health-care professionals' responsibility to patients' relatives in genetic medicine: a systematic review and synthesis of empirical research. Genet Med. 2016; 18(4):290–301

[12] Arbour L, Canadian Paediatric Society. Guidelines for genetic testing of healthy children. Paediatr Child Health. 2003; 8(1):42–52

[13] Association for Clinical Genetics Practice. Best Practice Guidelines. http://www.acgs.uk.com/committees/quality-committee/best-practice-guidelines/. Accessed April 2016

[14] The American Society of Human Genetics. Policy & Position Statement Archive. http://www.ashg.org/pages/policy_statements.shtml. Accessed April 2016

5 Corneal Dystrophies

Pablo Romero

Abstract
Corneal dystrophies are a group of inherited disorders characterized by loss of corneal transparency that affect different layers of the cornea. They are typically bilateral although onset may be sequential or asymmetric. Specific patterns of corneal deposition and morphological changes are seen. The International Committee for Classification of Corneal Dystrophies (IC3D) proposed a modified anatomic classification consisting of (1) epithelial and subepithelial dystrophies, (2) epithelial–stromal TGFBI (transforming growth factor-induced) dystrophies, (3) stromal dystrophies, and (4) endothelial dystrophies. Corneal dystrophies demonstrate both genetic and phenotypic heterogeneity.

Keywords: corneal dystrophies, corneal epithelial dystrophies, corneal subepithelial dystrophies, epithelial–stromal transforming growth factor-induced dystrophies, corneal stromal dystrophies, corneal endothelial dystrophies

---

Key Points

- Corneal dystrophies are a group of inherited, bilateral disorders of the cornea characterized by patterns of corneal deposition and morphological changes.
- The classification of corneal dystrophies is the International Committee for Classification of Corneal Dystrophies (IC3D).
- Corneal dystrophies demonstrate both genetic and phenotypic heterogeneity.

5.1 Overview

Corneal dystrophies are a group of inherited disorders characterized by loss of corneal transparency that affect different layers of the cornea. They are typically bilateral although onset may be sequential or asymmetric. The International Committee for Classification of Corneal Dystrophies (IC3D), Edition 2, proposed a modified anatomic classification consisting of (1) epithelial and subepithelial dystrophies, (2) epithelial–stromal transforming growth factor-induced (*TGFBI*) dystrophies, (3) stromal dystrophies, and (4) endothelial dystrophies (▶ Table 5.1).

5.1.1 Epithelial and Subepithelial Dystrophies

Epithelial basement membrane dystrophy (EBMD), also known as map-dot-fingerprint dystrophy, usually develops between the ages of 20 and 40 years. It is characterized by grayish epithelial fingerprint lines, dots (microcysts), and geographic maplike lines. Although it is usually asymptomatic, approximately 10% of patients develop painful, recurrent epithelial erosions and decreased vision. In some families, EBMD appears to segregate as an autosomal dominant (AD) disorder and point mutations in the *TGFBI* gene have been identified. EBMD is, however, present in up to 76% of persons over the age of 50 years, suggesting that most cases of this condition represent age-dependent degeneration of the cornea.

Table 5.1 The IC3D classification of corneal dystrophies

Epithelial and subepithelial dystrophies (OMIM)	Gene/loci	Inheritance
Epithelial basement membrane dystrophy (121820)	TGFBI (5q31.1)	AD
Epithelial recurrent erosion dystrophies (Franceschetti) (122400)	COL17A1 (10q25.1)	AD
Dystrophia Smolandiensis	Unknown	AD
Dystrophia Helsinglandica	Unknown	AD
Subepithelial mucinous corneal dystrophy (612867)	Unknown	AD
Meesmann's corneal dystrophy (122100)	KRT3 (12q13.13) KRT12 (17q21.2)	AD
Lisch's epithelial corneal dystrophy (300778)	Xp22.3	X-linked
Gelatinous droplike corneal dystrophy (204870)	TACSTD2 (1p32.1)	AR
Salzmann nodular degeneration	Unknown (nongenetic reactive forms)	Unknown
Epithelial–stromal corneal dystrophies (OMIM)	**Gene/Loci**	**Inheritance**
Reis–Bücklers corneal dystrophy (608470)	TGFBI (5q31.1)	AD
Thiel–Behnke corneal dystrophy (602082)	TGFBI (5q31.1)	AD
Granular corneal dystrophy, type 1 (121900)	TGFBI (5q31.1)	AD
Granular corneal dystrophy, type 2 (Avellino dystrophy) (607541)	TGFBI (5q31.1)	AD
Classic lattice corneal dystrophy (122200) Lattice variants (III, IIIA, I/IIIA, and IV)	TGFBI (5q31.1)	AD
Stromal dystrophies (OMIM)		
Macular corneal dystrophy (217800)	CHST6 (16q22)	AR
Schnyder's corneal dystrophy (21800)	UBIAD1 (1p36)	AD
Congenital stromal corneal dystrophy (610048)	DCN (12q21.33)	AD
Fleck corneal dystrophy (121850)	PIP5K3 (2q35)	AD
Posterior amorphous corneal dystrophy	Unknown	AD
Central cloudy dystrophy of François (217600)	Unknown	AD
Pre-Descemet corneal dystrophy	Unknown	Unknown
Endothelial dystrophies		
Fuchs' endothelial corneal dystrophy (136800)	COL8A1 (3q12.3) TCF4 (18q21.2) TCF8 (10p11.22) LOXHD1 (18q21.1) SLC4A11 (20p13) Early onset: COL8A2 (1p34.3–p32) Other loci: 13pTel –13q12.13; 1p34.3–p32; 5q33.1–q35.2; 9p24.1–p22.1; 15q25.	Some AD, most sporadic
Posterior polymorphous corneal dystrophies (122000; 609140; 609141)	Unknown (20p11.2–q11.2) COL8A2 (1p34.3–p32.3) ZEB1 (10p11.2)	AD
Congenital hereditary endothelial dystrophies (121700; 217700)	Unknown (20p 11.2–q11.2) SLC4A11 (20p13)	AD AR
X-linked endothelial corneal dystrophy	Unknown (Xq25)	X-linked dominant

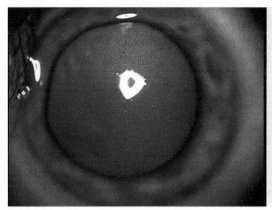

Fig. 5.1 Meesmann's corneal dystrophy, with multiple, small epithelial vesicles.

Meesmann's corneal dystrophy is a slowly progressive corneal dystrophy with early childhood onset, which presents with multiple, small epithelial vesicles that extend to the limbus (▶ Fig. 5.1). These are most numerous in the interpalpebral area. Coalescence of cysts may result in refractile linear opacities with intervening clear cornea. Corneal thinning and hypoesthesia may also be found. In the Stocker–Holt variant, the whole cornea shows fine grayish punctate, epithelial opacities that stain with fluorescein and linear opacities that may adopt a whorl pattern. Patients are usually asymptomatic, although some may have mild visual reduction, glare, photophobia, and recurrent painful punctiform epithelial erosions.

5.1.2 Epithelial–Stromal TGFBI Dystrophies

Symptoms of patients with Reis–Bücklers corneal dystrophy (RBCD) include painful recurrent corneal erosions and impaired vision, starting in the first decade of life. While recurrent corneal erosions tend to decrease with time, vision slowly deteriorates. In the early stages, discrete confluent irregular geographic-like opacities with varying densities develop at the level of the Bowman layer and superficial stroma. Subsequently, opacities extend to the limbus and deeper stroma.

Thiel–Behnke corneal dystrophy (TBCD) is also called corneal dystrophy of Bowman's layer type II, honeycomb-shaped corneal dystrophy, anterior limiting membrane dystrophy type II, and curly fiber corneal dystrophy. TBCD is an AD form of corneal dystrophy characterized by progressive honeycomb-like, subepithelial corneal opacities with recurrent erosions. It can be difficult to distinguish TBCD from RBCD in early or individual cases. In the early stage, RBCD shows more irregular diffuse opacities with clear interruptions, whereas TBCD exhibits multiple flecks with reticular formation. RBCD tends to have a more aggressive course. In patients with TBCD, the symptoms start at the first and second decades with painful recurrent corneal erosions. Gradually erosions become less frequent and characteristic solitary flecks or irregularly shaped scattered opacities at the level of the Bowman layer appear, followed by symmetrical subepithelial honeycomb opacities (▶ Fig. 5.2). The onset of visual impairment is noted at the second decade of life and gradually progresses, resulting from increase of corneal scarring. The peripheral cornea typically is not involved, but in older patient, opacities can progress to deeper stromal layers and affecting the corneal periphery. Anterior segment optical coherence tomography (OCT) demonstrates the sawtooth pattern of hyper-reflective material in the Bowman layer in patients with TBCD.

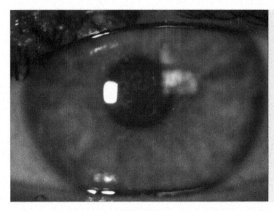

Fig. 5.2 Thiel–Behnke corneal dystrophy showing honeycomb central opacity affecting the Bowman's layer.

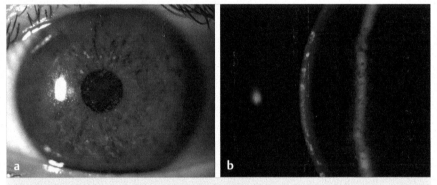

Fig. 5.3 (a) Granular corneal dystrophy type 1. **(b)** Note opacities in the anterior stroma.

Granular corneal dystrophy type 1 (GCD1), also called corneal dystrophy Groenouw type I, is characterized by multiple stromal opacities. Symptoms start as early as the age of 2 years. The initial symptoms are glare and photophobia. Visual acuity decreases as opacification progresses with age. Recurrent erosions are seen frequently. In children, a vortex pattern of brownish granules superficial to the Bowman layer can be observed. In later stages, well-defined granules appear white on direct illumination with clear intervening stroma (▶ Fig. 5.3). The size and number of granules increase, resulting in a "snowflake" appearance. On retroillumination, these granules are composed of extremely small, translucent dots that have been described to resemble vacuoles, glassy splinters, or crushed bread crumbs. Opacities do not extend to the limbus. In later life, granules extend into the deeper stroma approaching Descemet's membrane. With progression, opacities become more confluent in the superficial cornea and reduce visual acuity.

Granular corneal dystrophy type 2 (GCD2) is also called Avellino dystrophy and formerly Groenouw type I. The term combined granular–lattice dystrophy had been used because of the presence of an amyloid component on histology, but lattice lines are not seen clinically. Patients with GCD2 have fewer stromal opacities than those with GCD1. Initial signs are subtle superficial stromal tiny whitish dots, which typically

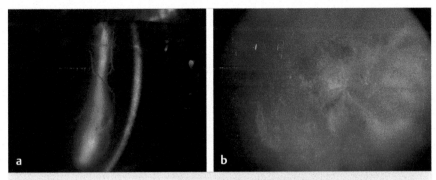

Fig. 5.4 (a) Lattice corneal dystrophy type 1 in a young patient. **(b)** Lattice corneal dystrophy type 1 in an older patient with progression of the condition. Note diffuse opacities associated with erosions.

develop small spokes or thorns. Later, patients develop spiky anterior to midstromal deposits that are star-, icicle-, or spider-shaped and partially translucent in retroillumination and superficial, whitish round patches that have moth-eaten centers, or discoid or ring shapes. Translucent short dashlike linear or dotlike deposits in the posterior stroma deep to the branching stromal opacities are also observed. The short lines or dashes are different from the more elaborate lattice lines. GCD2 opacities appear whiter and less refractile. Unlike lattice lines, these "dashes" rarely cross each other. Symptoms, such as painful recurrent corneal erosions, start as early as the age of 8 years. Vision slowly decreases with age as the central visual axis becomes involved. In later stages, consequent to epithelial erosions, spontaneous dropout of superficial granules results in clearing of the central zone of opacity, which also becomes thickened with recurrences.

Lattice corneal dystrophy (LCD) demonstrates variable clinical expression but a high degree of penetration. On initial stages, linear opacities associated with other smaller opaque spots and refractile lattice lines are present. In the second and third decade of life, a network of linear opacities associated with polymorphic anterior stromal opacities is seen (► Fig. 5.4). In advanced cases, corneal opacities are observed secondary to irregularity of the epithelial surface with subepithelial and anterior stromal scarring. A yellowish discoloration in the anterior stroma results in clouding of the central cornea.

5.1.3 Stromal Dystrophies

Macular corneal dystrophy (MCD) presents initially as a diffuse stromal haze extending to the limbus with later superficial, central, elevated, irregular whitish opacities called macules (► Fig. 5.5). There are no clear areas between corneal opacities, a feature that differentiates MCD from GCD. The cornea is thin in the early stages of MCD, but as the disease progresses, the corneal endothelium is affected and stromal edema develops. Patients usually present with severe visual impairment between the ages of 10 and 30 years. Other symptoms include corneal hypoesthesia, photophobia, and recurrent erosions. Based on the immunoreactivity of the macular deposits, there are three variants that are indistinguishable clinically: type I with no antigenic keratan sulfate reactivity in cornea or serum; type IA, with antigenic keratan sulfate reactivity in keratocytes; and type II, with keratan sulfate reactivity in the cornea deposits and serum normal or low levels of antigenic keratan sulfate.

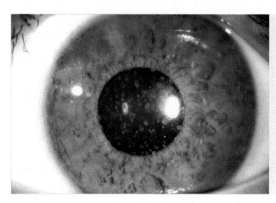

Fig. 5.5 Macular corneal dystrophy showing diffuse stromal opacities.

5.1.4 Endothelial Dystrophies

Congenital hereditary endothelial dystrophy (CHED)presents as diffuse bilateral corneal edema. The primary anomaly in CHED is thought to be a degeneration or maldevelopment of endothelial cells during gestation. According to a recent classification change, CHED (formerly CHED2) is most likely only an autosomal recessive condition. The autosomal dominant form (formerly CHED1) is no longer considered as a unique corneal dystrophy, as it appears to be similar to a type of posterior polymorphous corneal dystrophy linked to the same chromosome 20 locus. CHED is apparent at birth, often followed by nystagmus due to visual deprivation.

Posterior polymorphous corneal dystrophy (PPCD) has widely variable expression. Unilateral cases may or may not be heritable. Endothelial alterations often are asymptomatic, but visual impairment may develop secondary to corneal edema. The endothelia abnormalities have been described as "snail tracks" and can be confused with the longer scalloped parallel lines of Haab's striae seen in congenital glaucoma. Retroillumination may be required to visualize the changes that can occur anywhere on the endothelial surface. Approximately 20 to 25% of affected individuals require corneal transplantation.

Fuchs' endothelial corneal dystrophy (FECD) is perhaps the most common corneal dystrophy although prevalence varies according to population. For unknown reasons, women are more frequently affected, both in the early and in the later onset forms. Patients exhibit alterations in corneal endothelial cell morphology and progressive loss of corneal endothelial cells that eventually lead to corneal edema. The clinical appearance of diffuse dotlike opacities and elevations of the endothelium with or without pigmentation is known as cornea guttata, which starts centrally and spreads peripherally (stage 1). Some patients progress to endothelial decompensation and stromal edema (stage 2). Stromal edema may progress to involve the epithelium causing bullous keratopathy (stage 3). Subepithelial fibrosis, scarring, and peripheral superficial vascularization from chronic edema occur in long-standing cases (stage 4). Symptoms of FECD typically appear in patients older than 60 years and are characterized by intermittent reduced vision from epithelial/stromal edema, worse in the morning. Pain, photophobia, and epiphora due to epithelial erosions may also occur. Cataract surgery may worsen the disease by inducing further loss of corneal endothelial cells.

Molecular Genetics

TGFBI, 5q31, formerly called *BIGH3*, is mutated in several corneal dystrophies. This gene encodes an arginylglycylaspartic acid-containing protein that binds to types I, II, and IV collagens. This is found in many extracellular matrix proteins, where it modulates cell adhesion and serves as a ligand recognition sequence for integrins. The protein is induced by transforming growth factor-β and acts to inhibit cell adhesion. Rare alleles that result in Arg555Gln with other *TGFBI* mutations lead to variants of TBCD with atypical opacities. Homozygote and compound heterozygote *TGFBI* cases of GCD1 and GCD2 have earlier onset and more severe symptoms as compared with heterozygotes.

Differential Diagnosis

The corneal dystrophies must be distinguished from other causes of corneal deposition (e.g., metabolic disorders such as mucopolysaccharidoses or cystinosis), immune deposition (e.g., multiple myeloma), corneal edema (e.g., congenital glaucoma), corneal malformation (e.g., Peters anomaly), infection (e.g., subepithelial deposits following adenovirus, endotheliitis of congenital rubella), foreign bodies, and pseudophakic/aphakic bullous keratopathy.

Although glaucoma is rarely associated, the edema of CHED differs from that seen in congenital glaucoma in that Haab's striae are not present, the corneal diameter is normal, and the cornea has a very thick limbus-to-limbus "ground glass" appearance without dense white stromal opacification.

Uncommon Manifestations

In patients with epithelial–stromal corneal dystrophies, the corneal disease may be initiated or aggravated by laser refractive surgery. Superficial corneal opacities and irregularities treated by phototherapeutic keratectomy (PTK) can also relapse (▶ Fig. 5.6).

Salzmann's nodular degeneration of cornea with moderate dry eye has been seen in a girl with dermatopathia pigmentosa reticularis.

CHED corneal dystrophy with perceptive deafness (OMIM 217400) also known as Harboyan's syndrome is caused by *SLC4A11* mutations.

Dermochondrocorneal dystrophy (OMIM 221800), or François' syndrome, is a rare disease defined by the development of skin nodules, extremities deformities, and central and superficial corneal dystrophy characterized by whitish subepithelial opacities.

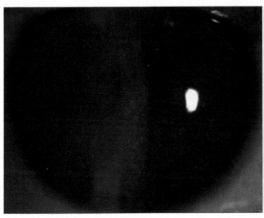

Fig. 5.6 Reis–Bücklers corneal dystrophy relapse, 3 years after treatment with phototherapeutic keratectomy.

A form of AR pontocerebellar hypoplasia has been associated with corneal dystrophy, underdevelopment of labioscrotal folds, and hairy nipples.

Clinical Testing

Confocal Microscopy

Confocal microscopy is capable of identifying corneal microstructural changes related to many corneal dystrophies in vivo, including deposits and reflectivity changes. Polymegethism, pleomorphism, decreased hexagonality, and reduced number of endothelial cells are also observed with confocal microscopy.

Anterior Segment Optical Coherence Tomography

Anterior segment OCT demonstrates abnormalities of corneal thickness and can help identify the layer and distribution of deposits.

Immunohistochemistry

Immunohistochemistry is helpful in many forms of corneal dystrophies, including epithelial recurrent erosion dystrophy, Reis–Bücklers and Thiel Behnke corneal dystrophies, LCD, macular dystrophy, and others.

Histopathology

Examples of histopathology are given in ▶ Table 5.2.

Table 5.2 Histopathology findings in corneal dystrophies

Corneal dystrophy	Histopathology findings
Reis–Bücklers corneal dystrophy	Intraepithelial basement membrane and microcysts
Meesmann's dystrophy	Intraepithelial microcysts
Thiel–Behnke dystrophy	Focal loss of epithelial basement membrane and Bowman's layer
Granular corneal dystrophy type 1	Discrete deposits of mutated protein appear red with Masson's trichrome stain
Granular corneal dystrophy type 2	Corneal deposits similar to granular corneal dystrophy type 1 plus amyloid
Lattice dystrophy	Birefringent amyloid that stains with Congo red
Macular corneal dystrophy	Deposits are positive for colloidal iron and Alcian blue
Familial subepithelial amyloidosis	Subepithelial amyloid deposits that contain lactoferrin
Central stromal crystalline dystrophy	Crystals of cholesterol ester in anterior stroma
Fleck dystrophy	Subepithelial and stromal amyloid deposits. Stains with colloidal iron and Alcian blue
Congenital hereditary endothelial dystrophy	Edematous epithelium with lack of Bowman's layer. Thickened stroma and Descemet's membrane. Diminished number of endothelial cells
Posterior polymorphous dystrophy	Abnormal Descemet's membrane. Multilayered epithelial cells in posterior cornea

Genetic Testing

Specific genes and inheritance patterns are described in ▶ Table 5.1. In patients with clinical findings compatible with EBMD, epithelial–stromal dystrophies and some stromal dystrophies, *TGFBI* sequencing can be performed. If endothelial dystrophies such as CDPD (corneal dystrophy and perceptive deafness), CHED, or FECD are found, *SLC4A11* sequencing should be considered. In early-onset FECD, *COL8A2* can be sequenced. Multigene array panels are becoming available for corneal dystrophies.

5.2 Problems

5.2.1 Case 1

A healthy but consanguineous couple with no previous history of eye disease present with their 2-week-old son who has cloudy corneas that began a few days after spontaneous vaginal delivery. Physical examination including intraocular pressure is otherwise normal. The corneas of the baby show limbus-to-limbus "ground glass" opacity with marked increase in thickness. Corneal diameters are 10.25 mm. Physical examination and hearing test are normal. Which of the following is the most likely diagnosis?

a) CHED.
b) Congenital glaucoma.
c) FECD.
d) Congenital rubella syndrome.

Correct answer is a.

CHED is causing diffuse bilateral corneal edema. The AR subtype is apparent at birth, often followed by nystagmus due to visual deprivation.

a) **Correct.**
b) **Incorrect.** Congenital glaucoma can produce corneal clouding from microcystic epithelial as well as stromal edema, but is accompanied by enlargement of the corneal diameter, Haab's striae, and usually a white stromal opacity.
c) **Incorrect.** FECD is usually adult onset.
d) **Incorrect.** The classic features of congenital rubella syndrome include cardiac malformations, chorioretinitis, cataract, corneal clouding, microphthalmia, strabismus, glaucoma, and deafness. It may present with endotheliitis.

5.2.2 Case 2

A 27-year-old woman is interested in knowing the risk to her offspring of the corneal disorder that causes her mother, brother, and her to suffer from painful recurrent corneal erosions. She would like to assess her chances of having a child with this disease. Based on her slit-lamp examination (see ▶ Fig. 5.4), what is the chance of her having a child with the same condition?

a) 66.6%.
b) 50%.
c) 25%.
d) 100%.

Correct answer is b.

Classic LCD is an AD disorder. This woman has 50% chance of having an affected child with each pregnancy.

a) **Incorrect.**
b) **Correct.**
c) **Incorrect.**
d) **Incorrect.**

5.2.3 Case 3

A 59-year-old woman complains of intermittent reduction of her vision, especially in the morning. She is not complaining of pain, photophobia, or epiphora. Anterior segment examination reveals mild bilateral corneal edema in the morning and central cornea guttata. Confocal microscopy shows polymegethism, pleomorphism, decreased hexagonality, and reduced number of endothelial cells. Which of the following factors is most responsible in the formation of her corneal edema?

a) Normal aging.
b) PPCD.
c) X-linked recessive corneal endothelial dystrophy.
d) FECD.

Correct answer is d.

This is a presentation of FECD stage 1. The symptoms start on average at the age of 60 years with intermittent reduced vision worse in the morning. Pain, photophobia, and epiphora are characteristic of stage 3.

a) **Incorrect.** Although guttata may be seen, aging, usually, does not produce polymegethism, pleomorphism, decreased hexagonality, and symptoms at the age of 59 years.
b) **Incorrect.** Endothelial alterations from PPCD are often asymptomatic, although visual impairment may develop secondary to corneal edema. The endothelia abnormalities are usually described as "snail tracks."
c) **Incorrect.** Patient is female. In addition, it presents as congenital ground glass corneal clouding or a diffuse corneal haze.
d) **Correct.**

5.2.4 Case 4

A 32-year-old woman complains of slowly worsening vision in both eyes over the last 5 years. She also complains of episodic eye pain since she was 3 years old. Her 59-year-old father and her 14-year-old daughter also have similar but milder symptoms. The cornea exam shows central subepithelial honeycomb opacity, while anterior segment OCT demonstrates the sawtooth pattern of hyper-reflective material in the Bowman layer. Which of the following gene mutations is most likely responsible in the formation of corneal opacity?

a) *SLC4A11*.
b) *TGFBI*.
c) *CHST6*.
d) *TACSTD2*.

Correct answer is b.

This is a presentation of TBCD, an AD disorder with a high degree of variable expression not necessarily correlated with age.

a) **Incorrect.** Mutations of *SLC4A11* are associated with Harboyan's syndrome.

b) **Correct.**

c) **Incorrect.** Mutations of *CHST6* are associated with MCD.

d) **Incorrect.** Mutations of *TACSTD2* are associated with gelatinous droplike corneal dystrophy.

5.2.5 Case 5

A 35-year-old woman presents with worsening vision over the last 10 years. Her 35-year-old dizygotic twin sister has similar symptoms. There are no other affected family members. Clinical and genetic study confirms a stromal cornea dystrophy. Which of the following is the most possible diagnosis in this case?

a) LCD.

b) RBCD.

c) MCD.

d) TBCD.

Correct answer is c.

This is a presentation of MCD that follows an AR pattern of inheritance.

a) **Incorrect.** LCD is an epithelial–stromal dystrophy that follows an AD pattern of inheritance.

b) **Incorrect.** RBCD is an epithelial–stromal dystrophy that follows an AD pattern of inheritance.

c) **Correct.**

d) **Incorrect.** TBCD is an epithelial–stromal dystrophy that follows an AD pattern of inheritance.

Suggested Reading

[1] Weiss JS, Møller HU, Lisch W, et al. The IC3D classification of the corneal dystrophies. Cornea. 2008; 27 Suppl 2:S1–S83

[2] Weiss JS, Møller HU, Aldave AJ, et al. IC3D classification of corneal dystrophies—edition 2. Cornea. 2015; 34 (2):117–159

[3] Aldave AJ, Sonmez B. Elucidating the molecular genetic basis of the corneal dystrophies: are we there yet? Arch Ophthalmol. 2007; 125(2):177–186

[4] Stone EM, Mathers WD, Rosenwasser GO, et al. Three autosomal dominant corneal dystrophies map to chromosome 5q. Nat Genet. 1994; 6(1):47–51

[5] Escribano J, Hernando N, Ghosh S, Crabb J, Coca-Prados M. cDNA from human ocular ciliary epithelium homologous to beta ig-h3 is preferentially expressed as an extracellular protein in the corneal epithelium. J Cell Physiol. 1994; 160(3):511–521

[6] Dighiero P, Niel F, Ellies P, et al. Histologic phenotype-genotype correlation of corneal dystrophies associated with eight distinct mutations in the TGFBI gene. Ophthalmology. 2001; 108(4):818–823

[7] Abramowicz MJ, Albuquerque-Silva J, Zanen A. Corneal dystrophy and perceptive deafness (Harboyan syndrome): CDPD1 maps to 20p13. J Med Genet. 2002; 39(2):110–112

[8] Desir J, Moya G, Reish O, et al. Borate transporter SLC4A11 mutations cause both Harboyan syndrome and non-syndromic corneal endothelial dystrophy. J Med Genet. 2007; 44(5):322–326

[9] Vithana EN, Morgan PE, Ramprasad V, et al. SLC4A11 mutations in Fuchs endothelial corneal dystrophy. Hum Mol Genet. 2008; 17(5):656–666

[10] Kannabiran C. Genetics of corneal endothelial dystrophies. J Genet. 2009; 88(4):487–494

6 Aniridia

Abstract

Patients with aniridia show a bilateral nearly complete or partial absence of iris. It is caused by abnormalities of the transcription factor *PAX6* gene, which is located on chromosome 11. These patients usually present nystagmus, corneal pannus, strabismus, refractive error, glaucoma, cataract, foveal hypoplasia, and optic nerve hypoplasia. The WAGR (Wilms tumor, aniridia, genitourinary malformation, mental retardation) syndrome is a contiguous gene deletion disorder due to del(11)(p13). Detection of WAGR deletions is essential to prevent morbidity and mortality due to renal malignancy.

Keywords: aniridia, *PAX6* gene, Wilms tumor, aniridia, genitourinary malformation, mental retardation, del(11)(p13), nystagmus, macular hypoplasia

Key Points

- Aniridia is an autosomal dominant panocular disorder typically caused by heterozygous point mutations or deletions in the *PAX6* gene.
- The WAGR (Wilms tumor, aniridia, genitourinary malformation, mental retardation) syndrome is a contiguous gene deletion disorder due to del(11)(p13).
- Detection of WAGR deletions is essential to prevent morbidity and mortality due to renal malignancy.

6.1 Overview

Patients with aniridia show a bilateral nearly complete or partial absence of iris (▶ Fig. 6.1). Estimated incidence varies between 1 in 40,000 and 100,000 people. It is caused by a mutation of the transcription factor *PAX6* gene, which is located on chr11p13. *PAX6* is the "master control gene" for eye development. Therefore, disruption of this gene's function results in abnormal expression of many downstream genes potentially causing abnormalities in virtually every part of the eye, including nystagmus, corneal pannus (▶ Fig. 6.2) ranging from peripheral avascular pannus due to limbal stem cell deficiency to severe pancorneal vascularization, strabismus, refractive error, glaucoma, cataract (especially anterior pyramidal; ▶ Fig. 6.3), foveal/macular hypoplasia (▶ Fig. 6.4 and ▶ Fig. 6.5) that results in varying degrees of visual impairment, and optic nerve hypoplasia.

6.2 Molecular Genetics

Aniridia is an autosomal dominant (AD) disorder. Most *PAX6* mutations (40%) are premature termination codons (nonsense). Missense mutations (25%) result in less severe forms of aniridia. Intragenic deletions may also occur and usually result in more severe disease. Some mutations in the gene will be expressed only as isolated parts of the disorder without iris malformation: AD macular hypoplasia, cataract, or keratitis. Homozygous or compound heterozygous disruption of *PAX6* function results in anophthalmia, brain malformation, and often death.

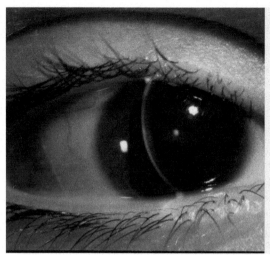

Fig. 6.1 Patient with "partial" aniridia due to *PAX6* gene mutation.

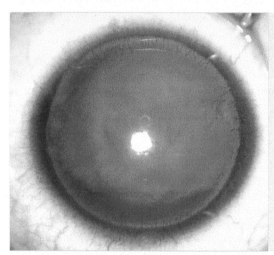

Fig. 6.2 Keratopathy in a patient with aniridia.

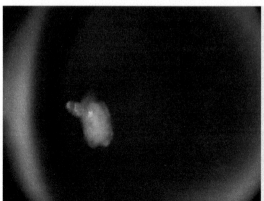

Fig. 6.3 Anterior pyramidal cataract in a patient with aniridia.

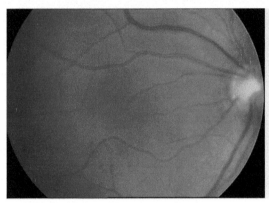

Fig. 6.4 Macular hypoplasia in a patient with aniridia. Note the absence of foveal reflex and vessels coursing through the central macula.

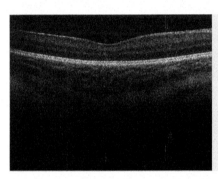

Fig. 6.5 Optical coherence tomography demonstrating foveal hypoplasia in a patient with aniridia.

If a heterozygous contiguous gene deletion occurs within the 11p13 region, encompassing *PAX6* as well as the nearby *WT1* gene, WAGR syndrome results, with a prevalence of 1 in 500,000. Patients with deletion of *PAX6* and *WT1* have a 45 to 50% risk of developing Wilms' tumor. These deletions vary in size from those large enough to be detected by karyotype to submicroscopic deletions requiring FISH (fluorescence in situ hybridization) or chromosomal microarray to detect. Even smaller deletions may not encompass *WT1* but still result in the other manifestations. Deletions may occur de novo or as a result of parental translocations. Very small deletions can rarely result in a history of familial aniridia with minimal associated systemic manifestations.

6.2.1 Differential Diagnosis

Axenfeld–Rieger Spectrum (OMIM 180500)

Axenfeld–Rieger spectrum (OMIM 180500) may be distinguished from aniridia by the presence of posterior embryotoxon and the absence of corneal vascularization or foveal hypoplasia. Rarely, an aniridic variant may occur due to deletion or duplication of 6p25, but these patients also have posterior embryotoxon and normal foveae.

Iris Coloboma

Iris coloboma is often accompanied by posterior coloboma. It may be unilateral. In the absence of fundus coloboma, there is no macular hypoplasia. Cornea is normal.

Albinism (OMIM 203100)

Albinism typically presents in early infancy with nystagmus but a structurally complete iris and the presence of iris transillumination, fundus hypopigmentation, gray optic nerve, and, in the case of oculocutaneous albinism, skin and hair hypopigmentation. In addition, a three-lead VEP (visual evoked potential) may show pattern reversal in albinism patients. Iris transillumination does not occur in aniridia.

Peters Anomaly (OMIM 604229)

The most common manifestation is corneal opacification at birth with posterior corneal scalloped defect seen on optical coherence tomography (OCT) or ultrasound biomicroscopy (UBM), often with iridocorneal adhesions. Various iris anomalies may occur, but foveae are usually normal, though other posterior segment anomalies can occur. This can be unilateral.

Trauma

It is usually unilateral with other findings of trauma and a positive history. It may also occur as a result of surgery.

Other Anterior Segment Dysgenesis

A wide variety of anterior segment dysgenesis may have aniridia variants, but these patients often have microphthalmia, other anterior segment findings atypical for aniridia, and normal foveae.

Persistent Fetal Vasculature (OMIM 221900)

It is typically unilateral, and usually associated with posterior cataract. It can be accompanied by significant retinal abnormalities. It may be seen in true aniridia as it is a developmental defect of the eye, but is usually seen in isolation or with many other anterior segment dysgenesis.

Gillespie Syndrome (OMIM 206700)

This is an AR condition characterized by aniridia, mental retardation, and cerebellar ataxia. Although it has been associated with *PAX6* mutations, many reports fail to demonstrate pathogenic variants in this gene.

6.3 Uncommon Manifestations

Other ocular abnormalities that can be found in patients with aniridia include ectopia lentis, tunica vasculosa lentis remnants, persistent pupillary membrane strands, ptosis, persistent fetal vasculature, microphthalmia, late-onset retinal degeneration, or Peters anomaly.

6.4 Clinical Testing

6.4.1 Macular Optical Coherence Tomography

Macular OCT can be used to demonstrate foveal hypoplasia, but test quality may be limited by nystagmus.

6.4.2 Anterior Segment OCT or High-Frequency Ultrasound Biomicroscopy

Anterior segment OCT or high-frequency UBM can be helpful in patients with corneal opacity.

6.4.3 Systemic Evaluation

Systemic findings in patients with WAGR syndrome include hypospadias and cryptorchidism, gait abnormalities, and developmental delay. Less commonly, patients may have reduced smell sensation, obesity, hearing abnormalities, cerebral or cerebellar hypoplasia, and absence of the pineal gland.

6.4.4 Renal Ultrasound

Renal ultrasound should be performed in all patients, every 6 months until age 7 to 8 years or until the presence of WAGR syndrome has been ruled out by genetic testing. In patients with deletions involving the *WT1* gene, renal ultrasound should be continued every 3 months until the age of 8 years.

6.5 Genetic Testing

Although aniridia is diagnosed by clinical examination, genetic testing in these patients is crucial. To identify a disease-causing mutation in patients with isolated aniridia, sequencing and/or deletion/duplication analysis of *PAX6* should be performed. Typically, gene sequencing is conducted first although some laboratories will automatically perform deletion/duplication analysis if no mutation is found. Sequencing detects a mutation in about 60 to 80% of cases, whereas deletion/duplication analysis identifies an additional 17% of cases. These numbers may vary between laboratories. If an intragenic abnormality is found, then there is no need to consider WAGR syndrome and clinical screening for Wilms' tumor may be abandoned. In addition, if no mutations are found by full *PAX6* gene sequencing, then a search for promoter mutations should be considered. Recently, two genes downstream to *PAX6* have been reported as *PAX6* "enhancer genes": *DCDC1* and *ELP4*. Partial or whole gene deletions of one or both of these genes, many of which may be too small for chromosomal microarrays to detect, have been found in some families with aniridia and should also be considered in *PAX6*-negative families. A recent study found that overexpression of *TRIM44* significantly reduced the expression of *PAX6* in human lens epithelial cells, which represents a novel pathogenic mechanism for aniridia.

As an alternate approach, especially when WAGR is suspected based on family history or clinical examination, a karyotype may be initiated. If the karyotype is normal, chromosomal microarray or FISH can detect smaller chromosomal deletions. Microarray detects 11p13 deletions in up to 20% of patients with no prior family history.

6.6 Problems

6.6.1 Case 1

An otherwise well 3-month-old girl with no family history presents with bilateral aniridia, nystagmus, buphthalmos, corneal edema, and macular hypoplasia. Which of the following tests should be done?
a) Echocardiogram.
b) Renal ultrasound.
c) Brain magnetic resonance imaging (MRI).
d) Chest radiograph.

Correct answer is b.
   Until genetic confirmation that the *WT1* gene is not involved, renal ultrasound is required to rule out manifestations of the WAGR syndrome, particularly in cases of aniridia with no prior family history.
a) **Incorrect.** Cardiac abnormalities are not associated with aniridia.
b) **Correct.**
c) **Incorrect.** Although brain malformation is a rare association, brain MRI is not indicated in an otherwise well child with aniridia.
d) **Incorrect.** Pulmonary abnormalities are not associated with aniridia.

6.6.2 Case 2

Two healthy parents had twins with WAGR syndrome due to del(11)(p13). The father reveals that he had a sibling and an uncle who died at young ages because of renal tumors. How can this be explained?
a) Coincidence. No further test needed.
b) Father is nonpenetrant. Do *PAX6* sequencing.
c) Father has a heterozygous mutation in the *WT1* gene and that gene should be sequenced.
d) Balanced translocation. Do karyotype on father.

Correct answer is d.
   Deletions causing WAGR syndrome may arise de novo or be inherited from an unaffected parent who has a balanced translocation involving 11q. It is likely that the deceased individuals also had WAGR.
a) **Incorrect.** Although possible, the chance of having two rare unrelated rare conditions is lower than one syndrome that explains both.
b) **Incorrect.** Nonpenetrance does not occur in chromosomal deletions such as WAGR. In addition, sequencing the *PAX6* gene may not detect WAGR if the gene is deleted.
c) **Incorrect.** Wilms' tumor usually occurs in childhood. If the father had a *WT1* mutation, he would have had renal findings. In addition, this would not explain the WAGR syndrome in his two sons.
d) **Correct.** Karyotype proved the balanced translocation in father and the resultant deletion in his children.

6.6.3 Case 3

Which of the following clinical presentations most likely correlates with a heterozygous mutation in the *PAX6* gene (c.299G > A)?
a) No expression of the disease.
b) Severe brain malformation and anophthalmia.
c) Aniridia.
d) WAGR syndrome.

Correct answer is c.

Heterozygous nonsense mutations of *PAX6* result in aniridia, especially nonsense mutations such as this, which create a truncated protein. *PAX6* missense mutations could have milder ocular phenotypes, including isolated keratitis, microcornea, Peters anomaly, ectopia pupillae, cataracts, isolated foveal hypoplasia, optic nerve hypoplasia, and macular hypoplasia as well as "partial" or full aniridia.

a) **Incorrect.** *Heterozygous PAX6* mutations produce dysfunctional transcription factors that affect eye development.
b) **Incorrect.** Patients with homozygous or compound heterozygous mutations have this severe phenotype.
c) **Correct.**
d) **Incorrect.** WAGR syndrome is due to a deletion in the 11p13 region. Point mutations in *PAX6* result in isolated ocular phenotype.

6.6.4 Case 4

A 4-year-old male patient with aniridia has negative *PAX6* sequencing and a normal male karyotype. Chromosomal microarray reveals a microdeletion that involves the *PAX6* gene but not *WT1*. Which from the following statements is correct?
a) Renal ultrasound is not needed.
b) FISH should be performed.
c) *PAX6* intronic sequencing is needed.
d) *WT1* sequencing is required.

Correct answer is a.

Microarray has detected a deletion that does not involve the *WT1* gene. Therefore, there is no elevated risk for Wilms' tumor.

a) **Correct.**
b) **Incorrect.** Both microarray and FISH detect deletions. If microarray reveals a deletion, then FISH is no longer needed.
c) **Incorrect.** Since the patient has aniridia, and the array shows a deletion involving the *PAX6* gene, we know that all or part of the *PAX6* gene is missing. This is the cause of the aniridia.
d) **Incorrect.** As WT1 is not involved in the deletion, there is no concern about an abnormality involving this gene.

Suggested Reading

[1] Azuma N, Hotta Y, Tanaka H, Yamada M. Missense mutations in the PAX6 gene in aniridia. Invest Ophthalmol Vis Sci. 1998; 39(13):2524–2528

[2] Brandt JD, Casuso LA, Budenz DL. Markedly increased central corneal thickness: an unrecognized finding in congenital aniridia. Am J Ophthalmol. 2004; 137(2):348–350

[3] Fischbach BV, Trout KL, Lewis J, Luis CA, Sika M. WAGR syndrome: a clinical review of 54 cases. Pediatrics. 2005; 116(4):984–988

[4] Gramer E, Reiter C, Gramer G. Glaucoma and frequency of ocular and general diseases in 30 patients with aniridia: a clinical study. Eur J Ophthalmol. 2012; 22(1):104–110

[5] Hingorani M, Williamson KA, Moore AT, van Heyningen V. Detailed ophthalmologic evaluation of 43 individuals with PAX6 mutations. Invest Ophthalmol Vis Sci. 2009; 50(6):2581–2590

[6] Glaser T, Walton DS, Maas RL. Genomic structure, evolutionary conservation and aniridia mutations in the human PAX6 gene. Nat Genet. 1992; 2(3):232–239

[7] Netland PA, Scott ML, Boyle JW, IV, Lauderdale JD. Ocular and systemic findings in a survey of aniridia subjects. J AAPOS. 2011; 15(6):562–566

[8] Shiple D, Finklea B, Lauderdale JD, Netland PA. Keratopathy, cataract, and dry eye in a survey of aniridia subjects. Clin Ophthalmol. 2015; 9:291–295

[9] Chang JW, Kim JH, Kim SJ, Yu YS. Congenital aniridia: long-term clinical course, visual outcome, and prognostic factors. Korean J Ophthalmol. 2014; 28(6):479–485

[10] Sadagopan KA, Liu GT, Capasso JE, Wuthisiri W, Keep RB, Levin AV. Anirdia-like phenotype caused by 6p25 dosage aberrations. Am J Med Genet A. 2015; 167A(3):524–528

[11] Zhang X, Qin G, Chen G, et al. Variants in TRIM44 cause aniridia by impairing PAX6 expression. Hum Mutat. 2015; 36(12):1164–1167

7 Peters Anomaly

Yu-Hung Lai

Abstract

Peters anomaly is a rare disorder characterized by corneal opacity with posterior corneal defects, and various degrees of iridocorneal and/or lenticulocorneal attachments. It is often caused by mutations of anterior segment development genes. It is a malformation sequence, primarily the result of failure of the lens to be created properly from surface ectoderm in response to the induction of the underlying optic vesicle. Neural crest migration to form the cornea and anterior segment structures is secondarily disrupted. Visual prognosis is usually based on location and size of the resulting scar. Most affected individuals are bilaterally involved and more likely to have associated systemic malformations. Patients have a lifetime risk of glaucoma with or without corneal surgery.

Keywords: Peters anomaly, glaucoma, Peters plus, cataract, anterior segment dysgenesis, posterior corneal defect, *PAX6, PITX2, FOXC1, CYP1B1, FOXE3, TFAP2A, FLNA, HCCS, NDP SLC4A11, B3GALTL*

Key Points

- Peters anomaly is characterized by corneal opacity with posterior corneal defect, and various degrees of iridocorneal and/or lenticulocorneal attachments.
- Mutations in anterior segment development genes can lead to Peters anomaly.
- Peters anomaly results from disruption of embryonic corneal/iris/lens formation.

7.1 Overview

Peters anomaly (OMIM 604229) is a rare disorder characterized by corneal opacity with posterior corneal defects, and various degrees of iridocorneal and/or lenticulocorneal attachments (▶ Fig. 7.1). It is often caused by mutations of anterior segment development genes, such as the *PAX6* gene. It is a malformation sequence primarily the result of failure of the lens to be created properly from surface ectoderm in response to the induction of the underlying optic vesicle. Neural crest migration to form the cornea and anterior segment structures are secondarily disrupted. Visual prognosis is usually based on location and size of the resulting scar. Most affected individuals are bilaterally involved and those with bilateral involvement are more likely to have associated systemic malformations. Treatment choices include corneal transplantation and/or lens extraction if cataract is present. For less severe cases, an optical iridectomy may be performed or pharmacologic dilation used. Patients have a lifetime risk of glaucoma with or without corneal surgery.

Rarely, patients with Peters anomaly may have associated systemic abnormalities including short stature, cleft lip/palate, characteristic facial features, and developmental delay, which are designated Peters plus syndrome (MIM 261540). In these individuals,

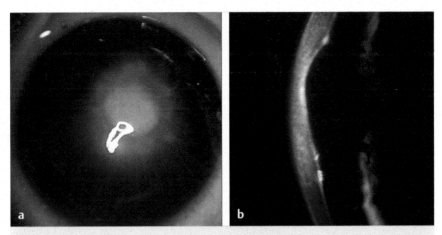

Fig. 7.1 Peters anomaly. (a) Note central corneal opacity with shallow anterior chamber and cataract. There are iridocorneal adhesions from the pupil to the corneal scar. (b) Posterior corneal defect. Note also the shallow anterior chamber and iridocorneal adhesions.

developmental delay is seen in approximately 80% of children. Peters may also present with a wide variety of other malformations in the absence of skeletal dysplasia with or without a defined syndromic diagnosis other than true Peters plus.

7.2 Molecular Genetics

Most cases are sporadic. Autosomal recessive and autosomal dominant inheritance has been reported. Mutations of anterior segment development genes can lead to Peters anomaly. Peters anomaly had been associated with mutations in the *PAX6* gene (autosomal dominant, 11p13, OMIM 607108). This gene is most commonly associated with aniridia, but Peters anomaly can occur without aniridia. The *PITX2* (autosomal dominant, 4q25, OMIM 601542) and *FOXC1* (copy number variations, autosomal dominant, 6p25, OMIM 601909) genes are reported more commonly with Axenfeld–Rieger spectrum. Mutations in the *CYP1B1* gene (autosomal recessive, 2p22.2, OMIM 601771) are more commonly associated with congenital glaucoma. The *FOXE3* gene (1p33, OMIM 601094) is also associated with primary aphakia. Other relevant genes include *TFAP2A* and *FLNA* when syndromic features such as facial dysmorphism, hearing loss, velopharyngeal insufficiency, short stature, kidney hypoplasia, and heart and skeletal abnormalities are present, and *HCCS*, *NDP*, and *SLC4A11* in patients with isolated Peters anomaly.

Beta-1,3-galactosyltransferase-like glycosyltransferase (*B3GALTL*) is the only gene in which mutations are known to produce Peters plus syndrome. Most affected individuals are homozygous for a splice-site mutation in intron 8 (c.660 + 1G > A). Peters plus syndrome is inherited in an autosomal recessive manner. Deletions and duplications of the gene's locus, 13q12.3, may also result in Peters plus syndrome.

7.3 Differential Diagnosis

7.3.1 Birth Trauma

Birth trauma of the cornea due to forceps may cause a break in Descemet's membrane with overlying stromal edema. Usually one can visualize vertically oriented, straight-edged, parallel lines on the endothelium. Forceps-related trauma usually presents with periorbital soft tissue injury, normal intraocular pressure, and normal corneal size.

7.3.2 Congenital Hereditary Endothelial/Stromal Dystrophy

Congenital hereditary endothelial/stromal dystrophy usually presents in infancy or early childhood with a completely and totally cloudy cornea, which is thick and has a "ground glass" appearance.

7.3.3 Corneal Dermoids

Corneal dermoids are rarely seen. Some syndromes, such as Lowe or Rubinstein–Taybi, can present with bilateral lesions.

7.3.4 Metabolic Disorders

Metabolic disorders in which substances are deposited in the cornea (e.g., mucopoly-saccharidoses) can present with cloudy corneas in infancy but rarely at birth. The anterior segment is otherwise normal.

7.3.5 Intrauterine Keratitis

Intrauterine keratitis such as herpetic or rubella may result in cloudy cornea in infants. Posterior synechia from uveitis may mimic the iris abnormalities of Peters anomaly.

7.3.6 Amniocentesis Perforation

Although reports of ocular damage from amniocentesis needles are rare, this event may be more frequent than reported. Reported findings include vascularized corneal leukoma, nonpigmented epithelial cyst of the anterior chamber, eyelid coloboma, retinal detachment, paralimbal scleral perforation with iris prolapse, distortion of the pupil, aphakia, and chorioretinal scarring. Only one eye is affected.

7.3.7 Congenital Glaucoma

Corneal edema is usually concentrated more centrally and may obscure a view of the anterior chamber. The eye is always enlarged. Iridocorneal adhesions would not be present.

7.3.8 Axenfeld–Rieger Spectrum

This is a heterogeneous condition with developmental anomalies of the anterior chamber including corectopia, polycoria, ectropion uveae, and posterior embryotoxon. Facial dysmorphism, abnormal teeth, and a redundant periumbilical skin may be seen. Glaucoma may occur.

7.3.9 Primary Aphakia

Patients present invariably with silvery corneal opacity and in the absence of a lens. Intraocular contents may be disorganized. It may be associated with Peters anomaly. Glaucoma is common.

7.4 Uncommon Manifestations

Peters anomaly may be a part of the phenotype in the anterior segment mesenchymal dysgenesis (OMIM 107250) or other developmental disorders such as aniridia, Axenfeld–Rieger, or persistent fetal vasculature. Posterior embryotoxon may be seen.

7.4.1 Walker–Warburg Syndrome

Walker–Warburg syndrome is a group of inherited disorders that affects development of the muscles, brain, and eyes. It is the most severe of the congenital muscular dystrophies, which cause muscle atrophy that begins in early infancy. Most affected patients do not survive past the age of 3 years. Neurological findings include cobblestone lissencephaly, hydrocephalus, severe developmental delay, seizures, and cerebellum/brainstem anomalies. Encephalocele may be seen. Eye abnormalities include microphthalmia, buphthalmos, cataracts, corneal opacities, retinal dysplasia, and the optic nerve anomalies. Peters anomaly may occur.

7.4.2 Congenital Corneal Ectasia

Congenital corneal ectasia is a severe form of Peters anomaly, often with significant microphthalmia, in which the central cornea at birth is ectatic or even perforated. It is usually bilateral and has a very guarded prognosis.

7.4.3 Jung Syndrome

Jung syndrome (OMIM 601427) consists of growth retardation, congenital hypothyroidism, narrow external auditory meatus, cerebellar hypoplasia, short neck, tracheal stenosis, hip dysplasia, genital abnormalities, and dense scalp hair. Deficiency of growth hormone, short feet, and shield thorax have also been described. Patients may have coloboma and/or anterior segment dysgenesis including Peters anomaly.

7.5 Clinical Testing

Key features on clinical examination often include an endothelial opacity that may have a very distinct circular edge. The anterior chamber may be shallow with iridocorneal or lenticulocorneal adhesion. The iris may even be completely adherent to the corneal endothelium. Glaucoma and/or cataract may or may not be present.

7.5.1 High-Frequency Ultrasound Biomicroscopy

High-frequency ultrasound biomicroscopy (UBM) may be used to investigate the contour of the posterior cornea (which often shows a posterior scallop previously known as the posterior ulcer of von Hippel), the severity of lens and iris anterior attachment, and anterior segment morphology.

Systemic malformations should also be evaluated.

7.6 Genetic Testing

Several laboratories offer gene panels for anterior segment disorders. Testing may be sculpted to target specific genes when particular clinical findings are present (e.g., posterior embryotoxon would lead one to suspect a mutation in *PITX2* or *FOXC1*).

Chromosomal microarray should be considered when gene sequencing is negative and, especially if systemic anomalies are present, as deletions and duplications may cause phenotypes with Peters anomaly. For a patient suspected to have Peters plus syndrome, *B3GALTL* gene (OMIM 610308) sequencing can be performed, but microarray is also indicated.

7.7 Problems

7.7.1 Case 1

A 2-month-old girl was noted with a bilateral corneal opacity. Ophthalmic examination reveals bilateral iridocorneal adhesion to the central endothelial corneal opacities without other findings. Birth history was unremarkable and there is no history of amniocentesis. Physical examination is normal. After counseling, parents would like to know the genetic cause. Which of the following tests would be the best first step in making a molecular diagnosis?

a) *PAX6* sequencing.
b) *PITX2* sequencing.
c) Whole exome sequencing.
d) Anterior segment gene disorder panel.

Correct answer is d.

In this case, there are no specific findings to suggest a single gene for sequencing. A reasonable approach would be an anterior segment gene disorder panel.

a) **Incorrect.** Although isolated Peters anomaly may rarely occur, the *PAX6* gene is most commonly associated with aniridia.
b) **Incorrect.** *PITX2* and *FOXC1* genes are reported more frequently with Axenfeld–Rieger spectrum.
c) **Incorrect.** Although it will likely find a mutated gene, it is not a usual first test because of cost, ethical concerns, and the availability of a more targeted strategy.
d) **Correct.**

7.7.2 Case 2

A 1-month-old girl was noted with a corneal opacity. Which of the following would suggest Peters anomaly?

a) Central corneal opacity with peripheral clear cornea.
b) Posterior embryotoxon.
c) A white mass at limbus with fine hairs on it.
d) Progressive corneal opacity.

Correct answer is a.

Peters anomaly is usually characterized by central corneal opacity with posterior corneal defects, and various degrees of iris and/or lens attachments to the cornea. The peripheral cornea is usually clear.

a) **Correct.**

b) **Incorrect.** This would suggest Axenfeld–Rieger spectrum.

c) **Incorrect.** This would suggest a limbal dermoid.

d) **Incorrect.** This would suggest infectious keratitis, metabolic diseases (e.g., mucopolysaccharidoses), or congenital hereditary endothelial dystrophy, all of which may not present until after birth.

7.7.3 Case 3

A newborn infant was referred to you for Peters anomaly. Which of the following examinations would be *least* appropriate for the baby?

a) Slit-lamp examination.

b) High-frequency UBM.

c) B-scan ultrasound if no view of the posterior segment.

d) Electroretinogram.

Correct answer is d.

Slit-lamp examination, UBM, and B-scan ultrasound are useful tools in the evaluation of Peters anomaly.

a) **Incorrect.**

b) **Incorrect.**

c) **Incorrect.**

d) **Correct.** The retina is usually normal in Peters anomaly. Visual loss stems from the corneal opacity, cataract, and amblyopia.

7.7.4 Case 4

An 11-month-old girl has bilateral Peters anomaly, short limbs, developmental delay, cleft lip, and cleft palate. Which of the following genetic test(s) is the most appropriate?

a) *B3GALTL* sequencing.

b) Chromosome microarray study.

c) Whole genome sequencing.

d) a + b.

Correct answer is d.

The description of the patient suggests Peters plus syndrome. The *B3GALTL* gene is the only currently known gene in which mutations would cause Peters plus syndrome. Deletions of this locus have also been reported.

a) **Correct.**

b) **Correct.** The *B3GALTL* gene could be the first step of a gene test. However, given the condition of multiple systemic abnormalities, chromosome microarray could also be arranged if the patient is not considered as typical Peters plus syndrome.

c) **Incorrect.** Whole genomic sequencing would only be appropriate if all other testing specific for the recognized clinical entity was negative.

d) **Correct answer is d.**

Suggested Reading

[1] Bhandari R, Ferri S, Whittaker B, Liu M, Lazzaro DR. Peters anomaly: review of the literature. Cornea. 2011; 30(8):939–944

[2] Reis LM, Semina EV. Genetics of anterior segment dysgenesis disorders. Curr Opin Ophthalmol. 2011; 22(5): 314–324

[3] Hanson IM, Fletcher JM, Jordan T, et al. Mutations at the PAX6 locus are found in heterogeneous anterior segment malformations including Peters anomaly. Nat Genet. 1994; 6(2):168–173

[4] Doward W, Perveen R, Lloyd IC, Ridgway AE, Wilson L, Black GC. A mutation in the RIEG1 gene associated with Peters anomaly. J Med Genet. 1999; 36(2):152–155

[5] Nishimura DY, Searby CC, Alward WL, et al. A spectrum of FOXC1 mutations suggests gene dosage as a mechanism for developmental defects of the anterior chamber of the eye. Am J Hum Genet. 2001; 68(2): 364–372

[6] Vincent A, Billingsley G, Priston M, et al. Phenotypic heterogeneity of CYP1B1: mutations in a patient with Peters anomaly. J Med Genet. 2001; 38(5):324–326

[7] Traboulsi EI, Maumenee IH. Peters anomaly and associated congenital malformations. Arch Ophthalmol. 1992; 110(12):1739–1742

[8] Weh E, Reis LM, Happ HC, et al. Whole exome sequence analysis of Peters anomaly. Hum Genet. 2014; 133 (12):1497–1511

8 Axenfeld–Rieger Syndrome

Yu-Hung Lai

Abstract

Axenfeld–Rieger spectrum is a form of anterior segment dysgenesis characterized by posterior embryotoxon and iridocorneal strands usually directly to the embryotoxon. Other findings may include iris malformations, corectopia, and/or polycoria. There is an approximately 50% lifetime risk for developing glaucoma at any age. Systemic findings include facial, dental, umbilical, and skeletal abnormalities. Axenfeld–Rieger spectrum is usually a bilateral, yet often asymmetric condition.

Keywords: Axenfeld–Rieger spectrum, posterior embryotoxon, iridocorneal strands, glaucoma, cataract, anterior segment dysgenesis, *PITX2, FOXC1, PAX6, JAG1, FOXC2, CYP1B1, LAMB2, PRDM5*

Key Points

- Typical findings of Axenfeld–Rieger spectrum are posterior embryotoxon, iridocorneal strands, iris anomalies, corectopia, and/or polycoria with or without dental or umbilical abnormalities.
- Approximately 50% of patients develop glaucoma.
- *PITX2* and *FOXC1* gene mutations account for 40% of cases. Mutations in *PAX6, JAG1, FOXC2, CYP1B1, LAMB2,* and *PRDM5* have also been associated.
- Patients with Axenfeld–Rieger spectrum may also have hearing deficits, maxillary hypoplasia, hydrocephalus, cryptorchidism, and/or kidney or heart anomalies.

8.1 Overview

Axenfeld–Rieger spectrum (ARS) is a form of anterior segment dysgenesis characterized by posterior embryotoxon (prominent and anteriorly displaced Schwalbe's line) and iridocorneal strands usually directly to the embryotoxon. Other findings may include iris malformations, corectopia, and/or polycoria (▶ Fig. 8.1). There is an approximately 50% lifetime risk for developing glaucoma at any age. Systemic findings may or may not be present. These include facial, dental (▶ Fig. 8.2), umbilical (▶ Fig. 8.3), and skeletal abnormalities. Previously, terms such as Axenfeld anomaly, Axenfeld syndrome, Rieger's anomaly, and Rieger's syndrome have been used to describe specific combinations of ocular and/or systemic findings. Molecular genetics has allowed the recognition of the wide spectrum of expression even with the same gene mutation and thus led to the use of the term ARS to include all patients. ARS is usually a bilateral, yet often asymmetric condition. Isolated posterior embryotoxon is not uncommon in the general population, perhaps as frequent as 15%.

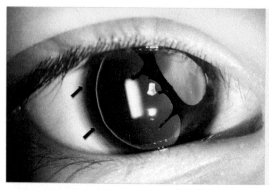

Fig. 8.1 Axenfeld–Rieger spectrum. There is polycoria, and marked iris dysgenesis. Arrows indicate posterior embryotoxon.

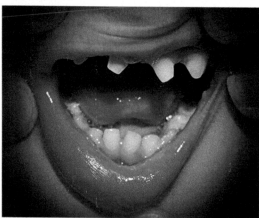

Fig. 8.2 Tooth anomalies in a patient with Axenfeld–Rieger spectrum. Note microdontia, oligodontia, and abnormal tooth shape.

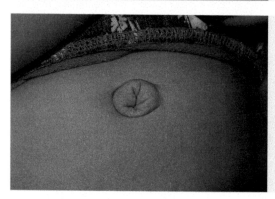

Fig. 8.3 Periumbilical redundant skin in a patient with Axenfeld–Rieger spectrum.

8.2 Molecular Genetics

ARS is genetically and phenotypically heterogeneous. Axenfeld–Rieger type 1 (RIEG1, OMIM 180500) is caused by *PITX2* gene mutation, while Axenfeld–Rieger type 3 (RIEG3, OMIM 602482) is caused by *FOXC1* gene mutation. Axenfeld–Rieger type 2

Table 8.1 Axenfeld–Rieger spectrum (ARS)

Gene	Findings
PAX6	Ectropion uvea, corectopia, iris hypoplasia, cataract
JAG1	Alagille syndrome; posterior embryotoxon
FOXC2	Lymphedema-distichiasis syndrome; iris hypoplasia, corectopia
CYP1B1	ARS associated with protruding umbilicus and dental anomalies
LAMB2	Pierson syndrome; iris hypoplasia, ectropion uvea, posterior embryotoxon
PRDM5	Congenital glaucoma, ectopia pupil, iris hypoplasia, corneal opacity, posterior embryotoxon, posterior subcapsular cataract
PIK3R1	SHORT syndrome; ARS
COL4A1	Brain small vessel disease with or without ocular anomalies, including ARS

Abbreviation: SHORT, Short stature, Hyperextensibility, Hernia, Ocular depression (enophthalmos), Rieger anomaly, and Teething delay.

(RIEG2, OMIM 601449) is linked to chromosome 13q14, but the gene has not been identified. *PITX2* (autosomal dominant, 4q25, OMIM 601542) and *FOXC1* (autosomal dominant, 6p25, OMIM 601090) genes account for approximately 40% of ARS cases. Type 1 is reported to be associated with dental and umbilical disorders, while type 2 is associated with heart and hearing defects, or with isolated ocular defects. Other genes that when mutated have ocular and systemic abnormalities that include features of ARS are listed in ▶ Table 8.1.

8.3 Differential Diagnosis

8.3.1 Peters Anomaly (OMIM 604229)

Peters anomaly (OMIM 604229) is characterized by central corneal opacity with posterior corneal defect, and iridocorneal and/or lenticular corneal adhesions. Some patients may also express signs of ARS, in particular posterior embryotoxon.

8.3.2 Congenital Glaucoma (OMIM 231300)

Although glaucoma at birth or in infancy may be a feature of ARS, in congenital glaucoma there are no anatomic anomalies of the anterior segment as seen in ARS. In congenital glaucoma, there may be heterochromia, radialization of the iris stroma, and/or peripheral iris stromal atrophy. Gonioscopy reveals patches of high iris insertion over the trabecular meshwork but neither anteriorization of Schwalbe's line nor iridocorneal adhesions.

8.3.3 Aniridia (OMIM 612469; 607108)

Aniridia (OMIM 612469; 607108) is distinguished by the partial or near total absence of iris. When partial iris is present, the disorder is distinguished from ARS by the absence of posterior embryotoxon. Cataract, foveal hypoplasia, and optic nerve hypoplasia are also common in aniridia but absent in ARS.

8.3.4 Iris Coloboma

Iris coloboma may manifest as a keyhole-shaped pupil and in the inferonasal quadrant of the iris. The pupil may also be drawn down toward that quadrant, thus mimicking the corectopia of ARS. Posterior embryotoxon and glaucoma do not occur. Unlike ARS, iris coloboma may be associated with cataract, lens notch, microphthalmia, and coloboma of the retina and/or optic nerve.

8.3.5 Iridocorneal Endothelial Syndrome

Iridocorneal endothelial syndrome is typically unilateral, occurring more in females, and manifested in adulthood. It is associated with the metaplastic transformation ("epithelialization") of corneal endothelium. Patients often have acquired iris atrophy, corectopia, iridocorneal adhesion, glaucoma, and/or iris nevus. They do not have posterior embryotoxon or congenital anterior segment dysgenesis.

8.3.6 Iris Stromal Cysts

Iris stromal cysts may lead to corectopia, iridocorneal adhesion, and glaucoma. Unlike ARS, they are almost always acquired, progressive, and not associated with posterior embryotoxon.

8.3.7 Isolated Normal Variant Posterior Embryotoxon

Isolated normal variant posterior embryotoxon is defined by the presence of a prominent and anteriorly displaced line of Schwalbe, which corresponds to the anatomical line seen on the interior surface of the cornea. It delineates the outer limit of the endothelium and represents the termination of Descemet's membrane. Depending on the population, 10 to 30% present posterior embryotoxon as an isolated normal variant.

8.3.8 Traumatic Corectopia

Traumatic corectopia can be easily differentiated from ARS by the patient's past history or ocular surgery. Perforation of the eye during amniocentesis may result in congenital corectopia with iridocorneal adhesion that can mimic ARS, although it is not associated with glaucoma or posterior embryotoxon.

8.4 Uncommon Manifestations

Less common manifestations of ARS include hearing defects, mild craniofacial dysmorphism, hydrocephalus, cryptorchidism, fetal lobulation of kidney, congenital heart defect, and congenital hip abnormalities.

8.4.1 Alagille Syndrome (OMIM 118450)

Alagille syndrome (OMIM 118450) is associated with *JAG1* gene mutations, and is characterized by varying degrees of biliary atresia, heart anomalies, vertebral anomalies, and a characteristic facies. Ocular features include posterior embryotoxon and occasionally iris hypoplasia, iridocorneal adhesion, and corectopia. Patients also may exhibit a pigmentary retinopathy. Angle closure glaucoma has been rarely reported.

8.4.2 Lymphedema-Distichiasis Syndrome (OMIM 153400)

Patients with this condition may have iris hypoplasia, and corectopia. The syndrome is associated with *FOXC2* gene mutations.

8.4.3 Pierson Syndrome (OMIM 609049; *LAMB2* Mutation)

Pierson syndrome (OMIM 609049; *LAMB2* mutation) is characterized by congenital nephrotic syndrome and neurological anomalies. Ocular features include miosis, iris hypoplasia, ectropion uvea, and/or posterior embryotoxon. Patients exhibit a pigmentary retinopathy and may have retinal detachment.

8.4.4 SHORT Syndrome (OMIM 269880)

Mutations in the *PIK3R1* gene are associated with SHORT (Short stature, Hyperextensibility, Hernia, Ocular depression [enophthalmos], Rieger anomaly, and Teething delay) syndrome, which is an autosomal dominant disorder. Contiguous deletion syndrome has also been described in this condition.

8.5 Clinical Testing

Slit-lamp examination, intraocular pressure, gonioscopy, and ultrasound biomicroscopy (UBM) may be useful to evaluate the clinical extent of the disease and identify the correct diagnosis. Periodic follow-up for the possibility of glaucoma is essential.

8.6 Genetic Testing

Since *PITX2* and *FOXC1* gene mutations account for 40% of the ARS cases, this may be a first-line testing target. Chromosomal microarray may be useful if the patient has multisystem involvement. Deletion or duplication of 6p25 is highly associated with ARS. Patients with ARS and dental and umbilical disorders are more likely to have *PITX2* gene mutations, while patients with heart and hearing defects are more likely associated with *FOXC1* gene mutations. Anterior segment dysgenesis panels and whole exome sequencing can also be considered in patients with unusual presentations as there may be phenotypic overlap with other genes. Additionally, there are research protocols that include genetic testing for anterior segment dysgenesis that can provide a far more affordable testing option for identifying the genetic cause in an individual.

8.7 Problems

8.7.1 Case 1

A 5-month-old male infant has ocular findings consistent with ARS disorder. He has no systemic findings. What is the best genetic testing strategy?
a) *PITX2* and *FOXC1* gene sequencing.
b) Retinal dystrophy panel.
c) Whole exome sequencing.
d) *PAX6* sequencing.

The most appropriate answer is a.

PITX2 and *FOXC1* gene mutations account for approximately 40% of the ARS cases.

a) **Correct.**

b) **Incorrect.** Retinal dystrophy is not a manifestation of ARS.

c) **Incorrect.** Whole exome sequencing is more appropriate for cases in which the testing of known causative genetic mutations is unrevealing or when a specific test is not available for the phenotype.

d) **Incorrect.** Mutations in *PAX6* are associated primarily with aniridia. Although phenotypes may mimic ARS, posterior embryotoxon is not present. ARS does not have findings seen in aniridia such as macular hypoplasia.

8.7.2 Case 2

A 2-month-old male infant was referred for an "abnormal pupil." What additional finding would most support a diagnosis of ARS?

a) Central corneal opacity with iridocorneal and lenticular corneal adhesions.

b) A teardrop-shaped pupil in the lower nasal quadrant of the iris associated with a lens notch.

c) Almost absent iris with anterior pyramidal cataract.

d) Corectopia and polycoria associated with posterior embryotoxon with attached iris strands.

The most appropriate answer is d.

a) **Incorrect**. This description would suggest Peters anomaly.

b) **Incorrect**. This description would suggest coloboma.

c) **Incorrect**. This description would suggest aniridia.

d) **Correct.**

8.7.3 Case 3

A 5-month-old male infant was found to have iris hypoplasia, and iris strands to posterior embryotoxon. What would be the least appropriate test for this baby?

a) Systemic evaluation.

b) Intraocular pressure.

c) *CYP1B1* gene analysis (sequencing, duplication, and deletion).

d) Slit-lamp examination.

Correct answer is c.

Mutations in the *CYP1B1* gene are typically associated with congenital glaucoma without features of ARS.

a) **Incorrect**. Patients with ARS can have abnormalities of the umbilicus, teeth, or limbs. There are also some systemic syndromes associated with ARS, such as Alagille syndrome, lymphedema-distichiasis syndrome, Pierson syndrome, and SHORT syndrome, which require systemic examination for detection.

b) **Incorrect**. Approximately 50% of ARS patient have glaucoma, so intraocular pressure measurement is appropriate.

c) **Correct.**

d) **Incorrect**. Slit-lamp examination is essential to identify the features of ARS.

8.7.4 Case 4

For the patient in Case 3, which of the following would be helpful?
a) Examine the parents.
b) Obtain pedigree.
c) Genetic testing.
d) All of the above.

Correct answer is d.

For patients with autosomal dominant ARS, there is variable expressivity of the phenotype within a family. If the parent(s) had a certain degree of anterior segment dysgenesis, it would also help us to sort out the inheritance pattern and associated diagnosis of the patient. Pedigree will provide the pattern of inheritance, associated diseases running in the family, or the possibility of concurrent diseases. Additionally, it would also provide the information for future genetic testing. Chromosomal microarray study is recommended for ARS patients with multiple systems involvement.
a) **Correct.**
b) **Correct.**
c) **Correct.**
d) **Correct and most appropriate.**

Suggested Reading

[1] Reis LM, Semina EV. Genetics of anterior segment dysgenesis disorders. Curr Opin Ophthalmol. 2011; 22(5): 314–324

[2] Reis LM, Tyler RC, Volkmann Kloss BA, et al. PITX2 and FOXC1 spectrum of mutations in ocular syndromes. Eur J Hum Genet. 2012; 20(12):1224–1233

[3] Berker N, Alanay Y, Elgin U, et al. A new autosomal dominant Peters anomaly phenotype expanding the anterior segment dysgenesis spectrum. Acta Ophthalmol. 2009; 87(1):52–57

[4] Micheal S, Siddiqui SN, Zafar SN, et al. Whole exome sequencing identifies a heterozygous missense variant in the PRDM5 gene in a family with Axenfeld-Rieger syndrome. Neurogenetics. 2016; 17(1):17–23

[5] Hashemi H, Khabazkhoob M, Emamian MH, Shariati M, Yekta A, Fotouhi A. The frequency of occurrence of certain corneal conditions by age and sex in Iranian adults. Cont Lens Anterior Eye. 2015; 38(6):451–455

[6] Rennie CA, Chowdhury S, Khan J, et al. The prevalence and associated features of posterior embryotoxon in the general ophthalmic clinic. Eye (Lond). 2005; 19(4):396–399

[7] Sowden JC. Molecular and developmental mechanisms of anterior segment dysgenesis. Eye (Lond). 2007; 21 (10):1310–1318

9 Primary Congenital Glaucoma and Juvenile Open Angle Glaucoma

Juan P. López

Abstract

Primary congenital glaucoma is characterized by elevated intraocular pressure due to dysgenesis of the trabecular meshwork. If left untreated, it leads to optic neuropathy with irreversible visual loss. It can be subdivided into neonatal, infantile, and late onset. Due to the increased elasticity of the cornea and sclera in children, elevated intraocular pressure results in buphthalmos and corneal enlargement with rupture of Descemet's membrane. The classic clinical presentation includes a triad of photophobia, blepharospasm, and epiphora due to corneal edema. The older the age of onset, the fewer the signs and symptoms. Mutations in the *CYP1B1* gene are currently the primary known etiology for primary congenital glaucoma, although genes at other loci have yet to be identified. Juvenile open angle glaucoma is an autosomal dominant disorder that usually affects individuals between the age of 4 and 40 years. Intrafamilial variation in age of onset is common. Early detection is difficult. Genetic testing of at-risk individuals may allow for appropriate screening. *MYOC* gene mutations are the only known cause at this time.

Keywords: primary congenital glaucoma, juvenile open angle glaucoma, *CYP1B1*, *MYOC*, intraocular pressure

---

Key Points

- Primary congenital glaucoma (PCG) includes neonatal onset (< 1 month), infantile onset (1–24 months), and late onset (> 2 years).
- The primary manifestation is elevated intraocular pressure resulting in enlargement of the globe.
- The *CYP1B1* gene is currently the primary known etiology for PCG. The genes for other PCG loci have not yet been identified.

9.1 Primary Congenital Glaucoma

9.1.1 Overview

Primary congenital glaucoma (PCG) is a potentially blinding disease characterized by elevated intraocular pressure (IOP) due to dysgenesis of the trabecular meshwork. If left untreated, it leads to optic neuropathy with irreversible visual loss. It can be subdivided into neonatal or newborn onset (0–1 month), infantile onset (1–24 months), and late onset or late recognized (> 2 years; ▸ Fig. 9.1). PCG occurs in 1 of 4,000 to 10,000 live births and is bilateral in more than two-thirds of patients. Incidence is higher in certain ethnic groups including gypsies and some countries of the Middle East. Due to the increased elasticity of the cornea and sclera in children, elevated IOP results in buphthalmos and corneal enlargement with rupture of Descemet's membrane (Haab's striae; ▸ Fig. 9.2). Although traditionally thought to be confined to children younger

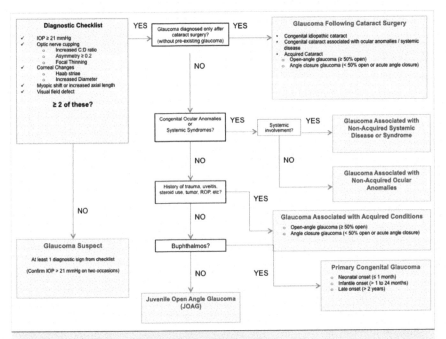

Diagnostic Checklist

✓ IOP ≥ 21 mmHg
✓ Optic nerve cupping
  ○ Increased C:D ratio
  ○ Asymmetry ≥ 0.2
  ○ Focal Thinning
✓ Corneal Changes
  ○ Haab striae
  ○ Increased Diameter
✓ Myopic shift or increased axial length
✓ Visual field defect

≥ 2 of these?

YES →

Glaucoma diagnosed only after cataract surgery? (without pre-existing glaucoma)

YES →

Glaucoma Following Cataract Surgery

• Congenital idiopathic cataract
• Congenital cataract associated with ocular anomalies / systemic disease
• Acquired Cataract
  ○ Open-angle glaucoma (≥ 50% open)
  ○ Angle closure glaucoma (< 50% open or acute angle closure)

NO

Congenital Ocular Anomalies or Systemic Syndromes?

YES →

Systemic involvement?

YES →

Glaucoma Associated with Non-Acquired Systemic Disease or Syndrome

NO

NO

Glaucoma Associated with Non-Acquired Ocular Anomalies

History of trauma, uveitis, steroid use, tumor, ROP, etc?

YES →

Glaucoma Associated with Acquired Conditions

  ○ Open-angle glaucoma (≥ 50% open)
  ○ Angle closure glaucoma (< 50% open or acute angle closure)

NO

NO

Buphthalmos?

Primary Congenital Glaucoma

  ○ Neonatal onset (≤ 1 month)
  ○ Infantile onset (> 1 to 24 months)
  ○ Late onset (> 2 years)

NO

Glaucoma Suspect

At least 1 diagnostic sign from checklist

(Confirm IOP > 21 mmHg on two occasions)

NO

YES

Juvenile Open Angle Glaucoma (JOAG)

Fig. 9.1 The Childhood Glaucoma Research Network (CGRN) algorithm for categorizing childhood glaucoma.

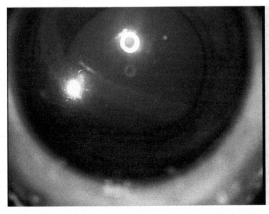

Fig. 9.2 Horizontal rupture of Descemet's membrane (Haab's striae) in a patient with congenital glaucoma.

than 2 years, this may occur rarely even up to the age of 7 years. Other findings may include anterior iris stromal atrophy, heterochromia, and axial myopia (or loss of normal-for-age hyperopia) as well as corneal epithelial and/or stromal edema. Anterior segment dysgenesis is absent. Gonioscopy typically reveals patchy high iris insertion. The classic clinical presentation includes a triad of photophobia, blepharospasm, and epiphora due to corneal edema. The older the age of onset, the fewer the signs and symptoms.

9.1.2 Molecular Genetics

PCG, known as GLC3 in the genetic nomenclature, is usually an autosomal recessive (AR) disorder, although autosomal dominant (AD) patterns have also been observed. Variable expression and nonpenetrance are also known. The GLC3A locus contains the cytochrome P450 subfamily I, polypeptide 1 (*CYP1B1*, 2p22-p21) gene which is currently the primary known etiology for primary congenital glaucoma. Mutations in this gene are responsible for 80% of PCG in Saudi Arabia but only up to 20% of PCG in North America. Neonatal onset PCG is more likely to be due to *CYP1B1* mutations. The genes for GLC3B (1p36) and GLC3C (14q24.3) have not yet been identified. All three loci are characterized by an AR pattern.

9.1.3 Differential Diagnosis

Although many disorders can mimic the epiphora, photophobia, and corneal clouding that characterize PCG, buphthalmos is the key distinguishing factor and a requisite for the diagnosis. The differential diagnosis here is restricted to conditions that cause true glaucoma with buphthalmos and/or macrocornea. Axial myopia, exorbitism (shallow orbits) due to craniofacial disorders, and upper lid retraction can give the illusion of an enlarged globe. Although Haab's striae are considered pathognomic for PCG, there are other causes of Descemet's breaks including trauma, in particular forceps-induced breaks. Congenital rubella endothelialitis, Descemet's folds, and syphilis may have corneal endothelial changes that mimic Haab's striae. Corneal enlargement is only seen with true Haab's striae due to PCG.

Megalocornea (OMIM 309300)

Megalocornea (OMIM 309300) is characterized by bilateral enlarged corneal diameter (> 13 mm) without increased IOP. Some authors refer to megalocornea as "anterior megalophthalmos," since the anterior segment may appear as larger than normal. Other findings include astigmatism, atrophy of the iris stroma sometimes with radial iris transillumination, miosis, iridodonesis, and lens subluxation. Affected individuals may exhibit cataract and secondary glaucoma due to lenticular dislocation. It is usually X-linked recessive, but there is an AR form, associated with developmental delay, known as Neuhauser syndrome (OMIM 249310). X-linked recessive carrier mothers may also have mildly enlarged corneas.

Microspherophakia and/or Megalocornea, with Ectopia Lentis and with or without Secondary Glaucoma (OMIM 251750)

This condition is caused by pathogenic mutations in latent transforming growth factor β binding protein 2 (*LTBP2*; GLC3D; 14q24.3). *LTBP2* mutations may present with primary enlarged corneas with or without increased IOP and ectopia lentis with subsequent risk of lens dislocation and acute angle closure glaucoma (► Fig. 9.3). Some of these patients have marfanoid habitus. It is usually an AR condition.

Overgrowth Syndrome

Both Sturge–Weber syndrome and neurofibromatosis may have a globe that looks bigger in the absence of glaucoma. This is usually associated with orbital involvement of the systemic disease.

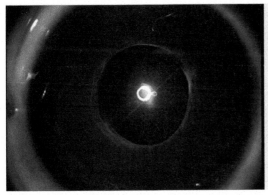

Fig. 9.3 Glaucoma associated with *LTBP2* mutation. Note ectopia lentis associated with megalocornea. Iris atrophy is often seen with a cryptless iris. (The oblique vertical line through the pupil is an artifact.)

9.1.4 Uncommon Manifestations

Some cases may present with normal IOP and optic discs but typical signs of PCG including buphthalmos and Haab's striae that are not progressive and do not show corneal edema. These cases may be classified as spontaneously arrested PCG.

Advanced buphthalmos may result in ectopia lentis.

9.1.5 Clinical Testing

Glaucoma management is beyond the scope of this chapter. Identification of the glaucoma etiology (▶ Fig. 9.1) is a key aspect of selecting the management plan.

9.1.6 Genetic Testing

Identification of biallelic pathogenic variants in *CYP1B1* confirms the diagnosis of PCG. Deletion/duplication analysis is recommended if only one or no pathogenic variant is found, given that other genes are yet to be discovered. A negative *CYP1B1* gene test does not rule out the diagnosis of PCG.

9.2 Juvenile Open Angle Glaucoma

Key Points

- Juvenile open angle glaucoma (JOAG) is an AD disorder usually affecting individuals between the age of 4 and 40 years. Intrafamilial variation in age of onset is common.
- Early detection is difficult. Genetic testing of at-risk individuals may allow for appropriate screening.
- *MYOC* gene mutations are the only known cause at this time.

9.2.1 Overview

JOAG (GLC1A) is a primary trabecular meshwork dysfunction that occurs in the absence of buphthalmos (▶ Fig. 9.1). This condition affects individuals between the ages of 4 and 40 years. JOAG has an estimated frequency of 1 in 50,000 individuals. Onset is often insidious and many times diagnosis is made only at late stages, with advanced optic nerve damage and elevated IOP, often ≥ 40 mm Hg. Genetic testing may identify at-risk individuals who then can undergo appropriate glaucoma screening for diagnosis before optic nerve damage. Gonioscopy is normal or may show an increase in the number of iris processes ("pectinate ligaments") crossing the trabecular meshwork, although this sign is nonspecific.

9.2.2 Molecular Genetics

JOAG is an AD condition. The primary known cause is myocilin (*MYOC*, 1q24.3) protein dysfunction (formerly known as trabecular meshwork inducible–glucocorticoid response protein [TIGR]). The myocilin protein is found in trabecular meshwork cells and juxtacanalicular connective tissue. *MYOC* gene mutations are identified in approximately 10% of patients with JOAG.

Compound heterozygous or heterozygous mutations in the *CYP1B1* gene have rarely been associated with JOAG. Mutations in *MYOC* along with *CYP1B1* have also been implicated via digenic inheritance. These individuals may present with even more severe disease. *CYP1B1* may act as a modifier of *MYOC* expression.

Four other loci have been associated with both primary open angle glaucoma (POAG) and JOAG: *GLC1J* (9q22), *GLC1K* (20p12), *GLC1M* (5q22.1q32), and *GLC1N* (15q22–24).

9.2.3 Differential Diagnosis

Physiologic Cupping

This is the most common diagnostic differential with JOAG. The optic nerve cup is usually round or slightly oval in shape with a very sharp edge. The neuroretinal rim usually has a relatively uniform width and a color (▶ Fig. 9.4). Nonglaucomatous black individuals and individuals with myopia have larger disc areas and larger cup-to-disc ratios. Physiologic cupping is AD so the presence of an affected parent is reassuring as is a normal optical coherence tomography (OCT) and visual field. In cases where the diagnosis is uncertain, longitudinal follow-up to ensure no JOAG is important.

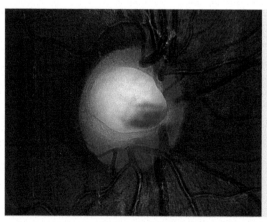

Fig. 9.4 Enlarged and deep optic cup with very sharp edges in the absence of glaucoma is characteristic of physiologic cupping. The child's father was similarly affected.

Steroid-Response Glaucoma

Steroid-response glaucoma will be revealed in a history of corticosteroid use.

Pseudoexfoliation Glaucoma

Patients may exhibit spokelike fibrillar material on the anterior lens capsule, pupillary transillumination, phacodonesis, or zonular weakness. This diagnosis is more common in older patients and has not been reported in children.

Pigmentary Glaucoma

Clinical findings include Krukenberg's spindle endothelial pigment deposits, myopic refraction, peripheral iris transillumination defects, and Sampaolesi's line on gonioscopy.

Uveitic Glaucoma

These patients may have anterior chamber reaction and evidence of chronic inflammation, such as synechiae or endothelial keratic precipitates.

Other Etiologies

Other etiologies include carotid-cavernous fistula, dural arteriovenous shunting, thyroid-associated ophthalmopathy, orbital tumor, Sturge–Weber syndrome, neurofibromatosis, nevus of Ota, or systemic high central venous pressure.

9.2.4 Clinical Testing

JOAG is an aggressive form of glaucoma that requires close monitoring and aggressive management. Although some patients may be managed medically, surgical intervention is often required.

9.2.5 Genetic Testing

Molecular genetic testing strategies include sequence analysis of *MYOC* or *CYP1B1* genes. If no pathogenic variants are found, deletion/duplication analysis should be considered.

9.3 Problems

9.3.1 Case 1

A 2-year-old healthy boy born by cesarean section comes for evaluation for an enlarged right globe size noticed by his parents. The right eye also has some mild epiphora and photophobia. Which of the following signs would be the most important for suspecting PCG?
a) Axial myopia OD (oculus dextrus) = –10.0 sph, OS (oculus sinister) = –2.0 sph.
b) Cup-to-disc ratio OD = 0.3, OS = 0.2.
c) Horizontal ruptures in Descemet's membrane OD.
d) IOP OD = 34, OS = 32, tested with Tonopen while crying.

Correct answer is c.

Even though IOP, optic nerve cupping, and myopic refraction are important signs to be taken into account for making the diagnosis of PCG, horizontal ruptures in Descemet in a child with no history of forceps trauma is almost pathognomonic of glaucoma.

a) **Less appropriate.** Progressive myopia or myopic shift is suspicious of glaucoma only if coupled with other signs of glaucoma such as corneal edema and optic nerve cupping.

b) **Incorrect.** Mild cup–disc asymmetry is not uncommon.

c) **Correct.**

d) **Incorrect.** Several conditions can cause artifactual elevation of IOP measurements, including crying and Valsalva maneuvers.

9.3.2 Case 2

A 3-week-old otherwise healthy girl presents with bilateral tearing, photophobia, and cloudy corneas. Her family history is negative for glaucoma and the examination under sedation shows IOP = 30 mm Hg and Haab's striae OU (oculus unitas). The family requests genetic testing for the baby and themselves in order to know the risk for future pregnancies. Which genetic testing would be the most appropriate for this scenario?

a) Molecular genetic testing for *CYP1B1* mutations.

b) Molecular genetic testing for *MYOC* mutations.

c) No genetic testing is indicated as this case is pathognomonic for *CYP1B1* mutations.

d) The case represents typical XL megalocornea.

Correct answer is a.

This case illustrates the typical signs of PCG. The neonatal type of PCG is more likely to be caused by mutation of *CYP1B1*. If gene testing for *CYP1B1* is normal, empiric data suggest an approximate 8% recurrence risk for parents of a child with PCG, and therefore *CYP1B1*-negative families should be advised that all future children be examined in the first 2 weeks of life. The same is true for parents who elect not to have any gene testing.

a) **Correct.**

b) **Incorrect.** Although a possible cause, *MYOC* is rarely involved in PCG.

c) **Incorrect.** Although the clinical picture allows for a diagnosis of PCG, molecular genetic testing is required for best counseling, especially since both AR and AD forms of CG have been reported.

d) **Incorrect.** X-linked recessive megalocornea is observed in males and does not present with increased IOP or other signs of PCG.

9.3.3 Case 3

A 1-year-old otherwise healthy boy presents with bilateral increased corneal diameters (14 OU), no corneal edema, and normal IOP. Axial length is approximately 21 in each eye. One eye shows lens subluxation without history of trauma. Family history is unremarkable. Systemic examination is normal. Axial length is within normal limits for his age. Which is the most probable genetic mechanism for this scenario?

a) *CYP1B1* mutations with secondary lens subluxation.

b) *LTBP2* mutations.

c) Marfan syndrome.

d) Neurofibromatosis.

Correct answer is b.

LTBP2 mutations are associated with primary enlarged corneas and lens subluxation with or without glaucoma.

a) **Incorrect.** Congenital glaucoma cases with extremely large axial lengths have been reported to show zonule fibers stretching and secondary ectopia lentis. This patient shows almost normal ocular dimensions for age.

b) **Correct.**

c) **Incorrect.** Although neonatal Marfan syndrome can be associated with early ectopia lentis, the corneas are not enlarged and patients have obvious signs of Marfan syndrome.

d) **Incorrect.** True enlargement of corneal diameters does not occur in neurofibromatosis in the absence of glaucoma. In addition, when glaucoma is present there is almost always obvious orbital and lid involvement.

9.3.4 Case 4

A 15-year-old otherwise healthy teenager was referred for glaucoma. Family history is unremarkable. His best corrected vision wearing –6.00 sph OU, slit-lamp examination, and gonioscopy are normal. Applanation tonometry is 19 mm Hg in both eyes. Cup-to-disc ratio is 0.7 in both eyes with sharp edges. OCT revealed normal thickness of the nerve fiber layer. The father is being followed for "large cups." Which is the most probably diagnosis?

a) Physiologic cupping.

b) JOAG.

c) PCG.

d) Pigmentary glaucoma.

Correct answer is a.

Physiologic cupping is the most common differential of JOAG. In this case, clinical examination and OCT were normal.

a) **Correct.**

b) **Incorrect.** Although longitudinal follow-up may be needed to be sure, the patient now does not seem to have glaucoma.

c) **Incorrect.** Gonioscopy is normal and there is no buphthalmos.

d) **Incorrect.** Clinical findings of pigmentary glaucoma include Krukenberg's spindle endothelial pigment deposits, peripheral iris transillumination defects, and Sampaolesi's line on gonioscopy.

Suggested Reading

[1] 9th Consensus Meeting: Childhood Glaucoma. World Glaucoma Association. http://www.worldglaucoma. org/consensus-9/. Accessed May 13, 2016

[2] Moller PM. Goniotomy and congenital glaucoma. Acta Ophthalmol (Copenh). 1977; 55(3):436–442

[3] Robin AL, Quigley HA, Pollack IP, Maumenee AE, Maumenee IH. An analysis of visual acuity, visual fields, and disk cupping in childhood glaucoma. Am J Ophthalmol. 1979; 88(5):847–858

[4] Lim S-H, Tran-Viet K-N, Yanovitch TL, et al. CYP1B1, MYOC, and LTBP2 mutations in primary congenital glaucoma patients in the United States. Am J Ophthalmol. 2013; 155(3):508–517.e5

[5] Plásilová M, Feráková E, Kádasi L, et al. Linkage of autosomal recessive primary congenital glaucoma to the GLC3A locus in Roms (Gypsies) from Slovakia. Hum Hered. 1998; 48(1):30–33

[6] Sarfarazi M, Stoilov I. Molecular genetics of primary congenital glaucoma. Eye (Lond). 2000; 14 Pt 3B:422–428

[7] Sarfarazi M, Stoilov I, Schenkman JB. Genetics and biochemistry of primary congenital glaucoma. Ophthalmol Clin North Am. 2003; 16(4):543–554, vi

[8] Kaur K, Reddy AB, Mukhopadhyay A, et al. Myocilin gene implicated in primary congenital glaucoma. Clin Genet. 2005; 67(4):335–340

[9] Kipp MA. Childhood glaucoma. Pediatr Clin North Am. 2003; 50(1):89–104

[10] Abu-Amero KK, Edward DP. Primary congenital glaucoma. In: Pagon RA, Adam MP, Ardinger HH, et al., eds. GeneReviews(®). Seattle, WA: University of Washington, Seattle; 1993

10 Childhood Cataract

Yu-Hung Lai

Abstract

Infantile cataract is a significant cause of childhood blindness. Isolated childhood cataract can be autosomal dominant or, less frequently, autosomal recessive. Syndromic cataract can occur by virtually any inheritance pattern or chromosomal aberration. Detailed evaluations are crucial in managing children with cataract. Recognizing the genetic etiology of a childhood cataract may be facilitated by careful attention to the cataract morphology. Next-generation sequencing gene panels and whole exome sequencing are promising tools to understand and diagnose the genetic etiology of childhood cataract.

Keywords: childhood cataract, anterior lenticonus, anterior pyramidal cataract, nuclear cataract, cerulean cataract, Coppock cataract, sutural cataract, posterior subcapsular cataract, cataract surgery

Key Points

- Isolated childhood cataract can be autosomal dominant or, less commonly, autosomal recessive. Syndromic cataract can occur by virtually any inheritance pattern or chromosomal aberration.
- Detailed ocular and systemic evaluations are important in managing children with cataract.
- Next-generation sequencing gene panels and whole exome sequencing are promising tools to understand and diagnose the genetic etiology of childhood cataract.

10.1 Overview

Infantile cataract is a significant cause of childhood blindness. The prevalence of congenital cataract is reported between 1 and 3 per 10,000 children. Early detection and prompt treatment are necessary to avoid severe visual loss. Depending on the severity of the cataract, treatment may include pharmacologic pupil dilatation, occlusion therapy, correction of refractive errors, and/or cataract surgery. Visual rehabilitation is required after the cataract surgery in young children. Recognizing the genetic etiology of a childhood cataract may be facilitated by careful attention to the cataract morphology such as anterior lenticonus in Alport syndrome, anterior pyramidal cataract in *PAX6* mutations, embryonal or fetal nuclear, cerulean, Coppock cataract, sutural, posterior subcapsular, and others. A unilateral cataract due to persistent fetal vasculature (PFV) is usually not due to a known germline genetic cause. Excellent reviews have been published on the systemic associations with cataract, which may also guide the genetic evaluation. One must also consider the nongenetic causes of cataract including intrauterine infection, trauma, steroids, uveitis, and radiation.

10.2 Molecular Genetics

Approximately 50% of congenital cataract cases have genetic causes. Autosomal dominant (AD), autosomal recessive (AR), and X-linked inheritance patterns have been described, with AD being the most frequent. Mutations in transcription factor genes, developmental genes, genes required in lens development, and lens crystallin genes can cause cataract. ▶ Table 10.1 illustrates examples from these categories. To date, for nonsyndromic cataract, at least 45 loci have been mapped and 38 genes identified.

The most important proteins found in lens are crystallins, which are water-soluble structural proteins that account for lens transparency. These proteins have many functions, including increasing the refractive index while not obstructing light, as well as evidence that suggests metabolic and regulatory functions (e.g., calcium binding proteins, interaction with alcohol dehydrogenase and quinone reductase). There are three subtypes: alpha, beta, and gamma crystallins. Cataracts can arise from dysfunction in any part of their complex functional and structural interaction. Multiple other genes serve additional functions in the lens such as *MIP* or *GJA8* genes. Cataract morphology depends on the location and timing of expression of the abnormal gene.

Some morphologies of cataract are linked to mutations in particular genes although there is usually much variability in expression even within the same family. For example, some anterior polar cataracts could be caused by mutations in *CRYGB* or *HSF4* genes. Anterior lenticonus is almost invariably caused by mutations in *COL4A3*, *COL4A4*, or *COL4A5* in the setting of Alport syndrome; some posterior polar cataracts could be caused by mutations in *EPHA2*, *PITX3*, *CRYAB*, or *CJA3*; mutations in *MIP*, *MAF*, *CRYAA*, or *CRYBB3* genes can lead to both anterior and posterior polar cataracts. Lamella cataract could be caused by mutations in *CRYGD*, *CRYGC*, *CRYGB*, *BFSP2*, *CRYAB**, *MIP**, *HSF4**, *MAF**, *CRYAA**, *CRYBA1*, *CRYBA4*, and *NHS* genes (those which also lead to other types of cataract are denoted by *).

10.3 Differential Diagnosis

10.3.1 Intrauterine Infection

Toxoplasmosis, rubella, cytomegalovirus, herpes zoster, syphilis, and herpes simplex may each result in congenital cataract.

10.3.2 Persistent Fetal Vasculature

PFV, formerly known as persistent hyperplastic primary vitreous (PHPV), refers to the unresorbed remnants of the fetal hyaloid vessels. It is usually unilateral and associated with microphthalmia, pulled in ciliary processes, poor pupillary dilatation, and a stalk from the optic nerve to the back of the lens where there is a plaque that may be avascular or vascularized. This cataract is almost always not due to germline mutation and therefore not heritable, although local genetic factors do play a role.

10.3.3 Cataract Due to Medications

Corticosteroid is the most well-known drug class leading to cataract. Many other drugs do so with a lower incidence.

Table 10.1 Summary of genes/loci associated with isolated cataract

Cataract description and morphology	Phenotype name (MIM number)	Gene/locus (MIM number)	Chromosome	Inheritance	Other association
Volkmann type (progressive, central, or zonular, with opacities in the embryonic, fetal, and juvenile nucleus and around the anterior and posterior Y-suture)	Cataract 8, multiple types; CTRCT8 (115665)	CTRCT8 (–)	1pter-p36.13	AD	
Posterior polar, congenital total, complete, age-related cortical	Cataract 6, multiple types; CTRCT6 (116600)	EPHA2[D] (176946)	1p36.13	AD	Myopia
Membranous and posterior capsular	Cataract 34, multiple types; CTRCT34 (612968)	CTRCT34 (–)	1p34.3-p32.2	AR	Corneal opacity, microcornea
Congenital, zonular pulverulent, nuclear, nuclear pulverulent, stellate nuclear, nuclear total, total, and posterior subcapsular	Cataract 1, multiple types; CTRCT1 (116200)	CX50, GJA8[G] (600897)	1q21.2	AD	Cataract-microcornea syndrome
Crystalline coralliform (multiple coral-like white opacities)	Cataract 29; CTRCT29 (115800)	CTRCT29 (–)	2pter-p24	AD	
Aculeiform, crystalline aculeiform, crystalline, crystal, frosted, needle-shaped, fasciculiform, congenital cerulean, nonnuclear polymorphic congenital, central nuclear, lamellar, and punctate	Cataract 4, multiple types; CTRCT4 (115700)	CRYGD[C] (123690)	2q33.3	AD	
Coppock-like; embryonic, fetal, infantile nuclear; zonular pulverulent; and lamellar	Cataract 2, multiple types; CTRCT2 (604307)	GRYGC (123680)	2q33.3	AD	Microcornea
Congenital lamellar, anterior polar, and complete	Cataract 39, multiple types; CTRCT39 (615188)	CRYGB[C] (123670)	2q33.3	AD	
Multifocal congenital	Cataract 42; CTRCT42 (115900)	CRYBA2[C] (600836)	2q35	AD	Eccentric pupil, myopia
Congenital and congenital nuclear	Cataract 18; CTRCT 18 (610019)	FYCO1[G] (607182)	3p21.31	AR	

83

Table 10.1 (continued)

Cataract description and morphology	Phenotype name (MIM number)	Gene/locus (MIM number)	Chromosome	Inheritance	Other association
Congenital nuclear, sutural, stellate cortical; juvenile-onset lamellar, cortical, nuclear embryonic, or Y-sutural; and adult-onset punctate cortical	Cataract 12, multiple types; CTRCT12 (611597)	BFSP2[G] (603212)	3q22.1	AD	
Progressive polymorphic anterior, posterior, or peripheral cortical, membranous	Cataract 20, multiple types; CTRCT20 (116100)	CRYGS[C] (123730)	3q27.3	AD	
Congenital nuclear	Cataract 41 (116400)	WFS1[G] (606201)	4p16.1	AD	
Congenital, total	Cataract 13 with adult i phenotype (116700)	GCNT2[G] (600429)	6p24.3-p24.2	AD	i-negative and i-positive red blood type
Cortical, age related	Cataract 28, age related, cortical, susceptibility to; CTRCT28 (609026)	ARCC1[G] (–)	6p12-q12	–	
Congenital	Cataract 38; CTRCT38 (614691)	AGK[C] (610345)	7q34	AR	Sengers syndrome
Cortical, pulverulent, nuclear, and posterior subcapsular	Cataract 26, multiple types; CTRCT26 (605749)	CAAR (–)	9q13-q22	AR	
Congenital, or juvenile cataract	Cataract 36; CTRCT36 (613887)	TDRD7[D] (611258)	9q22.33	AR	
Pulverulent, nuclear	Cataract 30, pulverulent; CTRCT30 (116300)	VIM[G] (193060)	10p13	AD	
Congenital total and posterior polar	Cataract 11, multiple types; cataract 11, syndromic; CTRCT11 (610623)	PITX3[T] (602669)	10q24.32	AD	Microphthalmia, neurodevelopmental abnormalities
Congenital posterior polar, congenital lamellar, nuclear, complete, and juvenile	Cataract 16, multiple types; CTRCT16 (613763)	CRYAB[C] (123590)	11q23.1	AR, AD	Myofibrillar myopathy, dilated cardiomyopathy

84

Table 10.1 (*continued*)

Cataract description and morphology	Phenotype name (MIM number)	Gene/locus (MIM number)	Chromosome	Inheritance	Other association
Polymorphic, progressive punctate lamellar, cortical, anterior and posterior polar, nonprogressive lamellar with sutural opacities, embryonic nuclear, and pulverulent cortical	Cataract 15, multiple types; CTRCT15 (615274)	MIP^G (154050)	12q13.3	AD	
Cerulean, cuneiform	Cataract 37; CTRCT37 (614422)	CCA5 (–)	12q24.2-q24.3	AD	
Zonular pulverulent, posterior polar, nuclear coralliform, embryonal nuclear, and Coppock-like	Cataract 14, multiple types; CTRCT14 (601885)	GJA3^G (121015)	13q12.11	AD	
Anterior polar, or posterior polar	Cataract 32, multiple types; CTRCT32 (115650)	CTAA1 (–)	14q22-q23	AD	
Central pouchlike cataract with sutural opacities	Cataract 25; CTRCT25 (605728)	CCSSO (–)	15q21-q22	AD	
Infantile, lamellar, zonular, nuclear, anterior polar, stellate, pulverulent and Marner type	Cataract 5, multiple types; CTRCT5 (116800)	HSF4^T (602438)	16q22.1	AD	
Juvenile cortical pulverulent and later progression of posterior subcapsular, congenital cerulean, lamellar, anterior polar, nuclear, poster polar, anterior subcapsular and stellate	Cataract 21, multiple types; CTRCT21 (610202)	MAF^T (177075)	16q23.2	AD	Microcornea, iris coloboma, macular hypoplasia (rare)
Anterior polar	Cataract 24, anterior polar; CTRCT24 (601202)	CTAA2 (–)	17p13	AD	
Congenital zonular with sutural opacities, congenital nuclear progressive, and progressive lamellar; Y-shaped sutural	Cataract 10, multiple types; CTRCT10 (600881)	CRYBA1^C (123610)	17q11.2	AD	
Posterior subcapsular and central	Cataract 43; CTRCT43 (616279)	UNC45B (611220)	17q12	AD	

Table 10.1 (continued)

Cataract description and morphology	Phenotype name (MIM number)	Gene/locus (MIM number)	Chromosome	Inheritance	Other association
Cerulean cataract	Cataract 7; CTRCT7 (115660)	CCA1 (–)	17q24	AD	
Congenital nuclear cataract	Cataract 35, congenital nuclear; CTRCT35 (609376)	CATCN1 (–)	19q13	AR	
Congenital dense white	Cataract 45; CTRCT45 (616851)	SIPA1L3 (616655)	19q13.1-q13.2	AR	
Late-onset cortical pulverulent; congenital total	Cataract 19, multiple types; CTRCT19 (615277)	LIM2ᴳ (154045)	19q13.41	AR	
Fluffy, cottonlike cortical; grapelike cysts in the anterior cortex	Cataract 33; CTRCT33 (611391)	BFSP1ᴳ (603307)	20p12.1	AR	
Posterior polar, progressive posterior subcapsular, nuclear, and anterior subcapsular	Cataract 31, multiple types; CTRCT31 (605387)	CHMP4Bᴳ (–)	20q11.22	AD	
Nuclear, zonular central nuclear, laminar, lamellar, anterior polar, posterior polar, cortical, embryonal, anterior subcapsular, fan shaped, and total	Cataract 9, multiple types; CTRCT9 (604219)	CRYAAᶜ (123580)	21q22.3	AD, AR	Cataract-microcornea syndrome, iris coloboma, microphthalmia
Congenital	Cataract 44; CTRCT44 (616509)	LSS (600909)	21q22.3	AR	Microcornea
Congenital nuclear cataract with cortical riders, nuclear, posterior polar, anterior polar, and cortical	Cataract 22; CTRCT22 (609741)	CRYBB3ᶜ (123630)	22q11.23	AR, AD	Glaucoma
Congenital cerulean, "blue dot," Coppock-like, sutural with punctate and cerulean opacities, pulverulent embryonal, pulverulent with cortical opacities, dense posterior star-shaped subcapsular with pulverulent opacities in the cortical and embryonal regions, and dense embryonal	Cataract 3, multiple types; CTRCT3 (601547)	CRYBB2ᶜ (123620)	22q11.23	AD	Microphthalmia

Table 10.1 (continued)

Cataract description and morphology	Phenotype name (MIM number)	Gene/locus (MIM number)	Chromosome	Inheritance	Other association
Congenital nuclear and pulverulent	Cataract 17, multiple types; CTRCT17 (611544)	CRYBB1^C (600929)	22q12.1	AD, AR	Microcornea
Congenital and congenital lamellar	Cataract 23; CTRCT23 (610425)	CRYBA4^C (123631)	22q12.1	AR	Microphthalmia
Lamellar, zonular, or perinuclear; posterior suture or posterior stellate cataracts in heterozygous females	Cataract 40; CTRCT40 (302200)	NHS^T (300457)	Xp22.2-p22.1	XL	Microcornea, microphthalmia, Nance–Horan syndrome
Anterior polar cataract	(–)	HMX1 (612109)	4p16	AR	Oculoauricular syndrome
Congenital nuclear cataract	(–)	PRX	19q13.2	AR	

Abbreviations: AD, autosomal dominant; AR, autosomal recessive; OMIM, Online Mendelian Inheritance in Man; ^{T}, transcription factor; ^{D}, developmental gene; ^{G}, gene required in lens development; ^{C}, lens crystallin gene.

Source: Adopted from OMIM: http://omim.org/phenotypicSeries/PS116200; accessed on April 23, 2016.

10.3.4 Metabolic Disorders

Metabolic disorders may be associated with cataract formation (▶ Table 10.2).

10.3.5 Trauma

Trauma as a cause for cataract is usually easily recognized by the history. Cataract due to covert trauma from physical abuse must also be considered. Traumatic cataracts may be delayed after the impact event.

10.3.6 Ocular Anomalies

Ocular anomalies may accompany cataract. Almost any congenital cataract may be associated with microphthalmia. Cataract-microcornea syndrome has been associated with mutations in several genes including *ABCA3*, *CRYAA*, *CRYBA4*, *CRYBB1*, *CRYBB2*, *CRYGC*, *CRYGD*, *GJA8*, and *MAF*. Cataract-microcornea syndrome can be inherited as AR and AD. Cataract may also be seen in ocular malformation syndromes such as Peters anomaly, aniridia, and ocular coloboma.

10.3.7 Cataracts Associated with Systemic Syndromes

The number of syndromes associated with cataract is beyond the scope of this book. The reader is referred to an excellent publication by Trumler on this topic. Some are also mentioned below as uncommon manifestations.

10.3.8 Chromosomal Aberrations

Chromosomal aberrations, in particular trisomy 21, 13, and 18, can be associated with cataract. Numerous aberrations have been reported in which cataract is a key component including 11q23 deletion and 10q25–10q26.1 deletion.

10.3.9 Uveitis

Uveitis may induce cataract. The cataract is typically posterior subcapsular but may progress rapidly to a total cataract with or without intumescence.

10.4 Uncommon Manifestations

10.4.1 Alport Syndrome (OMIM 301050)

Alport syndrome (OMIM 301050) is characterized by interstitial nephritis and hearing loss along with anterior lenticonus and/or posterior lenticonus. It can be AD, AR, or X-linked depending on which of the three collagen genes is mutated: *COL4A3*, *COL4A4*, and *COL4A5*. A maculopathy may also be seen.

10.4.2 Lowe Syndrome (OMIM 309000)

Lowe syndrome (OMIM 309000) is an X-linked recessive multisystemic disorder also known as the oculocerebrorenal syndrome. It is characterized by congenital cataract

Table 10.2 Examples of metabolic diseases leading to cataract

Disease	Cataract description	Gene	Inheritance	Phenotype
Galactosemia	Nuclear	GALT, GALK1, GALE	AR	Defect in galactose metabolization; lethargy; failure to thrive; jaundice, hepatomegaly; intellectual disability
Fabry disease	Most commonly stellate posterior subcapsular, also anterior subcapsular	GLA	XL	Excessive glycosphingolipids; acroparesthesias; angiokeratomas; hypohidrosis; progressive kidney damage, myocardial infarction, stroke, cornea verticillata
Wilson's disease	Sunflower	ATP7B	AR	Excessive copper accumulation; jaundice; nervous system or psychiatric problems; Kayser–Fleischer ring
Hypocalcemia	White punctuate opacities	–	–	Irritability; failure to thrive; seizure; hypoparathyroidism
Diabetes mellitus	Pleomorphic	–	–	Hyperglycemia, neuropathy, nephropathy, retinopathy
Alpha-mannosidosis	variable	MAN2B1	AR	Intellectual disability, skeletal abnormality, large head, protruding jaw, ataxia, hepatosplenomegaly

Abbreviations: AD, autosomal dominant; AR, autosomal recessive; XL, X-linked.

(usually posterior polar), intellectual disability, characteristic facies, and proximal renal tubular dysfunction (Fanconi's syndrome). Retinopathy may also be seen. The causative gene is *OCRL*. Female carriers may have radiating dot cortical opacities in their lenses.

10.4.3 Congenital Muscular Dystrophy (OMIM 615356)

Affected individuals with *TRAPPC11* mutations can have microcephaly, hypotonia, enlarged right cardiac ventricle, cataract, intellectual disability, and skeletal involvement.

10.4.4 Congenital Disorders of Glycosylation

Congenital disorders of glycosylation (CDG) are a genetically heterogeneous collection of AR disorders. Patients with CDG can present with developmental delay, dysmorphic features, skeletal anomalies, and neurological problems. Ophthalmic findings including retinitis pigmentosa, strabismus, and cataract have been reported.

10.4.5 Myotonic Dystrophy (OMIM 160900; 602668)

Myotonic dystrophy (OMIM 160900; 602668) is an AD disorder, characterized by "Christmas tree cataract": crystalline multicolored central nuclear deposits. Other features include progressive external ophthalmoplegia, ptosis, retinal pigmentary changes, progressive muscle weakness and wasting, gonadal atrophy, mental deterioration, and cardiac abnormalities. Mutations in *DMPK* and *CNBP* genes have been reported to lead to this disease.

10.4.6 Mowat–Wilson Syndrome (OMIM 235730)

Mowat–Wilson syndrome (OMIM 235730) is characterized by characteristic facial dysmorphism, microcephaly, intellectual deficiency, Hirschsprung's disease, short stature, and ocular anomalies including ocular coloboma, optic nerve hypoplasia/atrophy, cataract, and corectopia. Heterozygous *ZEB2* gene mutations or deletions are responsible for this syndrome.

10.4.7 Oculoauricular Syndrome (OMIM 612109)

Oculoauricular syndrome (OMIM 612109) is an AR disorder characterized by complex ocular anomalies including microphthalmia, coloboma, congenital cataract, anterior segment dysgenesis, and retinal dystrophy. Other features include malformed external ears but normal development. Mutation or deletion in *HMX1* is responsible for this syndrome.

10.4.8 Oculofaciocardiodental Syndrome

Oculofaciocardiodental (OFCD) syndrome is characterized by eye anomalies (congenital cataract, microphthalmia), facial abnormalities (long narrow face, high nasal bridge, cleft palate), cardiac anomalies (atrial or ventricular septal defect), and dental abnormalities. OFCD and Lenz's microphthalmia syndrome are allelic X-linked syndromes with *BCOR* gene mutations.

10.4.9 Warburg Micro Syndrome (OMIM 600118)

Warburg Micro syndrome (OMIM 600118) is an AR neurodevelopmental disorder characterized by microcephaly, microphthalmia, congenital cataract, cortical dysplasia, corpus callosum hypoplasia, intellectual disability, and hypogonadism. Patients with mutations in *RAB3GAP1*, *RAB3GAP2*, *RAB18*, or *TBC1D20* genes have been reported.

10.4.10 Rhizomelic Chondrodysplasia Punctate (OMIM 215100)

Rhizomelic chondrodysplasia punctate (OMIM 215100) is characterized by rhizomelic limb shortening, chondrodysplasia punctata, cervical dysplasia, congenital cataracts, dwarfism, intellectual disability, and seizures. It can be either AR, AD, or X-linked dominant (Conradi–Hünermann syndrome). It is associated with *FAR1*, *PEX7*, *GNPAT*, and *AGPS* mutations.

10.4.11 Rothmund–Thomson Syndrome (OMIM 268400)

Rothmund–Thomson syndrome (OMIM 268400) is an AR condition that presents with juvenile cataract, skin atrophy and hyper- and hypopigmentation with telangiectasias, congenital skeletal abnormalities, short stature, premature aging, and increased risk of malignant disease. Mutation in *RECQL4* is causative.

10.4.12 Other Genes

Other genes, such as *CTDP1* (AR), *KCNJ13* (AR), *RGS6* (AR), *STX3* (AR), *TRPM3* (AD), *TUBA1A* (AR), and *COL4A1* (AD) have been associated with cataract and systemic manifestations. Mutations in *CTDP1* present with facial dysmorphism and demyelinating neuropathy, and *RGS6* and *STX3* have intellectual disability. *COL4A1* mutations have been associated with small-vessel brain disease, porencephaly, cerebral aneurysms, retinal arterial tortuosity, Axenfeld–Rieger anomaly, kidney involvement, muscle cramps, Raynaud's phenomenon, and cardiac arrhythmia.

10.5 Clinical Testing

Cataract management is beyond the scope of this chapter. Diagnostic considerations with regard to identifying a possible genetic etiology include a history targeted to uncover possible nongenetic etiologies such as trauma or steroid use, family history, recognition of coexisting ocular malformations, medical history, and physical examination that may lead to a syndromic diagnosis. If there is no view of the posterior segment, B-scan ultrasound may be helpful. Early diagnosis, surgery, where indicated, and visual rehabilitation are critical to ensure the best visual outcomes.

10.6 Genetic Testing

There are next-generation sequencing cataract panels available, but their utility is challenged by the widely variable phenotypes of cataract morphology even within a family and the common occurrence of minor lens clarity changes in normal individuals, making it sometimes difficult to adjudicate if a family member is affected or not. This makes segregation analysis sometimes difficult. If coexisting ocular or systemic findings lead to a specific likely diagnosis (i.e., not isolated cataract), then genetic testing may be directed specifically to genes that when mutated cause the syndrome in question. Chromosome microarray (CMA) may find copy number variant (CNV) in up to 30% of patients with cataract and systemic abnormalities. Whole exome sequencing (WES) has also been suggested for patients with congenital cataract without a specific syndrome.

10.7 Problems

10.7.1 Case 1

A 6-month-old female infant has bilateral cataract and no identifiable affected family members. Physical examination reveals dysmorphism and microcephaly. Ocular examination shows nystagmus, normal corneal diameters, normal axial length, bilateral nuclear cataract, and normal intraocular pressure. No specific syndrome is apparent. The child appears to be thriving but with some hypotonia and developmental delay. Karyotype is normal. Which of the following tests would be most helpful?
a) Renal function studies.
b) WES.
c) *FOXE3* sequencing.
d) CMA.

Correct answer is d.
In the context of multiple affected systems and normal karyotype, CMA is the test of choice. A deletion or duplication that is submicroscopic may identify a region in which multiple genes are contributing to the phenotype.
a) **Incorrect**. The patient has no signs or symptoms referable to the renal system. If the CMA identified a CNV that is known to be associated with kidney disease, then further testing may be indicated.
b) **Less appropriate**. Although WES may be one strategy to identify a mutated gene, and perhaps indicated when no apparent syndrome leads to a specific genetic test, it may be more cost-effective to start with CMA that can identify an abnormality in a significant number of cases. If CMA is negative, then WES may be appropriate.
c) **Incorrect**. Mutations in *FOXE3* result in primary aphakia as well as other ocular anomalies.
d) **Correct**.

10.7.2 Case 2

You diagnosed a 2-month-old infant with a vascularized posterior plaque cataract in a microphthalmic eye with poor response to mydriatic agents, some unusual iris vessels, a slightly shallow anterior chamber, and pulled-in ciliary processes. Ultrasound reveals a stalk from the optic nerve to the back of the lens. Complete physical examination reveals no anomalies. Family history is negative. Which of the following would be most appropriate?
a) CMA.
b) No further workup is needed.
c) Brain MRI (magnetic resonance imaging).
d) *COL4A1* sequencing.

Correct answer is b.

PFV is a congenital condition that results from failure of the fetal hyaloid vascular system to regress. This child shows diagnostic ocular abnormalities. When unilateral (90%), it is considered not to be a germline genetic condition and no further systemic workup is needed.

a) **Incorrect.** CMA is most indicated when more than one body system is involved. There are no other systemic abnormalities in this patient with classic isolated PFV.

b) **Correct.**

c) **Incorrect.** PFV does not typically have systemic associations and the child has no signs or symptoms of central nervous system involvement.

d) **Incorrect.** Patients with *COL4A1* present with variable findings including small-vessel brain disease, porencephaly, cerebral aneurysms, retinal arterial tortuosity, Axenfeld–Rieger anomaly, kidney involvement, muscle cramps, Raynaud's phenomenon, and cardiac arrhythmia.

10.7.3 Case 3

A pediatrician calls you about a 1-week-old infant whose mother had surgery for bilateral infantile cataract. His physical examination reveals no other systemic association. Family history also reveals an affected maternal uncle and maternal grandfather with *HSF4* mutations. Which of the following would be most helpful?

a) Refer patient to genetics to obtain a more complete family history and pregnancy history.

b) A prompt thorough ocular examination of the new infant in the first 2 weeks of life.

c) Karyotype and/or chromosomal microarray before seeing the patient.

d) *HSF4* gene sequencing of the infant.

Correct answer is b.

This patient has a known family history of AD congenital cataract. Urgent examination is recommended to assess if the infant is affected as prompt intervention (usually at 4–6 weeks old) optimizes outcomes. If the initial examination is normal, the child should be re-examined, perhaps at 4 to 6 weeks old, 3 months old, 6 months old, and every 6 months for at least the first 2 years of life as the age of onset may be variable within a family.

a) **Incorrect.** Provided family history is enough to suspect AD cataract and risk (50%) for the infant to be affected.

b) **Correct.**

c) **Incorrect.** *HSF4* mutation will not be detected by karyotype or CMA. The child has no other body systems involved.

d) **Incorrect.** Although this may be of interest, the priority for this at-risk child is early examination and intervention if affected. Testing could be performed after the first negative clinical examination. If the test then came back showing the baby to be unaffected by the gene mutation, then clinical examination could be discontinued.

10.7.4 Case 4

An 11-month-old female child has nystagmus and bilateral anterior pyramidal cataract. Fundus examination shows mild macular hypoplasia. The pupils appear asymmetrically large and irregular as if some iris is missing. Physical examination is normal. Which of the following test would be most appropriate for her?

a) Next-generation sequencing cataract panel.

b) CMA.

c) WES.

d) *PAX6* sequencing.

Correct answer is d.

The presence of macular hypoplasia, iris anomalies, and anterior pyramidal cataract suggests a possibility of *PAX6* mutation. When specific ocular or systemic syndrome is suspected, and a gene(s) is known to be causative when mutated, then it is appropriate to sequence that gene(s) as the first test.

a) **Incorrect.** Although cataract panels typically include *PAX6*, the cost of the panel is usually more than the sequencing of one gene. In addition, other gene sequence variants would likely be found, the significance of which would be difficult to understand.

b) **Incorrect.** The patient has no systemic findings, though an infant may be young enough for some systemic involvement yet to be evident. The presence of aniridia does raise concern about a deletion of chr11p13, but these patients typically have more complete aniridia. If this patient had normal *PAX6* sequencing, then one should consider testing for a deletion. If the patient has a mutation in *PAX6*, then it becomes unnecessary to search for a deletion. One may consider ordering a baseline renal ultrasound to be safe while awaiting results of *PAX6* testing.

c) **Incorrect.** WES is indicated when there is not a specific testable gene that has a likelihood of being mutated.

d) **Correct.**

Suggested Reading

[1] Graw J. Eye development. Curr Top Dev Biol. 2010; 90:343–386

[2] Shiels A, Hejtmancik JF. Genetics of human cataract. Clin Genet. 2013; 84(2):120–127

[3] Amaya L, Taylor D, Russell-Eggitt I, Nischal KK, Lengyel D. The morphology and natural history of childhood cataracts. Surv Ophthalmol. 2003; 48(2):125–144

[4] Yuan L, Yi J, Lin Q, et al. Identification of a PRX variant in a Chinese family with congenital cataract by exome sequencing. QJM. 2016; 109(11):731–735

[5] Myers KA, Bello-Espinosa LE, Kherani A, Wei XC, Innes AM. TUBA1A mutation associated with eye abnormalities in addition to brain malformation. Pediatr Neurol. 2015; 53(5):442–444

[6] Morava E, Wosik HN, Sykut-Cegielska J, et al. Ophthalmological abnormalities in children with congenital disorders of glycosylation type I. Br J Ophthalmol. 2009; 93(3):350–354

[7] Bourchany A, Giurgea I, Thevenon J, et al. Clinical spectrum of eye malformations in four patients with Mowat-Wilson syndrome. Am J Med Genet A. 2015; 167(7):1587–1592

[8] Gillespie RL, Urquhart J, Lovell SC, et al. Abrogation of HMX1 function causes rare oculoauricular syndrome associated with congenital cataract, anterior segment dysgenesis, and retinal dystrophy. Invest Ophthalmol Vis Sci. 2015; 56(2):883–891

[9] Chograni M, Alkuraya FS, Maazoul F, Lariani I, Chaabouni-Bouhamed H. RGS6: a novel gene associated with congenital cataract, mental retardation, and microcephaly in a Tunisian family. Invest Ophthalmol Vis Sci. 2014; 56(2):1261–1266

[10] Khan AO, Bergmann C, Neuhaus C, Bolz HJ. A distinct vitreo-retinal dystrophy with early-onset cataract from recessive KCNJ13 mutations. Ophthalmic Genet. 2015; 36(1):79–84

[11] Buchert R, Tawamie H, Smith C, et al. A peroxisomal disorder of severe intellectual disability, epilepsy, and cataracts due to fatty acyl-CoA reductase 1 deficiency. Am J Hum Genet. 2014; 95(5):602–610

[12] Chen P, Dai Y, Wu X, et al. Mutations in the ABCA3 gene are associated with cataract-microcornea syndrome. Invest Ophthalmol Vis Sci. 2014; 55(12):8031–8043

[13] Zhao L, Chen XJ, Zhu J, et al. Lanosterol reverses protein aggregation in cataracts. Nature. 2015; 523(7562):607–611

[14] Trumler AA. Evaluation of pediatric cataracts and systemic disorders. Curr Opin Ophthalmol 2011 Sep; 22 (5):365-79. doi: 10.1097/ICU.0b013e32834994dc.

11 Microphthalmia

Abstract

Microphthalmia refers to a globe with a total axial length that is at least 2 standard deviations below the mean for age. Severe microphthalmia refers to a corneal diameter less than 4 mm and axial length less than 10 mm at birth or 12 mm after the first year of life. Orbital imaging such as computed tomography or magnetic resonance imaging can reveal remnants of ocular tissue, to rule out true anophthalmia, although pathology of orbital tissues have revealed remnant tissues not visible by imaging. Microphthalmia may be unilateral or bilateral. Coloboma is the most common associated malformation. Other concurrent findings may include persistent fetal vasculature, cataract, and a wide range of anterior segment dysgeneses. Glaucoma can enlarge a microphthalmic eye so that it becomes larger, thus misleading the examiner that microphthalmia is not part of the initial finding. Molecular causes of microphthalmia include chromosomal aberrations and many single genes.

Keywords: microphthalmia, anophthalmia, coloboma, microcornea, anterior segment dysgenesis

Key Points

- Microphthalmia is defined as a globe that has a total axial length that is at least 2 standard deviations below the mean for age.
- Coloboma is the most common intraocular malformation in microphthalmia.
- Molecular genetic testing can find a genetic cause in 80% of patients with bilateral severe microphthalmia.
- Clinical anophthalmia refers to the absence of an identifiable globe but the presence of globe remnants detectable by imaging or orbital tissue analysis. This is a severe form of microphthalmia and has a different genetic etiology than true anophthalmia.

11.1 Overview

Microphthalmia is defined when a globe has a total axial length that is at least 2 standard deviations (SDs) below the mean for age. Most postnatal growth of the eye happens in the first 3 years, primarily during the first year of life. In adults, the lower limit of axial length is approximately 21.0 mm, whereas in children this must be based according to age (► Table 11.1). Corneal diameter normally goes from 9.0 to 10.5 mm in neonates and 10.5 to 12.0 mm in adults.

Table 11.1 Mean axial length according to age

Age	Mean axial length (mm)
Premature infant	16.2
Term neonate	16.7
18 mo	20.3
5 y	21.4
13 y	22.7
Adult	24.4

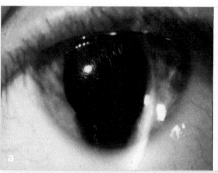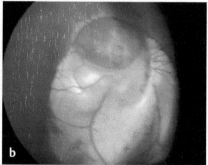

Fig. 11.1 Colobomatous microphthalmia. **(a)** Typical inferior iris coloboma. **(b)** Inferior chorioretinal coloboma involving the optic nerve.

Severe microphthalmia refers to a corneal diameter less than 4 mm and axial length less than 10 mm at birth or 12 mm after the first year of life. Orbital imaging such as computed tomography (CT) or magnetic resonance imaging (MRI) can reveal remnants of ocular tissue, to rule out anophthalmia, although pathology of orbital tissues reveals remnant tissues not visible by imaging.

Microphthalmia may be unilateral or bilateral, occurring in any degree of severity. Coloboma is the most common associated malformation (▶ Fig. 11.1). Other concurrent findings may include persistent fetal vasculature, cataract, and a wide range of anterior segment dysgeneses. Glaucoma can enlarge a microphthalmic eye so that it becomes larger, thus misleading the examiner that microphthalmia is not part of the initial finding.

Coloboma refers to those ocular abnormalities that result from failure of closure of the optic fissure during embryogenesis. This can be seen as fundus and/or iris coloboma. As the embryonic fissure closes between 5 and 7 weeks of gestation, abnormalities may occur anywhere along its distribution. The primary abnormality is failure of the (retinal pigment epithelium) RPE to close. Without RPE, the underlying choroid/uvea is not induced to form and the overlying sensory retina is maldeveloped (intercalary membrane). Clinically one observes a sharply demarcated white typically inferonasal lesion that may or may not encompass the optic nerve and/or fovea. Absence of a fovea portends a worse prognosis, whereas it is difficult to give a visual prognosis based on the appearance of the optic nerve. There is often hyperpigmentation at the edges of the fundus coloboma. Coloboma may also be isolated to the optic nerve or the iris. Heterotopic muscle and gliosis can rarely be observed within an optic nerve coloboma (ONC). Persistent fetal vasculature and ectopia lentis may be seen with coloboma, the latter due to involvement of the ciliary body with deficient zonules, which may also result in a lens notch. Retinal detachment may be a complication of fundus coloboma, seen in approximately 2% of patients.

The estimated prevalence of coloboma is 0.14%. This condition is usually sporadic. Around 50% of patients have bilateral involvement. Most patients with ONC alone are sporadic, although there are autosomal dominant (AD), autosomal recessive (AR), and X-linked (XL) recessive cases. Although the underlying molecular mechanism is often unknown, *PAX6* gene mutations have been identified in patients with large coloboma of the optic nerve, retina, and choroid, but most patients will not have *PAX6* mutations.

11.2 Molecular Genetics

Molecular genetic testing might begin with chromosomal microarray (CMA), particularly when systemic findings are present. Chromosome aberrations can be found in approximately 25 to 30% of patients with microphthalmia. The most frequent include trisomy of chromosome 9, trisomy of chromosome 12, trisomy of chromosome 18, Wolf–Hirschhorn syndrome (deletion of 4p), deletion of 13q, del(14)(q22.1–23.2), deletion of 18q, del(3)(q26), duplication of 3q, duplication of 4p, and duplication of 10q.

Single-gene causes of syndromic microphthalmia include *SOX2* (3q26; 15–20%), *OTX2* (14q22; 2–5%), *RAX* (18q21; 3%), *FOXE3* (1p33; 2.5%), *BMP4* (14q22; 2%), *PAX6* (11p13; 2%), *BCOR* (Xp11.4; 1%), *CHD7* (8q12.2; 1%), *STRA6* (15q24.1; 1%), and *GDF6* (8q22.1; 1%). Less common genetic causes include *CRYBA4*, *HCCS*, *HESX1*, *IKBKG*, and *SHH*, among other genes. Isolated microphthalmia known loci are shown in ► Table 11.2.

Patients with *SOX2* mutations or deletions of 3q27 region are characterized by microphthalmia that is often bilateral and severe. Other findings include brain malformations, esophageal atresia, cryptorchidism, micropenis, hypogonadotropic hypogonadism, pituitary hypoplasia, growth failure, delayed motor development, and learning disability. Molecular genetic testing finds a heterozygous *SOX2* mutation in approximately 40% of patients with bilateral severe microphthalmia. It is AD, but most cases are due to de novo mutations. Complete penetrance and variable expressivity are typically seen.

Individuals with *OTX2* mutations may have severe microphthalmia, with anterior segment dysgenesis, retinal dysplasia, and optic nerve hypoplasia. They may also have pituitary anomalies, brain anomalies, developmental delay, and autistic features. Patients with *RAX* gene mutations can present with microphthalmia, sclerocornea, and developmental delay.

Most ONC are sporadic. There are uncommon AD, AR, and XL recessive cases. In most patients, the underlying molecular mechanism is uncertain. *PAX6* gene mutations have been identified in patients with large coloboma of the optic nerve, retina, and choroid, a bilateral remnant of hyaloid vessel proliferation and growth, and mental retardation. Inversely, most patients with ONC do not have *PAX6* abnormalities.

Table 11.2 Isolated microphthalmia known loci

Microphthalmia subtype	Gene/Locus	Inheritance
MCOP1 (OMIM 251600)	14q32	AR
MCOP2 (OMIM 610093)	CHX10 (14q24)	AR
MCOP3 (OMIM 611038)	RAX (18q21.3)	AR
MCOP4 (OMIM 613094)	GDF6 (8q22.1)	Unknown
MCOP5 (OMIM 611040)	MFRP (11q23)	AR
MCOP6 (OMIM 613517)	PRSS56 (2q37.1)	AR
MCOP7 (OMIM 613704)	GDF3 (12p13.1)	Unknown
MCOP8 (OMIM 615113)	ALDH1A3 (15q26)	AR

Abbreviation: AR, autosomal recessive.

11.3 Differential Diagnosis

11.3.1 True Anophthalmia

This represents a failure of optic vesicle formation, leading to complete histologic absence of ocular tissues. Orbital imaging such as CT or MRI can reveal remnants only or complete aplasia of an optic nerve.

11.3.2 Microcornea

Microphthalmia needs also to be distinguished from microcornea. The axial length of the globe is normal. Refraction depends on axial length. Inheritance can be AR or AD.

11.3.3 Posterior Microphthalmia

When microphthalmia primarily affects the posterior segment, the term posterior microphthalmia is used. The anterior segment is clinically normal. Additional findings may include macular folds and high hyperopia. This disorder overlaps with nanophthalmia.

11.3.4 Nanophthalmia

True nanophthalmia is a rare condition, in which the eye is affected after the closure of the embryonic fissure. Findings include high hyperopia, small-sized to normal corneas, shallow anterior chamber, glaucoma, cataract, normal fundus or retinal abnormalities (macular hypoplasia, foveal cysts, pigmentary degeneration), and a predisposition to peripheral choroidal effusion. Scleral thickness is increased. Three loci have been identified: *NNO1* (11p), *NNO2* (*MFRP* gene; 11q23), and *NNO3* (2q11-q14). One mutation in *BEST1* has been associated with AD vitreoretinochoroidopathy and nanophthalmia.

11.3.5 Microphthalmia with Linear Skin Defects Syndrome (OMIM 309801)

Microphthalmia with linear skin defects (MLS) syndrome (OMIM 309801) is defined by unilateral or bilateral microphthalmia and/or anophthalmia and linear skin defects, frequently affecting the face and neck. These defects are present at birth and heal with time, leaving minimal residual scarring. Other findings may include developmental delay, heart defects, short stature, diaphragmatic hernia, nail dystrophy, preauricular pits, hearing loss, and genitourinary malformations. Linear skin defects have been reported in 95% of patients, and usually affect the face and neck. Xp22 monosomy or *HCCS* mutation are associated with MLS syndrome. It is inherited in an XL dominant (XLD) manner.

11.3.6 Gorlin–Goltz Syndrome (OMIM 305600)

Gorlin–Goltz syndrome is characterized by dermal hypoplasia and microphthalmia. Limb and skeletal malformations are commonly seen. The syndrome is caused by point mutations and deletions of *PORCN*.

11.3.7 Oculocerebrocutaneous Syndrome (OMIM 164180)

Oculocerebrocutaneous syndrome (OMIM 164180) is defined by orbital cysts and microphthalmia, focal skin defects, and brain malformations (polymicrogyria, periventricular nodular heterotopias, enlarged lateral ventricles, and agenesis of the corpus callosum).

11.3.8 Aicardi Syndrome (OMIM 304050)

Aicardi syndrome includes a triad of agenesis of the corpus callosum, typical chorioretinal lacunae, and infantile spasms. Microphthalmia, developmental delay, polymicrogyria, and costovertebral anomalies are also common. Refractory epilepsy and pigmentary lesions of the skin can be seen. This condition has been associated with the locus Xp22 and appears to be XLD by de novo mutations; however, the specific gene is unknown.

11.3.9 Lenz Microphthalmia Syndrome (OMIM 309800)

Lenz microphthalmia syndrome (LMS; OMIM 309800) is defined by unilateral or bilateral microphthalmia with malformations of the ears, teeth, fingers, skeleton, or genitourinary system. *BCOR* mutations have been associated with LMS. Inheritance is XL recessive. Most affected males have intellectual disability.

11.3.10 Oculofaciocardiodental Syndrome (Syndromic Microphthalmia-2, OMIM 300166)

Oculofaciocardiodental syndrome (syndromic microphthalmia-2, OMIM 300166) is caused by different mutations in BCOR (BCL-6 corepressor) (Xp11.4). This syndrome consists of eye, facial, cardiac, and dental anomalies. These include congenital cataract, microphthalmia, or secondary glaucoma; long narrow face, high nasal bridge, pointed nose, cleft palate, or submucous cleft palate; atrial septal defect, ventricular septal defect, or floppy mitral valve; and canine radiculomegaly, delayed dentition, oligodontia, persistent primary teeth, or variable root length. Inheritance is XLD, and lethal in males.

11.3.11 Klinefelters Syndrome

Klinefelters syndrome (gynecomastia, small testes, and infertility) is caused by the presence of one or more additional X chromosomes in an affected male (e.g., XXY). Microphthalmia, cataracts, and malformed pupils can rarely be seen.

11.4 Conditions That Can Mimic Optic Nerve Coloboma

Some syndromes in which coloboma has been reported are listed in ► Table 11.3.

11.4.1 Morning Glory Disc Anomaly (MGDA; OMIM 120430)

Morning glory disc anomaly (MGDA; OMIM 120430) is a term first used to describe the resemblance of the optic nerve head malformation to a morning glory flower. The optic nerve characteristically is enlarged with the retinal vessels emerging from a central excavation in a radiating straightened pattern, each emerging from the peripheral edges of the nerve. There is usually pigmentation surrounding the nerve head, and a characteristic central glial tuft. This condition is usually unilateral. Rarely there may be a more typical coloboma in the other eye. It is thought that an embryonic development alteration of the lamina cribrosa and the posterior sclera causes this malformation. No specific genetic defect has been described, although *PAX6* gene mutations have been identified in patients with bilateral morning glory disc anomaly. Visual acuity in

Table 11.3 Syndromes associated with coloboma

Clinical syndrome	Type of coloboma (ONC vs. macular)
CHARGE syndrome	Both ONC and macular coloboma
Basal cell nevus carcinoma syndrome	Macular
Congenital contractural arachnodactyly	Macular
Meckel–Gruber syndrome	Macular
Sjogren–Larsson syndrome	Macular
Humeroradial synostosis	Macular
Oral-facial-digital syndrome (type VIII)	Macular
Lenz microphthalmia syndrome	Macular
Aicardi syndrome	Both ONC and macular coloboma
MIDAS syndrome	Macular
Catel–Manzke syndrome	Macular
Trisomy 13 (Patau syndrome)	Both ONC and macular coloboma
Trisomy 18 (Edwards syndrome)	Macular
Wolf–Hirschhorn syndrome	Macular
Cat eye syndrome	Macular
Linear sebaceous nevus syndrome	Macular
Rubinstein–Taybi syndrome	Both ONC and macular coloboma
Kabuki syndrome	Macular
Oculo-auriculo-vertebral syndrome	Both ONC and macular coloboma
Verheij syndrome	Macular. Optic nerve hypoplasia can be seen

Abbreviation: CHARGE, Coloboma of the eye, Heart defects, Atresia of the nasal choanae, Retardation of growth and/or development, Genital and/or urinary abnormalities, and Ear abnormalities; MIDAS, microphthalmia, dermal aplasia, and sclerocornea; ONC, optic nerve coloboma.

patients with MGDA is usually poor, with only one-third achieving 20/40 or better. An afferent pupillary defect may be present. Associated ocular findings may include optic nerve calcifications, microphthalmos, and retinal detachment. Facial anomalies include hypertelorism; cleft lip or cleft palate may also be seen. A lower lip notch is an indicator of possible encephalocele. Other central nervous systemic findings include agenesis of corpus callosum, pituitary dysfunction, and Moyamoya's disease. It is also seen in PHACES (posterior fossa malformations–hemangiomas–arterial anomalies–cardiac defects–eye abnormalities–sternal cleft and supraumbilical raphe) syndrome. The characteristic appearance of the optic nerve as well as a funnel-shaped anterior optic nerve sheath at the junction to the globe on ultrasound distinguishes MGDA from ONC.

11.4.2 Renal Coloboma Syndrome (OMIM 120330, Also Known as Papillorenal Syndrome)

The optic nerve in this syndrome has a large central cup and absent cilioretinal vessel bilaterally. It is not associated with true ONC or fundus coloboma. Renal findings include renal hypodysplasia and oligomeganephronia. This syndrome is due to AD*PAX2* mutation (10q24).

11.4.3 CHARGE Syndrome (OMIM 214800)

The acronym stands for Coloboma of the eye, Heart defects, Atresia of the nasal choanae, Retardation of growth and/or development, Genital and/or urinary abnormalities, and Ear abnormalities with or without deafness. The estimated prevalence is 1:10,000. Mutations in *CHD7* are found in approximately 70% of cases. Some patients have del8q12, though other chromosome aberrations have been reported (del22q11, dup14q22-q24, and balanced translocation of chromosome 8).

11.4.4 Peripapillary Staphyloma

This condition typically manifests as a deep excavation surrounding the optic disc. The optic disc can appear as normal, but in some cases some pallor regions can be seen. Vessel configuration is usually normal. The optic nerve head may appear to be deeply set with an excavation in the sclera. It is considered to be sporadic, nonheritable, and unilateral. Visual acuity is usually low. It is rarely associated with other congenital defects or systemic diseases.

11.4.5 Megalopapilla

This anomaly consists in an enlarged optic disc with normal disc morphology. It is associated with bigger-than-normal physiologic blind spots and rarely reduced visual acuity. It may be confused with glaucoma because the cup area looks bigger in both conditions; however, this can be differentiated with optical coherence tomography (OCT).

11.4.6 Optic Pit

This term describes a localized round excavation or regional depression in the margin of the optic nerve head. Estimated frequency is less than 1 in 10,000 and it is bilateral in up to 15% of cases. There is often enlargement of the physiologic cup and a variable amount of prepapillary glial tissue. The size of the optic pit varies between a quarter and an eighth of the disc, and the color is usually gray but can be yellow or white. Vessels can also be seen emerging from the pit. Large temporal pits are associated with a higher risk of macular detachments, which are more frequent in the third and fourth decades of life. The most common visual defect seen in optic pits is arcuate scotoma.

11.4.7 Tilted Disc

In this condition, the optic nerve appears to enter the eye in an oblique angle. Its prevalence in the general population is up to 3.5%. Ocular associations include high myopia due to increased axial length, color vision alterations, situs inversus of the vessels, and retinal abnormalities, such as chorioretinal thinning, posterior staphyloma, and peripapillary atrophy. Glaucoma is not associated. The most common visual field defect is a scotoma in the superior temporal quadrant.

11.4.8 Doubling of the Optic Disc

This is a very rare anomaly in which two discs appear to be next to each other or overlapping as a bilobed disc. Each disc has its own vascular system. This condition is usually unilateral and is commonly associated with low vision.

11.5 Uncommon Manifestations

11.5.1 Cystic Eye

This is a cystic malformation that lacks normal ocular structures. At birth, this cyst can be small and be confused with anophthalmia. With time, this cyst can grow and bulge. Imaging studies can show an intraorbital cyst with attached extraocular muscles but no optic nerve. Colobomatous cysts are not associated with isolated ONC.

11.6 Clinical Testing

11.6.1 A- and B-Scan Ultrasonography

A- and B-scan ultrasonography is used to measure total axial length and evaluate the internal structures of the globe.

11.6.2 Orbital Computed Tomography or Magnetic Resonance Imaging

Orbital CT or MRI can reveal remnants of ocular tissue, helping differentiate anophthalmia from severe microphthalmia. These tests can also define brain anatomy and the presence of orbital cyst.

11.6.3 Exhaustive Physical Examination

Exhaustive physical examination is performed to rule out skin lesions, neurologic abnormalities, developmental assessment, hearing problems, or involvement of other organs (endocrine tests, dental evaluation, echocardiogram, renal ultrasound, spine radiographs).

11.7 Genetic Testing

After detailed family history, ophthalmologic examination, ocular/brain imaging studies, physical examination, and further study according to findings, testing can include CMA or single gene testing. Multiple genes can be tested with customized panels when available or when a specific gene is not suggested by the clinical findings. If none of these tests confirm a diagnosis, whole exome sequencing (WES) could be considered.

11.8 Additional Resources

11.9 Problems

11.9.1 Case 1

A 2-month-old male infant presents with bilateral severe microphthalmia without anterior segment dysgenesis other than the small size. He also has microtia, tracheoesophageal fistula, developmental delay, hypospadias, and Dandy–Walker malformation on MRI. Family history reveals two unaffected sisters and normal parents. The child's mother has not had prior miscarriages. Which from the following seems the most appropriate genetic testing?

a) *OTX2* sequencing.
b) *SOX2* sequencing.
c) *RAX* sequencing.
d) Cytogenetics microarray.

Correct answer is b.

Individuals with *SOX2* mutations are characterized by microphthalmia that is often bilateral and severe. Other findings include brain anomalies, esophageal atresia, genital abnormalities, endocrine dysfunction, and developmental delays. *SOX2* mutations are the most frequent found in patients with bilateral severe microphthalmia. It is AD, with complete penetrance and variable expressivity, although most of the cases are de novo mutations.

a) **Incorrect.** *OTX2* mutations are less frequent than *SOX2* mutations. In addition, patients with *OTX2* may present with anterior segment dysgenesis or severe retinal dysplasia.
b) **Correct.**
c) **Incorrect.** *RAX* mutations are even less frequent than *OTX2* mutations. Patients tend to have sclerocornea.
d) **Less appropriate.** With multiple organ systems involved, microarray testing would otherwise be indicated, but in this case the clinical signs strongly point to a specific gene abnormality.

11.9.2 Case 2

A 3-month-old female infant with confirmed trisomy 13 by karyotype presents for ophthalmologic evaluation. She also has holoprosencephaly, seizures, cleft lip and palate, and microcephaly. Ocular examination shows severe microphthalmia, bilateral chorioretinal coloboma, and retinal dysplasia. Which one from the following would be the best test to confirm the cause of this ocular malformation?

a) Cytogenetics microarray.
b) *SOX2* sequencing.
c) Microphthalmia panel.
d) There is no need of further genetic study.

Correct answer is d.

Ophthalmic malformations have been found in almost 80% of patients with trisomy 13. The ophthalmic findings in this patient are consistent with the diagnosis already established by karyotype. There is no need for further studies. These anomalies are frequently severe and incompatible with vision. Because of the poor life prognosis, treatment of ocular conditions must be carefully considered.

a) **Incorrect.** CMA would not provide more significant information as the complete trisomy is confirmed by the karyotype.
b) **Incorrect.** Although *SOX2* mutations are associated with bilateral severe microphthalmia, the systemic manifestations are different than those seen in trisomy 13.
c) **Incorrect.** The karyotype has sufficiently explained the ophthalmic manifestations.
d) **Correct.**

11.9.3 Case 3

A 2-month-old male patient presents for ophthalmic evaluation. Clinical examination revealed no identifiable globes and ultrasound failed to prove ocular remnants. He also had severe microcephaly with normal karyotype. In this context, which from the following alternatives seems to be more correct?
a) The patient has anophthalmia. There is no need for further testing.
b) Biopsy of orbital tissues should be conducted.
c) Before any additional clinical testing, *OTX2* sequencing can be done to orient future testing.
d) Further orbital imaging can be helpful to clarify the diagnosis.

Correct answer is d.
Orbital imaging such as CT or MRI can reveal remnants of ocular tissue even if ultrasound is negative. It will also identify the absence or presence of an optic nerve. The absence of an optic nerve supports a diagnosis of true anophthalmia as opposed to severe microphthalmia (clinical anophthalmia).
a) **Incorrect.** Without complete imaging, severe microphthalmia remains possible.
b) **Incorrect.** This invasive procedure is usually unnecessary.
c) **Incorrect.** Clarifying the phenotype is the first step in determining the appropriate genetic testing.
d) **Correct.**

11.9.4 Case 4

A 5-year-old boy was referred by a geneticist for evaluation of "small eyes." Physical examination is unremarkable. Ophthalmic findings under anesthesia include bilateral corneal diameters of 11 mm, normal anterior segment, normal lens, axial length of 18 mm, normal scleral thickness, mild macular folds, and cycloplegic refraction of 8 diopters. Which one of the following seems to be the most correct diagnosis?
a) Microcornea.
b) Posterior microphthalmia.
c) Microphthalmia.
d) Nanophthalmia.

Correct answer is b.
Posterior microphthalmia primarily affects the posterior segment, often with macular folds and hyperopia.
a) **Incorrect.** The corneal diameter is normal for age.
b) **Correct.**
c) **Incorrect.** The cornea size and anterior segment are normal.
d) **Incorrect.** Although nanophthalmia overlaps with posterior microphthalmia, there is no scleral thickening or shallowing of the anterior chamber.

11.9.5 Case 5

A 1-year-old girl was referred by a colleague for evaluation of ONC. Physical examination is unremarkable. Ophthalmic findings include bilateral corneal diameters of 11 mm, normal anterior segment, normal lens, normal axial length, normal retina, and cycloplegic refraction of + 2 diopters. Bilateral asymmetric ONC is present. Which one of the following seems to be the most appropriate next step?

a) Orbital B scan.

b) Sequence *PAX6*.

c) Order levels of cortisol and TSH (thyroid stimulating hormone).

d) None of the above.

Correct answer is d.

Isolated ONC with an otherwise normal eye examination usually does not require any of the listed tests. Neuroimaging might be considered.

a) **Incorrect.** Optic nerve coloboma is not associated with orbital cysts unless there is also fundus coloboma.

b) **Incorrect.** Most patients with isolated ONC do not have an underlying molecular cause.

c) **Incorrect.** Endocrine axis study is required in optic nerve hypoplasia (septo-optic dysplasia). Endocrine abnormalities are not typically associated with ONC.

d) **Correct.**

Suggested Reading

[1] Bakrania P, Robinson DO, Bunyan DJ, et al. SOX2 anophthalmia syndrome: 12 new cases demonstrating broader phenotype and high frequency of large gene deletions. Br J Ophthalmol. 2007; 91(11):1471–1476

[2] Gonzalez-Rodriguez J, Pelcastre EL, Tovilla-Canales JL, et al. Mutational screening of CHX10, GDF6, OTX2, RAX and SOX2 genes in 50 unrelated microphthalmia-anophthalmia-coloboma (MAC) spectrum cases. Br J Ophthalmol. 2010; 94(8):1100–1104

[3] Schilter KF, Reis LM, Schneider A, et al. Whole-genome copy number variation analysis in anophthalmia and microphthalmia. Clin Genet. 2013; 84(5):473–481

[4] Schneider A, Bardakjian T, Reis LM, Tyler RC, Semina EV. Novel SOX2 mutations and genotype-phenotype correlation in anophthalmia and microphthalmia. Am J Med Genet A. 2009; 149A(12):2706–2715

[5] Chassaing N, Causse A, Vigouroux A, et al. Molecular findings and clinical data in a cohort of 150 patients with anophthalmia/microphthalmia. Clin Genet. 2014; 86(4):326–334

[6] Choi A, Lao R, Ling-Fung Tang P, et al. Novel mutations in PXDN cause microphthalmia and anterior segment dysgenesis. Eur J Hum Genet. 2015; 23(3):337–341

[7] Jimenez NL, Flannick J, Yahyavi M, et al. Targeted "next-generation" sequencing in anophthalmia and microphthalmia patients confirms SOX2, OTX2 and FOXE3 mutations. BMC Med Genet. 2011; 12:172

[8] Reis LM, Tyler RC, Schneider A, Bardakjian T, Semina EV. Examination of SOX2 in variable ocular conditions identifies a recurrent deletion in microphthalmia and lack of mutations in other phenotypes. Mol Vis. 2010; 16:768–773

[9] Williamson KA, FitzPatrick DR. The genetic architecture of microphthalmia, anophthalmia and coloboma. Eur J Med Genet. 2014; 57(8):369–380

[10] Juhn AT, Nabi NU, Levin AV. Ocular anomalies in an infant with Klinefelter Syndrome. Ophthalmic Genet. 2012; 33(4):232–234

[11] Tucker S, Enzenauer RW, Morin JD, et al. Corneal diameter, axial length, and intraocular pressure in premature infants.. Ophthalmology. 1992; 99:1296–1300

[12] Nelson LB, Olitsky SE. Harley's Pediatric Ophthalmology. Philadelphia, PA: Lippincott Williams & Wilkins; 2013

[13] Hornby SJ, Adolph S, Gilbert CE, Dandona L, Foster A. Visual acuity in children with coloboma: clinical features and a new phenotypic classification system. Ophthalmology. 2000; 107(3):511–520

[14] Savell J, Cook JR. Optic nerve colobomas of autosomal-dominant heredity. Arch Ophthalmol. 1976; 94(3):395–400

[15] Brodsky MC. Congenital optic disk anomalies. Surv Ophthalmol. 1994; 39(2):89–112

[16] Lee BJ, Traboulsi EI. Update on the morning glory disc anomaly. Ophthalmic Genet. 2008; 29(2):47–52

[17] Parsa CF, Silva ED, Sundin OH, et al. Redefining papillorenal syndrome: an underdiagnosed cause of ocular and renal morbidity. Ophthalmology. 2001; 108(4):738–749

[18] Azuma N, Yamaguchi Y, Handa H, et al. Mutations of the PAX6 gene detected in patients with a variety of optic-nerve malformations. Am J Hum Genet. 2003; 72(6):1565–1570

12 Marfan Syndrome and Other Causes of Ectopia Lentis

Abstract

Many conditions are associated with ectopia lentis, including Marfan syndrome, Weill–Marchesani syndrome, and homocystinuria. Marfan syndrome is an autosomal dominant systemic condition of connective tissue with a high degree of phenotypic variability. Main findings involve the ocular, skeletal, and cardiovascular system, with increased risk of retinal detachment, glaucoma, ectopia lentis, myopia, scoliosis, tall stature, and aortic aneurysm. The *FBN1* gene encodes for fibrillin, a protein intimately involved in connective tissue integrity. *FBN1* mutations cause a wide clinical spectrum, ranging from isolated ectopia lentis to severe progressive neonatal Marfan syndrome.

Keywords: ectopia lentis, Marfan syndrome, Weill–Marchesani syndrome, homocystinuria, *FBN1*

Key Points

- Many conditions are associated with ectopia lentis, including Marfan syndrome (MFS), Weill–Marchesani syndrome, and homocystinuria.
- MFS is an autosomal dominant systemic condition of connective tissue with a high degree of phenotypic variability. Main findings involve the ocular, skeletal, and cardiovascular system, with increased risk of retinal detachment, glaucoma, ectopia lentis, myopia, scoliosis, tall stature, and aortic aneurism.
- *FBN1* encodes for fibrillin, a protein intimately involved in connective tissue integrity.
- *FBN1* mutations cause a wide clinical spectrum, ranging from isolated ectopia lentis to severe progressive neonatal MFS.

12.1 Overview

Marfan syndrome (MFS) is an autosomal dominant (AD) systemic condition of connective tissue that affects multiple organs, including the eye, skeleton, and cardiovascular system. The estimated prevalence of MFS ranges from 1 in 5,000 to 10,000. Clinical diagnosis is based on the revised Ghent criteria, which delineates minor and major criteria. Findings other than aortic root enlargement or ectopia lentis are considered in a systemic score. As many manifestations of MFS appear with age, it may take years for the systemic diagnosis of MFS to become clear.

Major skeletal features include pectus carinatum, pectus excavatum requiring surgery, reduced upper-to-lower body segment ratio, combination of both positive wrist and thumb signs, scoliosis of greater than 20 degrees or spondylolisthesis, and reduced extension at the elbows. The thumb sign is considered positive when the entire distal phalanx of the adducted thumb extends beyond the ulnar border. The wrist sign is positive when the tip of the thumb covers the entire fingernail of the fifth finger when wrapped around the contralateral wrist (▶ Fig. 12.1). Minor features include pectus excavatum of moderate severity, joint hypermobility, high arched palate

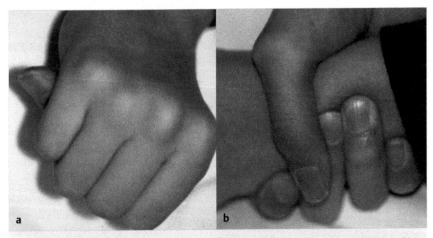

Fig. 12.1 (a) Positive thumb sign in a patient with Marfan syndrome. Part of the thumb is visible beyond the ulnar border of the hand. (b) Positive wrist sign in the same patient. The thumb is able to pass the distal phalangeal joint of the middle finger of the opposite hand when grasping the wrist.

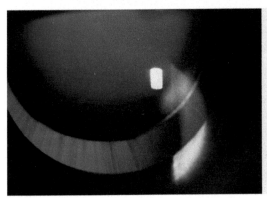

Fig. 12.2 Ectopia lentis in a patient with Marfan syndrome. Note zonules are stretched rather than broken.

with crowding of teeth, and facial appearance (dolichocephaly, malar hypoplasia, enophthalmos, retrognathia, downslanting palpebral fissures). Skeletal anomalies can appear even in infancy and tend to progress during growing periods. Patients with MFS are not necessarily tall as familial background is also a determinant. Many of the skeletal findings of MFS are frequently found in the normal general population.

The only major ocular finding is ectopia lentis (▶ Fig. 12.2). Minor features include flat cornea, increased globe axial length, and hypoplasia of pupillary dilator resulting in miosis. Myopia may be lenticular, due to ectopia lentis, or axial. It may progress rapidly during infancy due to progressive ectopia lentis. Ectopia lentis is only found in approximately 60% of patients. Although the typical lens subluxation is superotemporal, the lens can move in any direction. As flat keratometry may "counteract" myopia, measuring axial length and careful examination for subtle ectopia lentis is required. Patients with MFS are also at increased risk for retinal detachment (with or without lens surgery), adult-onset open angle glaucoma, and cataract within the ectopic lens.

Major cardiovascular findings include dilatation of the ascending aorta with or without aortic regurgitation or dissection of the ascending aorta. Minor features are mitral valve prolapse with or without mitral valve regurgitation, dilatation of the main pulmonary artery, calcification of the mitral annulus below the age of 40 years, and dilatation or dissection of the descending thoracic or abdominal aorta below the age of 50 years. Aortic root dilatation tends to progress over time, although the onset and rate are extremely variable. Medical and surgical advances have increased life expectancy.

Dural ectasia is considered a major criterion, and can lead to low back pain, proximal leg pain, weakness and numbness, headache, and genital/rectal pain. Pulmonary and skin abnormalities are minor features. Pulmonary findings include spontaneous pneumothorax and apical blebs. Skin features are striae atrophicae (not associated with marked weight changes, pregnancy, or repetitive stress), and recurrent or incisional hernias.

12.2 Molecular Genetics

MFS is caused by mutation of *FBN1* (15q21.1), which can be detected by thorough sequencing in over 95% of patients. Intron mutations, large deletions, and promoter mutations may occur. Even in the presence of an *FBN1* mutation, clinical confirmation by the revised Ghent criteria is recommended. *TGFBR1*, *TGFBR2*, or *TGFB2* mutations have also been seen in patients with clinical MFS although ectopia lentis is rarely seen with these genes.

Approximately 25% of MFS is due to de novo mutation. Because of variable expression, in the absence of genetic testing, both parents should have a comprehensive clinical examination and echocardiogram. Few genotype–phenotype correlations exist in MFS. Severe early-onset MFS usually presents alterations in exons 24 and 32, although some patients with mutations in this region have classic or even mild MFS. Nonsense mutations result in rapid degradation of mutated transcripts and can be associated with mild conditions.

12.3 Differential Diagnosis

12.3.1 Homocystinuria (OMIM 236200)

Homocystinuria (OMIM 236200) is an autosomal recessive (AR) disorder associated with cystathionine β-synthase (21q22.3) deficiency, and affects the transsulfuration pathway, resulting in elevated serum and urine homocysteine and plasma methionine. 5,10-Methylenetetrahydrofolate reductase (MTHFR) deficiency can also result in homocystinuria, usually with more mild ectopia lentis. Frequency of cystathionine β-synthase is variable, ranging from 1:30,000 to 60,000 live births. Unlike MFS, approximately 50% of patients have a variable degree of intellectual disability. Ectopia lentis is seen in up to 40% of children and almost all patients by adulthood. Whereas the zonules are stretched in MFS, they are broken in homocystinuria and often seen clumped on the lens edge with crenulations of lens edge (▶ Fig. 12.3). Other findings that differentiate this disorder from MFS include coarse hair with premature graying, and most importantly, the increased risk of thromboembolic events. As the latter is aggravated by general anesthesia, and can result in significant stroke or death, all patients should have serum and urine homocysteine levels measured preoperatively unless another cause of their ectopia lentis is clear. The phenotype may overlap with MFS, because individuals with homocystinuria may have Marfanoid habitus, myopia,

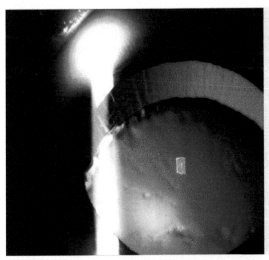

Fig. 12.3 Ectopia lentis in a patient with homocystinuria. Note the broken lens zonules resulting in crenulations of the lens edge.

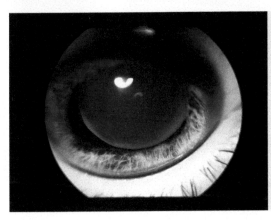

Fig. 12.4 Microspherophakia with progressive anterior movement of the lens and iris in a patient with autosomal recessive Weill–Marchesani syndrome. This may result in angle closure glaucoma and iris atrophy.

pectus deformity, scoliosis, mitral valve prolapse, and highly arched palate although their wrist and thumb signs are negative. Although the lens usually luxates down and nasally (approximately half of individuals), posteriorly in 20%, and anteriorly in 10% of patients, any direction is possible. If the lens dislocates into the anterior chamber, pupillary block, acute glaucoma, and secondary corneal decompensation may occur. Approximately half of patients with homocystinuria are responsive to vitamin B_6 supplementation.

12.3.2 Weill–Marchesani Syndrome (OMIM 277600; 608328; 614819)

This condition includes microspherophakia with progressive anterior movement of the lens (▶ Fig. 12.4) resulting in angle closure glaucoma and iris atrophy. Other features include short stature, brachydactyly, joint stiffness, and lack of vascular manifestations of MFS. Mutation in *FBN1* can cause AD Weill–Marchesani Syndrome (WMS). Mutations in *ADAMTS10* and *ADAMTS17* are known to cause AR WMS. The AD form is less severe. Mild cardiac abnormalities, not including aneurysm, can occur in the AR form.

12.3.3 Autosomal Dominant Isolated Ectopia Lentis (OMIM 129600)

Caused by heterozygous mutation in *FBN1*, these patients lack the systemic features of MFS, although, as a fibrillinopathy, some have later shown signs of aortic root enlargement. It has been argued that the presence of ectopia lentis and an identified *FBN1* mutation meets criteria for diagnosis of MFS and therefore ongoing screening with echocardiography is recommended.

12.3.4 Autosomal Recessive Isolated Ectopia Lentis (OMIM 225100)

This entity can be caused by mutations in *ADAMTSL4* and is not associated with systemic manifestations. Mutations in this gene may also result in **ectopia lentis et pupillae**, which presents with corectopia in the opposite direction of the subluxed lens. It is also associated with persistent pupillary membranes that may be best appreciated after pupillary dilatation.

12.3.5 *ADAMTS18* Mutations Associated with Ectopia Lentis (OMIM 225200)

Patients present with ocular developmental abnormalities including microcornea, corectopia, ectopia lentis, myopic chorioretinal atrophy, rhegmatogenous retinal detachment, and early onset of cone–rod dystrophy.

12.3.6 Loeys–Dietz Syndrome (OMIM 609192; 610168)

Patients with heterozygous mutation in either *TGFBR1* or *TGFBR2* may present aortic aneurysm associated with arachnodactyly, joint laxity, pectus deformity, scoliosis, and dural ectasia. These patients do not have ectopia lentis, but do have long face, downward-slanting palpebral fissures, high arched palate, malar hypoplasia, micrognathia, and retrognathia.

12.3.7 Ehlers–Danlos Syndrome

Ehlers–Danlos syndrome is a group of disorders that present with joint hypermobility. The classic type (OMIM 130000) is an AD condition characterized by skin hyperextensibility, abnormal wound healing, and joint hypermobility. Approximately half of patients with classic Ehlers–Danlos syndrome have a mutation in *COL5A1* or *COL5A2* genes. Among the other Ehlers–Danlos subtypes, the vascular type (OMIM 130050) is particularly relevant because of the tendency for aneurysm or dissection of any medium to large muscular artery. In addition, the tissues can be extremely friable, increasing significantly the surgical risk. This disorder is confirmed by identification of a mutation in *COL3A1*. Only type VI, the oculoscoliotic form, due to biallelic mutations in *PLOD1* (1p36.22), has significant ocular manifestations: spontaneous corneal rupture ("brittle" cornea). Ectopia lentis occurs only secondary to ocular rupture.

12.3.8 Shprintzen–Goldberg Syndrome (OMIM 182212)

This condition demonstrates many skeletal findings of MFS but with the additional findings of hypertelorism, craniosynostosis, cognitive impairment, Chiari malformation, and proptosis. Aortic root enlargement is rarer and milder than in MFS. *FBN1* mutation has been associated with Shprintzen–Goldberg syndrome in some patients. More commonly patients have mutation in *SKI* (1p36). Ectopia lentis is not seen.

12.3.9 Stickler Syndrome (OMIM 108300)

This condition presents with myopia, cortical cataract, radial retinal lattice, retinal detachment, hearing loss, midfacial hypoplasia, cleft palate, spondyloepiphyseal dysplasia, and arthropathy. Inheritance can be AD or AR. Ectopia lentis is rarely seen.

12.3.10 Knobloch Syndrome (OMIM 267750)

Knobloch syndrome (OMIM 267750) is characterized by high myopia, with a characteristic myopic appearance of the fundus and geographic macular atrophy. Patients have an increased incidence of retinal detachment. They may also show ectopia lentis, abnormal vitreous, and a featureless iris. The cardinal feature is occipital defects, which can range from occipital encephalocele to cutis aplasia, although the occiput is normal in some patients. It is due to biallelic mutation in the *COL18A1* gene.

12.3.11 MASS Syndrome (OMIM 604308)

The AD syndrome of Mitral valve prolapse, Myopia, borderline and nonprogressive Aortic enlargement, and nonspecific Skin and Skeletal (MASS) manifestations overlaps with MFS. It is due to *FBN1* mutation. Ectopia lentis is not present.

12.3.12 Lens Subluxation Associated with *VSX* Mutation

A single patient from a consanguineous family presented superior lens subluxation, cone–rod dysfunction, and high myopia without vitreous condensations.

12.3.13 Traboulsi Syndrome (OMIM 601552)

This condition is characterized by facial dysmorphism (flat cheeks and beaked nose), ectopia lentis, anterior segment abnormalities, and spontaneous filtering blebs (nontraumatic conjunctival cysts presumably caused by abnormal thinning of the sclera). It is caused by homozygous mutation in the *ASPH* gene (8q12).

12.3.14 Sulfite Oxidase Deficiency (OMIM 272300)

This AR condition, also known as sulfocysteinuria, is caused by *SUOX* mutations (12q13.2). It is characterized by variable neurologic findings and possible bilateral ectopia lentis. The clinical spectrum ranges from fatal presentation to milder forms of developmental delay, ataxia, dystonia, choreoathetosis, and language delay. Milder forms cannot be distinguished from combined molybdenum cofactor deficiency clinically.

12.3.15 Hyperlysinemia (OMIM 238700)

This condition is an AR disease with variable clinical features. Some patients can present with nonspecific seizures, hypotonia, or mildly delayed psychomotor development, but many are asymptomatic. There are sporadic cases of bilateral ectopia lentis. Biallelic mutations in *AASS* (7q31.32) are causative.

12.3.16 Cornea Plana (OMIM 121400; 217300)

Cornea plana presents with reduced corneal curvature leading in most cases to hyperopia, hazy corneal limbus, and arcus at an early age. There are two types: CNA1 (AD; 12q21.33) and CNA2 (AR; *KERA* gene; 12q21.33). CNA1 is usually mild, whereas CNA2 is severe and frequently associated with additional ocular manifestations, such as microcornea, posterior corneal stromal haze, posterior embryotoxon, iridocorneal adhesions, iris nodules, iris atrophy, and pupillary irregularities. Conjunctival xerosis has been described in CNA1. The mean keratometry value for CNA2 is approximately 30 and for CNA1 it is 38.

Ectopia lentis may also occur with the wide range of ocular developmental anomalies such as persistent fetal vasculature, aniridia, and coloboma. Any cause of early childhood glaucoma that results in buphthalmos may also result in ectopia lentis. Even in the absence of glaucoma, congenital rubella syndrome may be associated with ectopia lentis. Trauma is the most common cause of ectopia lentis, although almost always unilateral.

12.4 Uncommon Manifestations

Uncommon findings in MFS include total dislocation of the lens onto the retina and cataract. Midperipheral iris transillumination can also occur as a sign of dilator aplasia.

12.5 Clinical Testing

12.5.1 Echocardiography

It is recommended that all patients suspected to have MFS have echocardiography to assess for aortic root dilatation and valvular anomalies.

12.5.2 Axial Length and Keratometry

These tests are used to distinguish the source of myopia.

12.5.3 Homocysteine Testing

Homocystinuria is characterized by raised urinary homocysteine excretion. All patients should have appropriate testing to rule out homocystinuria unless an alternate diagnosis is confirmed.

12.5.4 Ultrasound Biomicroscopy

Ultrasound biomicroscopy may be required to assess lens position in some cases, especially when there is severe miosis.

12.6 Genetic Testing

The most frequent strategy for molecular diagnosis of a patient suspected of having MFS is sequencing *FBN1* exons and flanking intronic regions followed by deletion/duplication if a mutation is not identified. If initial *FBN1* sequencing fails, deep intronic sequencing should also be considered. There are multigene testing panels available for MFS and disorders that include aortic aneurysms and dissections.

12.7 Additional Resources

The Marfan Foundation (www.marfan.org) and Genetic Aortic Disorders Association of Canada (http://www.gadacanada.ca/), formerly known as the Canadian Marfan Association.

12.8 Problems

12.8.1 Case 1

A 7-year-old boy comes for ophthalmic evaluation. He failed a vision screening at school. Initial examination shows myopia (−6.00 sph OU [oculi uterque]) and bilateral superotemporal lens subluxation. Further study reveals aortic root enlargement. Physical examination shows positive wrist and thumb signs and pectus carinatum. He is the tallest in his class. Family history is unrevealing. Which from the following candidate genes seems more appropriate to sequence first?
a) *FBN1*.
b) *ADAMTSL4*.
c) *ADAMTS18*.
d) *TGFBR1*.

Correct answer is a.
   Clinical presentation strongly suggests MFS. Approximately 25% of cases are due to spontaneous mutation.
a) **Correct.**
b) **Incorrect.** *ADAMTSL4* is associated with AR isolated ectopia lentis or ectopia lentis et pupillae. Patients do not have systemic findings.
c) **Incorrect.** *ADAMTS18* mutations are associated with ectopia lentis in the presence of other ocular findings such as microcornea, corectopia, and retinal abnormalities.
d) **Incorrect.** Patients with Loeys–Dietz syndrome do not show ectopia lentis.

12.8.2 Case 2

A 9-year-old girl presents with bilateral ectopia lentis, mild pectus excavatum, and scoliosis, but otherwise normal physical examination, echocardiogram, serum homocysteine, and plasma methionine. Family history is unrevealing. Which from the following is most correct?
a) Patient has isolated AR ectopia lentis.
b) Patient could still have MFS.
c) Weill–Marchesani syndrome.
d) Shprintzen–Goldberg syndrome.

Correct answer is b.

The patient does not fulfill the revised Ghent criteria for a clinical diagnosis now, but many manifestations of MFS can appear with age.

a) **Less appropriate.** Although possible, the presence of scoliosis and pectus deformity at this young age suggests emerging MFS.

b) **Correct.**

c) **Incorrect.** Patient lacks other manifestations such as microspherophakia, short stature, and brachydactyly

d) **Incorrect.** Patient does not have clinical findings of Shprintzen–Goldberg syndrome.

12.8.3 Case 3

A 35-year-old woman presents with history of bilateral ectopia lentis and high myopia. She has many affected family members, including her father, two paternal aunts, and one sister. There is no history of sudden death in her family. Her physical examination and echocardiogram were normal. Which from the following tests seems most appropriate?

a) *COL2A1* sequencing.

b) *COL18A1* sequencing.

c) *CBS* sequencing.

d) *FBN1* sequencing.

Correct answer is d.

This patient has isolated ectopia lentis and AD transmission. She is at an age when other manifestations of MFS would have been expected to manifest in her family or her. Her diagnosis is isolated AD ectopia lentis most likely due to *FBN1* mutation.

a) **Incorrect.** Physical examination is normal. Other findings would be expected, such as hearing loss, midfacial underdevelopment, cleft palate, micrognathia, or **arthropathy.**

b) **Incorrect.** Physical examination is normal and she does not have a characteristic retina described. An occipital defect would be expected.

c) **Incorrect.** AD pattern of inheritance and lack of systemic features rule out homocystinuria.

d) **Correct.**

12.8.4 Case 4

A 9-year-old girl presented with vomiting, headache, lethargy, Marfanoid habitus, and left eye pain and redness. The patient has some learning challenges in school. Ophthalmic examination reveals inferior ectopia lentis in one eye and, in the other eye, a lens in the anterior chamber with an intraocular pressure of 45 and corneal edema. Which from the following tests seems most appropriate to order?

a) Quantitative tests for homocysteine in urine and blood.

b) MRI (magnetic resonance imaging) of the brain.

c) Echocardiography.

d) Hand radiographs.

Correct answer is a.

The combination of ectopia lentis, lens dislocation into the anterior chamber (due to broken zonules), marfanoid habitus, and learning disability (or developmental delay) strongly suggests homocystinuria.

a) **Correct.**

b) **Incorrect.** Although patients with homocystinuria have an increased prevalence of cerebral stroke, neuroimaging is not indicated if there are no neurologic symptoms. Spontaneous stroke in a young child in the absence of anesthesia or prolonged bed rest would be very unusual.

c) **Incorrect.** Lens dislocation into the anterior chamber is very rare in MFS. Patients with MFS have normal cognition. Mild cardiac anomalies can however be seen in homocystinuria, but first this diagnosis must be confirmed.

d) **Incorrect.** Although the lens migrates forward in Weill–Marshesani syndrome, it rarely comes through the pupil. Patients generally have short stature and characteristic contractures. Therefore, a search by radiograph for brachydactyly is not warranted in this case.

Suggested Reading

[1] Ahram D, Sato TS, Kohilan A, et al. A homozygous mutation in ADAMTSL4 causes autosomal-recessive isolated ectopia lentis. Am J Hum Genet. 2009; 84(2):274–278

[2] Brooke BS, Habashi JP, Judge DP, Patel N, Loeys B, Dietz HC, III. Angiotensin II blockade and aortic-root dilation in Marfan's syndrome. N Engl J Med. 2008; 358(26):2787–2795

[3] Erkula G, Jones KB, Sponseller PD, Dietz HC, Pyeritz RE. Growth and maturation in Marfan syndrome. Am J Med Genet. 2002; 109(2):100–115

[4] Faivre L, Collod-Beroud G, Loeys BL, et al. Effect of mutation type and location on clinical outcome in 1,013 probands with Marfan syndrome or related phenotypes and FBN1 mutations: an international study. Am J Hum Genet. 2007; 81(3):454–466

[5] Faivre L, Gorlin RJ, Wirtz MK, et al. In frame fibrillin-1 gene deletion in autosomal dominant Weill-Marchesani syndrome. J Med Genet. 2003; 40(1):34–36

[6] Judge DP, Dietz HC. Marfan's syndrome. Lancet. 2005; 366(9501):1965–1976

[7] Kosaki K, Takahashi D, Udaka T, et al. Molecular pathology of Shprintzen-Goldberg syndrome. Am J Med Genet A. 2006; 140(1):104–108, author reply 109–110

[8] Loeys B, De Backer J, Van Acker P, et al. Comprehensive molecular screening of the FBN1 gene favors locus homogeneity of classical Marfan syndrome. Hum Mutat. 2004; 24(2):140–146

[9] Couser NL, McClure J, Evans MW, et al. Homocysteinemia due to MTHFR deficiency in a young adult presenting with bilateral lens subluxations. Ophthalmic Genet. 2016; 38(1):91–94

[10] Zhang L, Lai YH, Capasso JE, Han S, Levin AV. Early onset ectopia lentis due to a FBN1 mutation with non-penetrance. Am J Med Genet A. 2015; 167(6):1365–1368

[11] Khan AO, Aldahmesh MA, Noor J, Salem A, Alkuraya FS. Lens subluxation and retinal dysfunction in a girl with homozygous VSX2 mutation. Ophthalmic Genet. 2015; 36(1):8–13

[12] Guo H, Wu X, Cai K, Qiao Z. Weill-Marchesani syndrome with advanced glaucoma and corneal endothelial dysfunction: a case report and literature review. BMC Ophthalmol. 2015; 15:3

[13] Chandra A, Arno G, Williamson K, et al. Expansion of ocular phenotypic features associated with mutations in ADAMTS18. JAMA Ophthalmol. 2014; 132(8):996–1001

[14] Longmuir SQ, Winter TW, Gross JR, Boldt HC. Primary peripheral retinal nonperfusion in a family with Loeys-Dietz syndrome. J AAPOS. 2014; 18(3):288–290

[15] Loeys BL, Dietz HC, Braverman AC, et al. The revised Ghent nosology for the Marfan syndrome. J Med Genet. 2010; 47(7):476–485

13 Familial Exudative Vitreoretinopathy

Abstract

Familial exudative vitreoretinopathy is a group of disorders characterized by failure of peripheral retinal vascularization, which leads to further retinal vascular complications. Expressivity within the same family may be highly variable. The disorder can rarely be asymmetric or even unilateral. Individuals may be entirely asymptomatic or present with severe visual loss, usually due to retinal detachment. Laser photocoagulation of the ischemic areas is useful to inhibit neovascularization and induce regression of new vessel formation, preventing retinal detachment. The disorder may be autosomal dominant, autosomal recessive, or X-linked recessive.

Keywords: familial exudative vitreoretinopathy, retinal nonperfusion, retinal detachment, *FZD4, LRP5, TSPAN12, ZNF408, NDP*

Key Points

- Familial exudative vitreoretinopathy (FEVR) is a genetically heterogeneous family of disorders characterized by incomplete vascularization of the retinal periphery leading to peripheral retinal vascular incompetency and neovascularization.
- FEVR may be autosomal dominant, autosomal recessive, or X-linked recessive.
- Early diagnosis and treatment are critical to prevent vision loss.

13.1 Overview

Familial exudative vitreoretinopathy (FEVR) can be defined as a group of disorders characterized by failure of peripheral retinal vascularization, which leads to further retinal vascular complications. Expressivity within the same family may be highly variable. The disorder can rarely be asymmetric or even unilateral. Most patients are affected bilaterally and symmetrically. Individuals may be entirely asymptomatic or present with severe visual loss usually due to retinal detachment. The incidence of FEVR is unknown as so many individuals are asymptomatic. Retinal findings may be subtle and only detectable by intravenous fluorescein angiography showing peripheral nonperfusion. More obvious signs include peripheral nonperfusion with or without a demarcation zone characterized by exudate, hemorrhage or neovascularization, peripheral fibrovascular mass, traction with possible macular drag, vessel straightening, retinal detachment, posterior retinal exudates, and falciform folds (▶ Fig. 13.1).

Laser photocoagulation of the ischemic areas is useful to prevent and induce regression of new vessel formation and prevent retinal detachment. In case of significant retinal traction, vitreoretinal surgery may be needed. The role of intravitreal antivascular endothelial growth factor (anti-VEGF) drugs is not fully known for this condition.

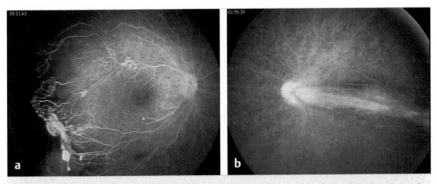

Fig. 13.1 Familial exudative vitreoretinopathy. **(a)** Peripheral avascular retina with abnormal vessels and neovascularization. **(b)** Falciform retinal fold extending temporally through the macula.

13.2 Molecular Genetics

Mutations in one of five genes are known to be associated with this phenotype: *FZD4* (11q14.2; encodes protein frizzled-4), *LRP5* (11q13.2; encodes low-density lipoprotein receptor-related protein 5), *TSPAN12* (7q31.31; encodes tetraspanin-12), *NDP* (Xp11.3; encodes norrin), and *ZNF408* (11p11.2; encodes zinc finger protein 408). These genes are all involved in the Wnt pathway, which determines retinal vascular development. Mutations of these genes are responsible for FEVR in approximately 70% of cases. Reported mutations include missense, nonsense, small deletions, and small insertions. The mutation prevalence is 20 to 40% for *FZD4*, 10 to 25% for *LRP5*, and 3 to 10% for *TSPAN12*. *FZD4* and *TSPAN12* are associated with autosomal dominant (AD) FEVR. Mutations of *LRP5* are usually associated with autosomal recessive (AR) FEVR but can also be seen with AD inheritance. The gene also has phenotypic heterogeneity as do *NDP* mutations which can cause osteoporosis-pseudoglioma syndrome (OPPG; OMIM 259770) and Norrie disease (OMIM 310600), respectively. Recently, *KIF11* mutations have been identified as a common cause of AD FEVR (up to 8% in one cohort). Individuals with *KIF11* mutations presented typical but variable signs of FEVR, with or without systemic findings, such as microcephaly, lymphedema, and mental retardation.

13.3 Differential Diagnosis

13.3.1 Retinopathy of Prematurity

Retinopathy of prematurity (ROP) is considered a sporadic condition, although there is some evidence that genetic changes in the Wnt receptor signaling pathway may be associated with the development of advanced ROP stages. ROP is also characterized by failure of development of the peripheral retinal vasculature. Two of the most important risk factors are premature birth and low weight at birth.

13.3.2 Coats' Disease

Coats' disease usually presents with severe retinal telangiectasia, typically in the periphery and often unilaterally in only one quadrant of retina. It may represent a sporadic intraretinal mutation of a Wnt pathway gene. It is usually sporadic with variable age of onset. These abnormal vessels can produce massive exudates that lead to retinal detachment. Male-to-female ratio is 10:1. Age of onset ranges from birth to milder presentations in adulthood.

13.3.3 Persistent Fetal Vasculature

Persistent fetal vasculature (formerly persistent hyperplastic primary vitreous) is associated with failure of regression of the hyaloid vasculature. It is usually (90%) unilateral and sporadic. Eyes are often microphthalmic with cataract. Persistent hyaloid artery has been described in AR FEVR. Although peripheral retinal vascular abnormalities may occur, nonperfusion is unusual.

13.3.4 Peripheral Granulomatous Toxocariasis

Peripheral granulomatous toxocariasis may resemble FEVR because of retinal traction and retinal folds. Nevertheless, uveitis associated with toxocariasis is not seen in FEVR. Toxocara is not present in infancy and is almost always unilateral.

13.3.5 Incontinentia Pigmenti

Incontinentia pigmenti is a rare X-linked dominant disease that affects multiple organs, including skin, hair, teeth, nails, and eyes. The eye findings resemble FEVR and are present in 30% of patients.

13.3.6 Morning Glory Disc

Morning glory disc is a rare congenital disc anomaly. The optic nerve is large with a posterior conical excavation. There is glial tissue over the disc and the vessels are splayed outward to the edges of the disc. These eyes may have peripheral nonperfusion of the retina.

13.3.7 Wyburn–Mason Syndrome

Wyburn–Mason syndrome is a rare disorder that presents with arteriovenous malformations of the midbrain and retina. Retinal peripheral nonperfusion has been reported.

13.3.8 Adams–Oliver Syndrome (OMIM 100300)

Adams–Oliver syndrome (OMIM 100300) is a rare condition defined by the combination of aplasia cutis congenita usually of the scalp vertex and terminal transverse limb defects. Patients may have vascular anomalies including pulmonary hypertension, portal hypertension, and retinal hypervascularization with peripheral nonperfusion.

13.3.9 Facioscapulohumeral Muscular Dystrophy (OMIM 158900)

Facioscapulohumeral muscular dystrophy (OMIM 158900) presents with weakness of the facial muscles and the stabilizers of the scapula or the dorsiflexors of the foot. It may have retinal vasculopathy, defined by failure of vascularization of the peripheral retina, telangiectatic blood vessels, and microaneurysms.

13.3.10 Norrie Disease (OMIM 310600)

Norrie disease is also caused by mutation in *NDP* and is an X-linked recessive condition. Although family members, in particular female carriers, may show FEVR, this disorder in males presents with retinal dysplasia with total retinal nonattachment (also known as pseudoglioma). Findings are usually bilateral, symmetric, and present at birth. Approximately half of individuals also have developmental delay and may develop psychotic disease. Approximately one-third develop sensorineural deafness by around 20 years of age. Affected individuals may also have growth failure and seizures.

13.3.11 Osteoporosis-Pseudoglioma Syndrome (OMIM 259770)

This condition is caused by homozygous or compound heterozygous pathogenic variants in the *LRP5* gene (11q13). Affected individuals present with osteoporosis, multiple fractures, and total retinal nonattachment due to retinal dysplasia (pseudoglioma).

13.4 Uncommon Manifestations

Infrequent findings in patients with FEVR are retinoschisis and giant retinal tears. Spinal muscular atrophy with *SMN1* deletion has been described in patients with severe retinal detachment and *FZD4* mutation causing FEVR. β-catenin signaling is dysregulated in both disorders, so the co-occurrence may have affected the vitreoretinal phenotype.

13.5 Clinical Testing

13.5.1 Fundus Fluorescein Angiography

Intravenous fundus fluorescein angiography (IVFA) confirms peripheral ischemia. This is particularly helpful in mildly affected patients and relatives. Diagnosis of subtle characteristic abnormalities can allow early treatment. Female carriers of *NDP* mutations should have this test, although they are usually less affected than their male relatives and often do not require treatment.

13.5.2 Periodic Fundus Examination

Children who are at risk based on a positive family pedigree should undergo regular examination to evaluate for the development or progression of the condition.

13.6 Genetic Testing

Unless family history demonstrates a clear pattern of inheritance that rules in or out a particular gene, FEVR gene panels are available to simultaneously sequence known genes.

13.7 Problems

13.7.1 Case 1

A developmentally normal 2-year-old male patient is referred because of progressive strabismus. Examination reveals normal vision in the right eye but poor fixation in the left eye. Dilated fundus examination shows bilateral macular traction with vessel straightening in the right eye and a falciform fold in the left eye extending to the temporal periphery. Clinical retinal examination of his mother seems normal. Which of the following diagnostic alternatives seems most cost-effective?

a) Intravenous fluorescein angiography in the mother.
b) *FZD4* sequencing.
c) Toxocara antibodies.
d) Brain magnetic resonance imaging (MRI).

Correct answer is a.

IVFA is a crucial test to determine the presence of ischemia in asymptomatic carriers. In a 2-year-old child, the test would require general anesthesia and may not be readily available, as special equipment is needed. It can detect subclinical retinal vascular abnormalities in carriers of FEVR, in particular female carriers of X-linked recessive FEVR due to *NDP* gene mutation.

a) **Correct.**
b) **Incorrect.** The clinical information is insufficient to propose molecular diagnostic testing without considering the presence of the condition in other family members. Having a positive IVFA in the mother increase the chances of having a positive genetic testing by aiding gene test selection, but it will also help with interpretation of gene test results. Gene sequencing is also expensive and may not be covered by insurance, unlike IVFA.
c) **Incorrect.** Toxocara is typically unilateral. The absence of a peripheral granuloma makes this diagnosis very unlikely.
d) **Incorrect.** Although MRI can be rarely abnormal in Norrie disease, it is usually normal in isolated FEVR.

13.7.2 Case 2

A 1-year-old boy comes for unilateral leukocoria evaluation. Retinal evaluation reveals peripheral retinal telangiectasia associated with exudative retinal detachment. Fellow eye examination is normal and angiography of the unaffected eye shows normal perfusion and vessels. IVFA of the affected eye shows a quadrant of "lightbulb deformities" of the retinal vessels. Examination of his parents is normal. Which of the following genes will most likely reveal a mutation?

a) *TSPAN12*.
b) *FZD4*.
c) *LRP5*.
d) There is no need to confirm with genetic testing.

Correct answer is d.

This case depicts a clinically typical Coats' disease, a sporadic condition. The gene mutation, which research suggests may be in any FEVR gene, may be a somatic mutation (isolated to the affected tissue) occurring just in the retina of the affected eye and therefore not detectable by blood testing. In the absence of family history or any finding that suggests familial transmission, no further genetic workup is needed.

a) **Incorrect.** Blood testing of any of the genes known to cause FEVR when mutated is unnecessary.

b) **Incorrect.** See explanation above.

c) **Incorrect.** See explanation above.

d) **Correct.**

13.7.3 Case 3

A 4-year-old female patient comes for ophthalmic evaluation. Family history reveals a paternal grandmother with "cataract and retinal surgeries" in her 30s. The child's father has an "undiagnosed retinal condition." Examination of the child's eyes is otherwise normal, except for subtle bilateral vessel straightening in the temporal periphery. Paternal examination shows bilateral retinal folds extending temporally with macular traction. IVFA of the father shows severe peripheral nonperfusion. Which from the following alternatives is the most correct?

a) Yearly examination of the child until traction develops.

b) IVFA of the child to identify possible peripheral nonperfusion amenable to treatment.

c) Bilateral VEGF inhibitor injection for the child.

d) Patient is asymptomatic. Discharge with instructions to come back if vision gets worse.

Correct answer is b.

IVFA is the definitive means of evaluation in a child for FEVR. The temporal straightening of vessels is a worrisome sign that raises the possibility of more peripheral disease that can be invisible to the indirect ophthalmoscope. Even if the clinical examination was normal, one might consider IVFA if the pedigree or genetic testing shows the child to be at risk. The need for general anesthesia to perform the IVFA should not preclude its consideration and performance.

a) **Incorrect.** The natural history of FEVR is well known, especially in a scenario where two relatives present with severe complications. Once traction develops, it may be too late to prevent vision loss. The goal is early identification and prevention of this complication.

b) **Correct.**

c) **Incorrect.** Any treatment must be withheld until IVFA confirms the presence of the disease. Anti-VEGF remains off-label for use in the treatment of FEVR.

d) **Incorrect.** See explanation in a.

Suggested Reading

[1] Ai M, Heeger S, Bartels CF, Schelling DK, Osteoporosis-Pseudoglioma Collaborative Group. Clinical and molecular findings in osteoporosis-pseudoglioma syndrome. Am J Hum Genet. 2005; 77(5):741–753

[2] Boonstra FN, van Nouhuys CE, Schuil J, et al. Clinical and molecular evaluation of probands and family members with familial exudative vitreoretinopathy. Invest Ophthalmol Vis Sci. 2009; 50(9):4379–4385

[3] Downey LM, Bottomley HM, Sheridan E, et al. Reduced bone mineral density and hyaloid vasculature remnants in a consanguineous recessive FEVR family with a mutation in LRP5. Br J Ophthalmol. 2006; 90(9): 1163–1167

[4] Jia LY, Li XX, Yu WZ, Zeng WT, Liang C. Novel frizzled-4 gene mutations in Chinese patients with familial exudative vitreoretinopathy. Arch Ophthalmol. 2010; 128(10):1341–1349

[5] Kondo H, Kusaka S, Yoshinaga A, et al. Mutations in the TSPAN12 gene in Japanese patients with familial exudative vitreoretinopathy. Am J Ophthalmol. 2011; 151(6):1095–1100.e1

[6] Dickinson JL, Sale MM, Passmore A, et al. Mutations in the NDP gene: contribution to Norrie disease, familial exudative vitreoretinopathy and retinopathy of prematurity. Clin Experiment Ophthalmol. 2006; 34(7):682–688

[7] Drenser KA, Fecko A, Dailey W, Trese MT. A characteristic phenotypic retinal appearance in Norrie disease. Retina. 2007; 27(2):243–246

[8] Junge HJ, Yang S, Burton JB, et al. TSPAN12 regulates retinal vascular development by promoting Norrin- but not Wnt-induced FZD4/beta-catenin signaling. Cell. 2009; 139(2):299–311

[9] Khan AO, Aldahmesh MA, Meyer B. Correlation of ophthalmic examination with carrier status in females potentially harboring a severe Norrie disease gene mutation. Ophthalmology. 2008; 115(4):730–733

[10] Gilmour DF. Familial exudative vitreoretinopathy and related retinopathies. Eye (Lond). 2015; 29(1):1–14

[11] Hu H, Xiao X, Li S, Jia X, Guo X, Zhang Q. KIF11 mutations are a common cause of autosomal dominant familial exudative vitreoretinopathy. Br J Ophthalmol. 2016; 100(2):278–283

14 Stickler Syndrome

Abstract

Stickler syndrome is a connective tissue disorder characterized by hearing loss, facial dysmorphism, cleft palate, spondyloepiphyseal dysplasia, and arthropathy. Ocular findings include high myopia, cataract, characteristic vitreous changes, lattice degeneration, and a high risk for retinal detachment. Focal and circumferential laser treatment, as well as 360-degree cryotherapy, have been evaluated as prophylactic treatment to prevent retinal detachment in type 1 Stickler syndrome. Myopia is usually greater than 3 diopters at the time of diagnosis. Vitreous abnormalities include "membranous," "beaded," syneretic, "afibrillar," and "optically empty" vitreous. The facial appearance includes midface hypoplasia, broad or flat nasal bridge, possible telecanthus, and epicanthal folds. Micro/retrognathia is usual and can be associated with cleft palate as part of the Pierre Robin sequence (micrognathia, cleft palate, and glossoptosis).

Keywords: Stickler syndrome, high myopia, cleft palate, vitreous anomalies, *COL2A1*, *COL11A1*, *COL11A2*, *COL9A1*, *COL9A2*, *COL9A3*

> **Key Points**
>
> - Stickler syndrome is a multisystem connective tissue disorder that may also affect the eye.
> - Patients have a high risk of retinal detachment.
> - Six genes have been associated to this syndrome: *COL2A1*, *COL11A1*, or *COL11A2* (autosomal dominant) and *COL9A1*, *COL9A2*, or *COL9A3* (autosomal recessive).

14.1 Overview

The approximate incidence of Stickler syndrome among newborns is 1:9,000. It is a connective tissue disorder characterized by sensorineural and/or conductive hearing loss, facial dysmorphism (▶ Fig. 1.2), cleft palate, spondyloepiphyseal dysplasia, and arthropathy. Ocular findings include high myopia, cataract (▶ Fig. 14.1), characteristic vitreous changes, lattice degeneration (▶ Fig. 14.2), and a high risk for retinal detachment. Focal and circumferential laser treatment, as well as 360-degree cryotherapy have been evaluated as prophylactic treatment to prevent retinal detachment in type 1 Stickler syndrome. Although the methodology was retrospective and perhaps with high-risk bias, recommendations for prophylactic treatment are widely accepted. Myopia is usually greater than −3 diopters at the time of diagnosis. Vitreous abnormalities include "membranous" (type 1), "beaded" (type 2), syneretic, "afibrillar," and "optically empty" vitreous. The types may coexist and may show some genotype–phenotype correlations.

The facial appearance includes midface hypoplasia, broad or flat nasal bridge, possible telecanthus, and epicanthal folds. The myopic eyes often look exophthalmic. There is also small and upturned nasal tip, and long philtrum. Micro/retrognathia is usual and can be associated with cleft palate as part of the Pierre Robin sequence (micrognathia, cleft palate, glossoptosis). About 50% of patients with Pierre Robin sequence have an

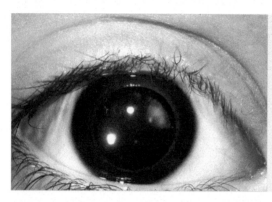

Fig. 14.1 Cortical wedge cataract in a patient with Stickler syndrome.

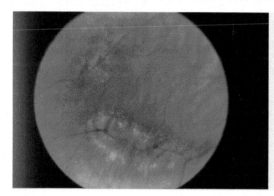

Fig. 14.2 Perivascular lattice degeneration in a patient with Stickler syndrome.

underlying syndrome, of which Stickler syndrome is the most frequent (up to 30%). Craniofacial findings characteristic of Stickler syndrome may become less distinctive with age.

The sensorineural hearing impairment mechanism is unknown, although it has been proposed that it is related to the expression of type II and IX collagen in the inner ear. Conductive hearing loss may also occur secondary to recurrent ear infections associated with craniofacial structure and middle ear anomalies. Mitral valve prolapse has been reported in up to 50% of patients with Stickler syndrome. Early-onset arthritis is common and may be severe, but frequently the arthropathy is mild.

14.2 Molecular Genetics

Mutations have been described in *COL2A1* (12q13.11), *COL11A1* (1p21.1), *COL11A2* (6p21.32), *COL9A1* (6q13), *COL9A2* (1p34.2), and *COL9A3* (20q13.33), although there are patients with the typical phenotype but without a mutation in those genes. *COL2A1*, *COL11A1*, or *COL11A2* mutations are autosomal dominant (AD). Penetrance is complete, with variable expression. *COL9A1*, *COL9A2*, or *COL9A3* mutations are typically autosomal recessive (AR). The majority of patients with Stickler syndrome have a *COL2A1* nonsense mutation resulting in haploinsufficiency. A specific *COL2A1* variant (p.Leu667Phe) has been associated with "afibrillar" vitreous gel. Mutations involving exon 2 of *COL2A1* affect predominantly the eye, with mild or no systemic findings as this exon is not expressed in nonocular tissues. These patients have optically empty vitreous, perivascular pigmentary changes, and early-onset retinal detachment.

Sequence variants and deletions in the *COL11A1* gene lead to Stickler syndrome with significant hearing loss and type 2 vitreous anomaly ("beaded"). Pathogenic variants of *COL11A2* are associated with nonocular Stickler syndrome.

Biallelic pathogenic variants in *COL9A1* are associated with AR Stickler syndrome. Affected patients have moderate to severe hearing loss, myopia with vitreoretinopathy, cortical cataracts, and epiphyseal dysplasia. Biallelic mutations in *COL9A2* are associated with mild to moderate hearing loss, high myopia, and vitreoretinopathy. Biallelic pathogenic variants in *COL9A3* are also associated with AR Stickler syndrome. These patients may have intellectual disability.

14.3 Differential Diagnosis

14.3.1 Knobloch Syndrome (OMIM 267750)

Knobloch syndrome (OMIM 267750) is a developmental disorder characterized by typical eye abnormalities, including high myopia, ectopia lentis, vitreoretinal anomalies, and retinal detachment, associated with occipital skull defects, which can range from occipital encephalocele to occipital cutis aplasia. It is due to biallelic mutation in the *COL18A1* gene.

14.3.2 Spondyloepiphyseal Dysplasia Congenita (OMIM 183900)

Phenotypically very similar to Stickler syndrome, although patients also have short stature. Retinal findings are usually severe. Myopia is frequently present. It is caused by *COL2A1* mutation.

14.3.3 Kniest Dysplasia (OMIM 156550)

Kniest dysplasia is characterized by severe short stature, flat facial profile, myopia, vitreoretinal degeneration, cleft palate, and kyphoscoliosis. It is due to *COL2A1* mutations, which are frequently de novo.

14.3.4 Marshall Syndrome (OMIM 154780)

This is an AD disorder associated with *COL11A1* mutations, particularly splice site changes. These patients have hypertelorism, hypoplasia of the nasal bones and maxilla, flat nasal bridge, and upturned nasal tip. The flat facial appearance of Marshall syndrome is usually more obvious in adulthood, as opposed to the Stickler facies, which is seen from infancy. Patients with Marshall syndrome also have high myopia, vitreous syneresis, and early-onset cataracts. Sensorineural hearing loss is frequent. Other findings include cleft palate, Pierre Robin sequence, short stature, arthropathy, and hypotrichosis. There is also a Marshall/Stickler overlap due to mutations in *COL11A1*.

14.3.5 Weissenbacher–Zweymuller Syndrome (OMIM 277610)

This AD disorder is due to *COL11A2* mutations. It has been reported as "neonatal" Stickler syndrome because of the similar facial appearance. In contrast, myopia is not a manifestation of this syndrome, although there are reports in some patients. The characteristic finding is short stature and "dumbbell"-shaped femurs.

14.3.6 Wagner Syndrome (OMIM 143200)

Wagner syndrome (OMIM 143200) is defined by the presence of ocular findings similar to those seen in Stickler and Marshall syndromes (high myopia, optically empty vitreous, avascular strands, chorioretinal atrophy, and cataract) but without the systemic manifestations. The ocular findings are typically progressive. Retinal detachment and glaucoma are also found. Scotopic electroretinogram (ERG) is typically altered. Erosive vitreoretinopathy, an allelic disorder of Wagner syndrome, is also a differential diagnosis, allelic to Wagner syndrome. *VCAN* gene mutation is causative.

14.3.7 High Myopia

High myopia can also be confused in patients with mild facial findings, particularly when of Asian descent with flat midface. The refractive error is greater than or equal to -6 diopters. Many loci for myopia have been reported (MYP1–25; updated July 2017).

14.3.8 Snowflake Vitreoretinal Degeneration (OMIM 193230)

Snowflake vitreoretinal degeneration (OMIM 193230) is defined by cataract, vitreous fibrillar degeneration, and typical retinal abnormalities that appear as shiny crystalline-like deposits resembling snowflakes. Patients have a low incidence of retinal detachment as opposed to Stickler syndrome.

14.3.9 Pierson Syndrome (OMIM 609049)

Pierson syndrome (OMIM 609049) is an AR disorder due to mutation in *LAMB2*, which presents with congenital nephrotic syndrome and ocular abnormalities, including microcoria, hypoplasia of the ciliary and pupillary muscles, as well as pigmentary retinopathy and recurrent retinal detachment. Many patients die young, and those who survive tend to have increased incidence of neurodevelopmental delay and visual loss.

14.3.10 High Myopia with Cataracts and Vitreoretinal Degeneration (OMIM 614292)

This AR condition is due to mutations in *LEPREL1*. It is seen in Bedouins. It has variable expressivity of cataract and vitreoretinal degeneration. Axial lengths range from 25.1 to 30.5 mm. Lens subluxation has also been described. These patients are not dysmorphic.

14.3.11 Other

There are many other rare dysplasias that are beyond the scope of this book, such as spondyloperipheral dysplasia, platyspondylic lethal skeletal dysplasia, fibrochondrogenesis types 1 and 2, various subtypes of multiple epiphysial dysplasias, and others.

14.4 Uncommon Manifestations

Posterior chorioretinal atrophy has been described in patients with pathogenic variants of *COL2A1*. Late retinal degeneration may occur in Stickler syndrome. ERG would be helpful to differentiate patients with Wagner disease.

14.5 Clinical Testing

14.5.1 Comprehensive Examination by a Multidisciplinary Team

Comprehensive examination by a multidisciplinary team to detect mandibular anomalies, sensorineural or conductive hearing loss, mitral valve prolapse, airway stenosis, malocclusion, or arthropathy should be conducted. Echocardiogram should be considered to detect mitral valve prolapse.

14.5.2 Auditory Testing

Hearing impairment is common (up to 40%). The degree of hearing impairment is variable and may be progressive, although typically mild in type I Stickler syndrome. Repeat testing every 6 months through age 5 years, and annually thereafter is recommended.

14.5.3 Serial Ocular Examination

Serial ocular examination is appropriate. Examination under anesthesia in young children may be considered to identify early at-risk lesions such as peripheral lattice that may warrant prophylactic treatment.

14.6 Genetic Testing

The diagnosis of Stickler syndrome is confirmed in individuals with a heterozygous mutation in *COL2A1*, *COL11A1*, or *COL11A2* or biallelic mutation in *COL9A1*, *COL9A2*, or *COL9A3*. *COL2A1* mutations are found in 80 to 90% of individuals with Stickler syndrome. *COL11A1* mutations more often result in "beaded" vitreous anomaly and significant hearing loss. This gene is mutated in 10 to 20% of patients. If craniofacial findings, joint manifestations, and hearing loss are present without ocular findings, *COL11A2* could be sequenced first. *COL9A1*, *COL9A2*, and *COL9A3* are seen in typical AR patterns. Gene panels are available for all of these scenarios.

14.7 Problems

14.7.1 Case 1

A 5-year-old boy and his twin sister come for ophthalmic evaluation because his mother says that they are holding things "too close." Both children have sensorineural hearing loss and micrognathia. Ophthalmic examination reveals high myopia and vitreous abnormalities. The family comes from China with many affected by high myopia. There is parental consanguinity, but neither parent has vitreous or hearing anomalies. Which from the following genes is more likely to be affected?

a) *COL2A1.*
b) *COL11A1.*
c) *COL9A1.*
d) *COL11A2.*

Correct answer is c.

COL2A1, COL11A1, or *COL11A2* mutations are AD. With unaffected consanguineous parents and dizygotic offspring who show features of Stickler syndrome, an AR form is more likely. *COL9A1,* as well as *COL9A2* and *COL9A3,* mutations are typically AR.

a) **Incorrect.** Typically AD.
b) **Incorrect.** Typically AD.
c) **Correct.**
d) **Incorrect.** Typically AD and no ocular involvement.

14.7.2 Case 2

A 7-year-old female comes for routine examination. Her uncorrected vision is 20/200 in both eyes. Cycloplegic refraction is −5.50 + 0.50 @ 90 degrees both eyes. Fundus examination shows optically empty vitreous, midperipheral perivascular pigmentary changes, and multiple areas of peripheral lattices. Family history is unremarkable. Comprehensive physical examination reveals no abnormalities with a normal facies and palate. Hearing is normal. Which one from the following genes is more likely to be affected?

a) *COL2A1.*
b) *COL11A1.*
c) *COL9A1.*
d) *COL11A2.*

Correct answer is a.

This patient may have ocular Stickler syndrome. Mutations affecting exon 2 of *COL2A1* create a phenotype predominantly involving the eye, characteristically with no systemic findings, as this exon is not expressed in nonocular tissues. These patients have optically empty vitreous, perivascular pigmentary changes, and early-onset retinal detachment.

a) **Correct.**
b) **Incorrect.** *COL11A1* is associated with systemic AD Stickler syndrome.
c) **Incorrect.** *COL9A1* is associated with systemic AR Stickler syndrome.
d) **Incorrect.** *COL11A2* is associated with systemic AD Stickler syndrome usually without ocular involvement.

14.7.3 Case 3

An 11-year-old male is experiencing nyctalopia. His ophthalmic evaluation reveals high myopia (–7.00 sph both eyes), optically empty vitreous, vitreous veils, chorioretinal atrophy, and a unilateral mild cortical wedge cataract. He is otherwise healthy. Scotopic ERG, adjusted for axial length, is moderately reduced in amplitude with delayed latencies. Which from the following seems to be the most likely diagnosis?

a) Stickler syndrome.
b) Marshall syndrome.
c) Erosive vitreoretinopathy.
d) Wagner syndrome.

Correct answer is d.

The presence of high myopia, optically empty vitreous, vitreous veils, chorioretinal atrophy, and cataract, but without the systemic manifestations raises the possibility of Wagner syndrome (*VCAN* gene mutation). The hallmark in this case is that the scotopic ERG is subnormal.

a) **Incorrect.** Although many of the features overlap with ocular Stickler syndrome (exon 2, *COL2A1*), the ERG is usually normal until much later in life and vitreous veils are uncommon.

b) **Incorrect.** This patient does not demonstrate the typical hearing loss, short stature, and facies of Marshall syndrome.

c) **Less likely.** Although erosive vitreoretinopathy is an allelic disorder to Wagner syndrome, the most characteristic finding, severe peripheral retinal abnormalities, is not present in this case. A history or progression and possible examination under anesthesia would assist in making the differential diagnosis.

d) **Correct.**

14.7.4 Case 4

A 5-year-old female with a diagnosis of Stickler syndrome due to heterozygous *COL2A1* mutation not involving exon 2 comes for a second opinion. She has mild sensorineural hearing loss, repaired cleft palate in infancy, and spondyloepiphyseal dysplasia. Her ocular examination revealed high myopia (–10.00 sph both eyes), membranous vitreous changes and a myopic appearance of the retina. She does not allow examination of the far retina periphery. Which from the following seems to be the most appropriate next step?

a) Examination under anesthesia for evaluation of retinal detachment risk.
b) ERG to rule out Wagner syndrome.
c) Observe over time for retinal detachment.
d) Prophylactic scleral buckle surgery.

Correct answer is a.

Laser treatment and cryotherapy have been evaluated as prophylactic treatment to prevent retinal detachment in type 1 Stickler syndrome. Although the reported literature is retrospective, recommendations for prophylactic treatment are widely accepted. Examination under anesthesia would allow a search for peripheral lattice that may increase the risk for detachment and perhaps raise the indication for prophylactic treatment.

a) **Correct.**

b) **Incorrect.** Wagner syndrome does not present with systemic findings.

c) **Incorrect.** Retinal detachment can be difficult to repair. Prevention is much preferred.

d) **Incorrect.** Scleral buckle has not been evaluated as a prophylactic treatment and would not address the predisposition to retinal breaks.

Suggested Reading

[1] Annunen S, Körkkö J, Czarny M, et al. Splicing mutations of 54-bp exons in the COL11A1 gene cause Marshall syndrome, but other mutations cause overlapping Marshall/Stickler phenotypes. Am J Hum Genet. 1999; 65 (4):974–983

[2] Go SL, Maugeri A, Mulder JJ, van Driel MA, Cremers FP, Hoyng CB. Autosomal dominant rhegmatogenous retinal detachment associated with an Arg453Ter mutation in the COL2A1 gene. Invest Ophthalmol Vis Sci. 2003; 44(9):4035–4043

[3] Lee MM, Ritter R, III, Hirose T, Vu CD, Edwards AO. Snowflake vitreoretinal degeneration: follow-up of the original family. Ophthalmology. 2003; 110(12):2418–2426

[4] Nikopoulos K, Schrauwen I, Simon M, et al. Autosomal recessive Stickler syndrome in two families is caused by mutations in the COL9A1 gene. Invest Ophthalmol Vis Sci. 2011; 52(7):4774–4779

[5] Vu CD, Brown J, Jr, Körkkö J, Ritter R, III, Edwards AO. Posterior chorioretinal atrophy and vitreous phenotype in a family with Stickler syndrome from a mutation in the COL2A1 gene. Ophthalmology. 2003; 110(1):70–77

[6] Liu MM, Zack DJ. Alternative splicing and retinal degeneration. Clin Genet. 2013; 84(2):142–149

[7] Carroll C, Papaioannou D, Rees A, Kaltenthaler E. The clinical effectiveness and safety of prophylactic retinal interventions to reduce the risk of retinal detachment and subsequent vision loss in adults and children with Stickler syndrome: a systematic review. Health Technol Assess. 2011; 15(16):iii–xiv, 1–62

15 *VCAN* Vitreoretinopathies (Erosive Vitreoretinopathy and Wagner Syndrome)

Abstract

VCAN vitreoretinopathies are characterized by "optically empty vitreous" with avascular vitreous strands and veils at the equatorial vitreoretinal interface. *VCAN* vitreoretinopathies include Wagner syndrome and erosive vitreoretinopathy. They are autosomal dominant with full penetrance but variable expression. Myopia is a typical finding, ranging from mild to severe. Approximately 50% of patients have cataract surgery before the fourth decade. Retinal detachment is either tractional or rhegmatogenous. Systemic abnormalities are not associated.

Keywords: VCAN gene, vitreoretinopathies, erosive vitreoretinopathy, Wagner syndrome, high myopia, retinal detachment

Key Points

- The key findings in the *VCAN* vitreoretinopathies are "optically empty" vitreous, myopia, and progressive chorioretinal atrophy, with an increased risk of retinal detachment.
- Systemic abnormalities are not found in these conditions.
- *VCAN*-related vitreoretinopathies are autosomal dominant with complete penetrance.

15.1 Overview

These conditions are characterized by several clinical findings, the hallmark being "optically empty vitreous" on slit-lamp examination with avascular vitreous strands and veils at the equatorial vitreoretinal interface. *VCAN*-related vitreoretinopathies include Wagner syndrome (WS) and erosive vitreoretinopathy (ERVR). They are autosomal dominant (AD) with full penetrance but variable expression. Myopia is a typical finding, ranging from mild to severe. Early cataract can also be found, with no particular type described. Approximately 50% of patients have cataract surgery before the fourth decade. Microphthalmia, ectopia lentis, and persistent fetal vasculature have rarely been associated with WS. One significant feature is the absence of systemic abnormalities. ERVR is characterized by pronounced vitreous abnormalities, complicated retinal detachments, and a progressive pigmentary retinopathy, in particular with thinning and progressive "erosion" in the equatorial periphery. The most distinctive feature is the progressive change in retinal pigment epithelium (RPE) associated with visual field constriction and rod and cone dysfunction.

In WS, progressive chorioretinal atrophy associated with night blindness and retinal detachment can occur. Night blindness and visual field constriction are not as severe as those seen in patients with retinitis pigmentosa. Retinal detachment can be caused by shrinkage of the preretinal membranes, vitreous strands, and veils, and therefore is either tractional or rhegmatogenous. Reported incidence varies from 15 to 50% of affected patients, especially in ERVR. It has been associated with increasing age, although it can occur at young ages. Other findings include outer retinal layer and choroidal thinning and abnormal dark adaptation.

15.2 Molecular Genetics

The *VCAN* gene (5q14.3; previously known as *CSPG2*) encodes a large proteoglycan called versican. Versican is found in the extracellular matrix, facilitating the assembly of the extracellular matrix and ensuring its stability. Within the eye, versican plays a role in maintaining the vitreous structure. Other additional functions include cell growth regulation and division, cell adhesion, and migration. Angiogenesis, scarring, and inflammation regulation have also been described. The *VCAN* gene produces four different isoforms of the versican protein: V0, V1, V2, and V3. *VCAN* is the only known gene in which mutations cause WS or ERVR. WS and ERVR are allelic disorders, which mean they are both caused by different mutations in the same gene.

15.3 Differential Diagnosis

15.3.1 Stickler Syndrome (OMIM 108300)

Stickler syndrome (OMIM 108300) is a systemic disorder associated with a skeletal dysplasia and craniofacial abnormalities, particularly cleft palate. Retinal detachment and myopia are frequent (up to 50%), but unlike *VCAN*-related vitreoretinopathies, abnormal dark adaptation has not been described in Stickler syndrome. For certain pathogenic variations in *COL2A1*, an ophthalmic nonsyndromic phenotype can be present. Some authors have described this form as WS type II.

15.3.2 Snowflake Vitreoretinal Degeneration (OMIM 193230)

Snowflake vitreoretinal degeneration (OMIM 193230) shows vitreous abnormalities, but avascular strands and veils are not observed. Retinal abnormalities affect the superficial retinal layers, whereas in *VCAN*-related vitreoretinopathy the outer retinal layers and choroid are more affected. Mutations in *KCNJ13* are associated.

15.3.3 Autosomal Dominant Vitreoretinochoroidopathy (OMIM 193229)

AD vitreoretinochoroidopathy (OMIM 193229) is a rare disease due to *VMD2* splicing defects, characterized by fibrillar condensation of the vitreous, but not optically empty vitreous. Patients have a characteristic well-demarcated peripheral band of chorioretinal hyperpigmentation and variable electroretinographic (ERG) findings.

15.3.4 Goldmann–Favre Syndrome

Goldmann–Favre syndrome is due to mutations in *NR2E3*. Patients experience night blindness and visual field constriction. Progressive vitreous changes and chorioretinal atrophy with pigmentary retinal degeneration occur in association with retinoschisis in the periphery and macula, which are not typically seen in *VCAN* vitreoretinopathies.

15.3.5 Knobloch Syndrome (OMIM 267750)

Knobloch syndrome (OMIM 267750) is characterized by high myopia, a typical fundus appearance with geographic macular atrophy occipital scalp/skull defects even ranging to encephalocele. Mutations in *COL18A1* are causative.

15.3.6 Marshall Syndrome (OMIM 154780)

Marshall syndrome (OMIM 154780) overlaps with Stickler syndrome, but is distinguished by flat midface, thick calvaria, abnormal frontal sinuses, shallow orbits, and intracranial calcifications. It is also associated with hearing loss and joint alterations. It is caused by *COL11A1* mutations.

15.3.7 Choroideremia

Sometimes, chorioretinal atrophy in *VCAN* vitreoretinopathies is so severe that it can resemble this condition.

15.4 Uncommon Manifestations

A family with WS had intraocular inflammatory manifestations associated with a novel splice site *VCAN* mutation. Spherophakia, ectopic fovea, optic atrophy, and congenital glaucoma have been reported rarely.

15.5 Clinical Testing

15.5.1 Electroretinogram

Full-field ERG becomes attenuated, but not severely depressed, differentiating WS from RP. Typically, a-waves and b-waves are reduced. Both scotopic and photopic responses are disturbed to varying degrees.

15.5.2 Optical Coherence Tomography

Optical coherence tomography is used to evaluate the vitreoretinal interface and atrophic retinal changes.

15.6 Genetic Testing

Most reported *VCAN* mutations associated with WS and ERVR are found in the splice acceptor or splice donor site of introns 7 and 8. Five-point mutations are more commonly associated with WS phenotype. A mutation in intron 7 (c.4004–5T > C) has been reported in both phenotypes. Sequencing of this region is recommended first. If no pathogenic variation is found, the entire coding regions and flanking intronic sites of *VCAN* can be sequenced. Deletions or duplications have not been reported.

15.7 Problems

15.7.1 Case 1

A 12-year-old patient with high myopia was referred to rule out Stickler syndrome. Physical examination was normal. Biomicroscopy confirmed vitreous abnormalities, equatorial chorioretinal atrophy, vitreous veils, and "optically empty vitreous." Full-field ERG, adjusted for axial length, revealed moderate attenuation of scotopic responses. *VCAN* sequencing showed intron 7 (c.4004–5T > C) mutation. Which of the following is the correct diagnosis?
a) Knobloch syndrome.
b) Stickler syndrome.
c) ERVR.
d) Isolated pathologic high myopia.

Correct answer is c.
The absence of systemic findings along with the vitreous and "erosive" chorioretinal changes and a known pathogenic mutation confirm a diagnosis of ERVR.
a) **Incorrect.** Patients with Knobloch syndrome have characteristic macular changes and may have occipital scalp or skull abnormalities.
b) **Incorrect.** The absence of typical systemic findings of Stickler syndrome, such as cleft palate, hearing deficits, typical facies, or micrognathia, makes this diagnosis less likely.
c) **Correct.**
d) **Incorrect.** High myopia is not associated with these vitreous abnormalities (although vitreous syneresis may occur at later ages) or significant ERG alteration when the ERG is appropriately calibrated for axial length.

15.7.2 Case 2

A 20-year-old female patient presents with retinal detachment in one eye. The vitreo-retinal surgeon asks for ocular genetics consultation because the patient's brother, mother, and maternal grandfather have also had retinal detachment in the last 10 years. Your examination of the unoperated eye reveals pronounced vitreous abnormalities, and a pigmentary retinopathy with thinning in the equatorial periphery plus many areas of chorioretinal atrophy. Scotopic ERG shows markedly reduced amplitudes and delayed implicit times. Physical examination was normal. Head computed tomography (CT) scan and hearing tests were normal. Which one of the following is the most likely diagnosis?
a) Stickler syndrome.
b) ERVR.
c) Marshall syndrome.
d) Knobloch syndrome.

Correct answer is b.
This pedigree is consistent with an AD pattern. The clinical findings described are compatible with ERVR.
a) **Incorrect.** Although the pedigree is suggestive of an AD disorder and Stickler syndrome has a high risk of retinal detachment, a normal physical examination suggests an alternate diagnosis.

b) **Correct.**
c) **Incorrect.** Normal hearing and normal neuroimaging rule out the clinical diagnosis.
d) **Incorrect.** Without an occipital defect, either by clinical examination or by neuroimaging, Knobloch syndrome is less likely. The fundus in this disorder is not characterized by progressive chorioretinal atrophy or pigmentary retinopathy.

15.7.3 Case 3

A 24-year-old male patient with vitreous abnormalities and a recurrent family history of retinal detachment comes with a "genetic test" result for WS that was negative. The report states, "all exons of *VCAN* gene were sequenced." Your clinical examination reveals "optically empty vitreous," peripheral RPE abnormalities, normal physical examination, and mildly attenuated scotopic ERG. Which from the following alternatives might explain the result?
a) Deep intron sequencing is needed.
b) Deletion/duplication analysis is needed.
c) An exon point mutation was missed.
d) Exonic–intronic boundaries should be sequenced.

Correct answer is d.

Most *VCAN* mutations that explain WS or ERVR are found in the splice acceptor or splice donor site of introns 7 and 8. Therefore, sequencing of this region is recommended first. If no pathogenic variation is found, the entire coding regions and flanking intronic sites of *VCAN* can then be sequenced.
a) **Incorrect.** Deep intronic mutations have not been reported.
b) **Incorrect.** Deletions or duplications have not been reported.
c) **Incorrect.** Although possible, certified laboratories have procedure in place to reduce the likelihood of a missed mutation.
d) **Correct.**

Suggested Reading

[1] Bennett SR, Folk JC, Kimura AE, Russell SR, Stone EM, Raphtis EM. Autosomal dominant neovascular inflammatory vitreoretinopathy. Ophthalmology. 1990; 97(9):1125–1135, discussion 1135–1136
[2] Brézin AP, Nedelec B, Barjol A, Rothschild PR, Delpech M, Valleix S. A new VCAN/versican splice acceptor site mutation in a French Wagner family associated with vascular and inflammatory ocular features. Mol Vis. 2011; 17:1669–1678
[3] Brown DM, Graemiger RA, Hergersberg M, et al. Genetic linkage of Wagner disease and erosive vitreoretinopathy to chromosome 5q13–14. Arch Ophthalmol. 1995; 113(5):671–675
[4] Brown DM, Kimura AE, Weingeist TA, Stone EM. Erosive vitreoretinopathy. A new clinical entity. Ophthalmology. 1994; 101(4):694–704
[5] Graemiger RA, Niemeyer G, Schneeberger SA, Messmer EP. Wagner vitreoretinal degeneration. Follow-up of the original pedigree. Ophthalmology. 1995; 102(12):1830–1839
[6] Hejtmancik JF, Jiao X, Li A, et al. Mutations in KCNJ13 cause autosomal-dominant snowflake vitreoretinal degeneration. Am J Hum Genet. 2008; 82(1):174–180
[7] Keren B, Suzuki OT, Gérard-Blanluet M, et al. CNS malformations in Knobloch syndrome with splice mutation in COL18A1 gene. Am J Med Genet A. 2007; 143A(13):1514–1518
[8] Kloeckener-Gruissem B, Bartholdi D, Abdou MT, Zimmermann DR, Berger W. Identification of the genetic defect in the original Wagner syndrome family. Mol Vis. 2006; 12:350–355
[9] Kloeckener-Gruissem B, Neidhardt J, Magyar I, et al. Novel VCAN mutations and evidence for unbalanced alternative splicing in the pathogenesis of Wagner syndrome. Eur J Hum Genet. 2013; 21(3):352–356

[10] Richards AJ, Martin S, Yates JR, et al. COL2A1 exon 2 mutations: relevance to the Stickler and Wagner syndromes. Br J Ophthalmol. 2000; 84(4):364–371

[11] Rothschild PR, Brézin AP, Nedelec B, et al. A family with Wagner syndrome with uveitis and a new versican mutation. Mol Vis. 2013; 19:2040–2049

[12] Mukhopadhyay A, Nikopoulos K, Maugeri A, et al. Erosive vitreoretinopathy and Wagner disease are caused by intronic mutations in CSPG2/Versican that result in an imbalance of splice variants. Invest Ophthalmol Vis Sci. 2006; 47(8):3565–3572

[13] Black GC, Perveen R, Wiszniewski W, Dodd CL, Donnai D, McLeod D. A novel hereditary developmental vitreoretinopathy with multiple ocular abnormalities localizing to a 5-cM region of chromosome 5q13-q14. Ophthalmology. 1999; 106(11):2074–2081

16 Incontinentia Pigmenti

Abstract

Incontinentia pigmenti is a rare condition with X-linked dominant inheritance that affects the skin, eye, and central nervous system. It occurs primarily in females. The diagnosis is established in a proband with compatible clinical findings and a heterozygous mutation in *IKBKG*. Tooth abnormalities are the most frequent noncutaneous finding. The phenotype is usually present in the first months of life. Penetrance is high, but expressivity is variable. Central nervous anomalies are present in one-third of patients and include seizures, intellectual disability, and other rare anomalies. Eosinophilia may be present, particularly in the early dermatologic stages. Up of 75% of patients have eye involvement, of which 60 to 90% have retinal findings. The most common is retinal peripheral nonperfusion, which may be complicated by retinal neovascularization, hemorrhage, and/or exudate. If peripheral ischemia is left untreated, retinal detachment may rapidly develop.

Keywords: Incontinentia pigmenti, *IKBKG*, eosinophilia, retinal ischemia, retinal detachment

Key Points

- X-linked dominant condition affecting the skin, hair, teeth, nails, eyes, and central nervous system. It is usually lethal in males.
- Cardinal sign on eye examination is peripheral retinal nonperfusion.
- Most affected individuals have a mutation or deletion in the *IKBKG* gene.

16.1 Overview

Incontinentia pigmenti (IP) is a rare condition with X-linked dominant inheritance that affects the skin (▶ Fig. 16.1), eye, and central nervous system. It occurs primarily in females and infrequently in males. Female-to-male ratio is 20:1. Most of the affected males that survive show a somatic mosaicism for a 47,XXY karyotype. The estimated frequency of IP is 0.7 per 1,000,000 newborns. IP diagnosis is established in a proband with compatible clinical findings and a heterozygous mutation in *IKBKG*. Diagnostic criteria are listed in ▶ Table 16.1. At least one major criterion is needed to confirm IP. Minor criteria are usually seen in the presence of major criteria, and just support the diagnosis. Tooth abnormalities are the most frequent noncutaneous finding (approximately 80% of cases; ▶ Fig. 16.2 and ▶ Table 16.1).

The phenotype is usually present in the first months of life. Penetrance is high, but expressivity is variable. For females without major systemic or neonatal complications, life expectancy is considered to be normal.

Central nervous anomalies are present in one-third of patients with IP and include seizures, intellectual disability, and, rarely, primary brain abnormalities such as agenesis of the corpus callosum, periventricular leukomalacia, cystic changes, myelination delays, ventricular dilatation, spastic paresis, occipital encephalocele, or polymicrogyria. Affected males are more likely to have neurologic anomalies. It is thought that

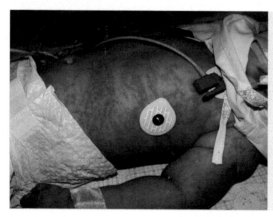

Fig. 16.1 Incontinentia pigmenti. Swirling cutaneous hyperpigmentation. (This image is provided courtesy of Ximena Fajre, MD.)

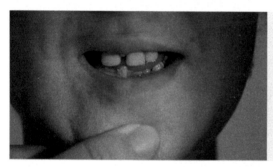

Fig. 16.2 Tooth anomalies in a patient with incontinentia pigmenti. Note peg-shaped tooth and other tooth anomalies. Note that top tooth are implants following reconstructive dental surgery.

Table 16.1 Incontinentia pigmenti diagnostic criteria

Major criteria	Minor criteria
1. Erythema followed by vesicles that follows a linear distribution[a] (within first 2 years of life; stage 1[b])	1. Tooth abnormalities: hypodontia, adontia, microdontia
2. Verrucous lesions that do not affect Blaschko's lines, occurring mostly on the limbs (within first 2 y of life; stage 2[b])	2. Alopecia or "woolly" hair
	3. Nail anomalies: ridging, pitting, or onychogryphosis
3. Hyperpigmented streaks and whorls that respect Blaschko's lines, occurring mostly on the trunk (up to 16 y old, then fades; stage 3[b])	4. Retinal peripheral nonperfusion
	5. X-linked inheritance
	6. Multiple male miscarriages
4. Pale, hairless, atrophic linear streaks or patches (adulthood; stage 4[b])	7. Breast aplasia or supernumerary nipples

[a]Except face.
[b]Incontinentia pigmenti skin alterations manifest in stages that evolve sequentially. The onset and duration of each stage is variable among patients, and not all affected individuals present with each stage. The skin anomalies can resolve to nonspecific minor abnormalities.

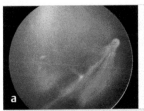
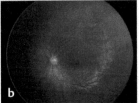
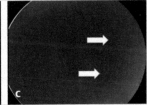

Fig. 16.3 (a) Peripheral retinal fold in a patient with incontinentia pigmenti (right eye) (b) Left eye from the same patient is apparently normal, but angiography (c) reveals peripheral nonperfusion with abrupt vessel endings (arrows).

central nervous system dysfunction is associated with microvasculature anomalies, resulting in ischemia. Neurovascular abnormalities are most frequently seen in the first year of life. There is evidence that in patients with neurological symptoms and multiple cerebral infarctions, corticosteroid therapy may be helpful.

Eosinophilia may be present, particularly in the first IP stages. Nevertheless, eosinophilia is not typically associated with any clinical manifestations and frequently resolves spontaneously. Eosinophilic infiltration may be helpful in confirming IP in a female patient with borderline clinical findings in whom molecular genetic testing has not identified a mutation.

Up of 75% of individuals have eye involvement, of which 60 to 90% have retinal findings. The most common is retinal peripheral nonperfusion (▶ Fig. 16.3), which may be complicated by retinal neovascularization, hemorrhage, and/or exudate. If peripheral ischemia is left untreated, retinal detachment may rapidly develop. Asymmetric retinal disease between eyes in the same individual and variable retinal findings within a family can occur. These differences can be explained by random X chromosome inactivation or epigenetic factors. One study found that the long-term follow-up risk of retinal detachment is approximately 22%, although they did not compare treated eyes to those without treatment. Significant risk factors are retinal neovascularization or ischemic optic neuropathy on initial examination. Most tractional detachments occur before the age of 3 years, whereas most rhegmatogenous detachments are seen in adults. Most retinal tears occur at the border of vascular and avascular retina. Sequelae also include optic atrophy and retinal pigmentary abnormalities.

Patients with IP require multidisciplinary care including pediatric neurology, dentistry, developmental care, dermatology, and ophthalmology. All patients with IP retinopathy should be closely monitored throughout adulthood for the development of retinal complications. If initial intravenous fluorescein angiography (IVFA) in infancy is normal, then there is little, if any, long-term risk. Patients with peripheral retinal ischemia benefit from early ablation of the nonperfused retina by laser or cryotherapy. Retinal detachment can develop rapidly and therefore, especially if treatment is deferred, frequent follow-up is essential to identify early retinal traction, neovascularization, and hemorrhage.

16.2 Molecular Genetics

The *IKBKG* gene (Xq28) encodes nuclear factor-kappa B essential modulator (NEMO). When mutated, it predisposes cells to apoptosis from intrinsic factors. It is estimated that 65% of patients have a de novo mutation. The most common abnormality is an

11.7-kb deletion that affects exons 4 to 10. This is seen in 60 to 80% of affected females. Approximately 10% of parents of patients with IP carry two *IKBKG* benign variants, suggesting recombination as a possible pathologic mechanism that generates the 11.7-kb pathologic deletion. When IP occurs as the result of a de novo event, the paternal allele is more frequently affected. Exon 10 mutations are associated with milder IP manifestations in females and a lower risk of miscarriage.

There are two rare *IKBKG* allelic disorders that affect males exclusively. These are X-linked hypohidrotic ectodermal dysplasia and immunodeficiency (HED-ID) and HED-ID with osteopetrosis and lymphedema. These two conditions are caused mostly by missense mutations in the gene. Another *IKBKG*-related phenotype is X-linked atypical mycobacteriosis (*AMCBX1*, OMIM 300636), a condition with immunodeficiency and susceptibility to both pyogenic bacteria and mycobacterial diseases.

16.3 Differential Diagnosis

As skeletal involvement, body asymmetry, severe neurologic deficits, severe alopecia, or hyperpigmentation that follows the lines of Blaschko are all uncommon findings in IP, these findings should raise consideration of other diagnoses. Nongenetic disorders with peripheral retinal nonperfusion include morning glory optic nerve, shaken baby syndrome, and retinopathy of prematurity (ROP). Although sickle cell disease may cause nonperfusion of the peripheral retina, it is extremely uncommon to do so in the first decade of life.

16.3.1 Herpes Simplex, Varicella, Bullous Impetigo, or Epidermolysis Bullosa

Herpes simplex, varicella, bullous impetigo, or epidermolysis bullosa should be considered in the differential diagnosis of stage 1 skin changes. These infectious diseases are associated with fever or inflammatory systemic symptoms. Scrapings and cultures of the lesions are diagnostic. Vesicles that appear after light trauma are distinctive of epidermolysis bullosa. IP diagnosis, besides molecular testing, is established by skin biopsy, electron microscopy, or immunofluorescence. These disorders do not have the peripheral retinal nonperfusion or dental abnormalities seen in IP and they are not familial.

16.3.2 Warts or Molluscum Contagiosum

These conditions may resemble stage 2 IP skin lesions but are not associated with dental or ophthalmic manifestations. Skin biopsy may be helpful.

16.3.3 Hypomelanosis of Ito (OMIM 300337)

IP stage 3 can be differentiated from this condition because it is the hyperpigmented areas that are abnormal in IP. Hypomelanosis of Ito is usually due to chromosomal mosaicism, which can be detected by skin biopsy and fibroblast analysis for karyotype as chromosomal aberration is the most common etiology. Although ocular manifestations may occur, to our knowledge peripheral retinal nonperfusion has not been reported.

16.3.4 Scarring, Vitiligo, and Alopecia

Scarring, vitiligo, and alopecia can resemble the stage 4 atrophic skin lesions of IP. Vitiligo is usually a progressive condition, but areas of hyperpigmentation, usually surrounding the hypopigmented areas, are unusual and the hypopigmented areas are distinctly amelanotic compared to normal skin, unlike the usually normal skin in non-hyperpigmented areas of IP. Vitiligo is not preceded by the other IP stages. Although vitiligo may be associated with peripheral serous retinal effusion, which can lead to a band of peripheral retinal hypo- or hyperpigmentation, it is not associated with peripheral retinal nonperfusion or dental abnormalities.

16.3.5 Naegeli Syndrome (OMIM 161000)

Also known as Naegeli–Franceschetti–Jadassohn syndrome, it is a rare AD condition characterized by reticular cutaneous pigmentation starting at approximately the age of 2 years without a preceding inflammatory stage, discomfort provoked by heat with diminished sweat gland function, and tooth anomalies. Males and females are equally affected. Hyperhidrosis and punctate hyperkeratosis of the palms and soles differentiate it from IP. Also unlike IP, the cutaneous findings do not evolve. Mutations of the *KRT14* gene are causative.

16.3.6 Familial Exudative Vitreoretinopathy (OMIM 133780)

This disorder is characterized by incomplete development of the retinal vasculature with peripheral nonperfusion. Clinical presentation is variable, even among families, ranging from severely affected individuals with retinal detachment to mildly affected patients with asymptomatic mild peripheral retinal nonperfusion. The disorder may be autosomal dominant (*FZD4, LRP5, TSPAN12, ZNF408*), autosomal recessive (*LRP5*), or X-linked recessive (*NDP*). Dental, neurologic, or skin abnormalities are not found.

16.3.7 Facioscapulohumeral Muscular Dystrophy (OMIM 158900)

This disorder presents with weakness that starts from infancy to later in life. In general, the disease initially involves the face and the scapulae. Typical findings are muscle asymmetry with sparing of bulbar extraocular and respiratory muscles. Peripheral retinal nonperfusion may be associated with neovascularization and exudative retinal detachment. Individuals may have hearing loss. It is associated with contraction of the *D4Z4* macrosatellite repeat in the subtelomeric region of 4q35. There are no dermatologic or dental findings.

16.3.8 Adams–Oliver Syndrome (OMIM 100300)

Also known as aplasia cutis congenita, this developmental disorder is defined by the combination of aplasia cutis congenita of the scalp vertex and terminal transverse limb defects. In addition, vascular anomalies such as cutis marmorata telangiectatica congenita, pulmonary hypertension, portal hypertension, and peripheral retinal nonperfusion are seen. Heterozygous mutation in the *ARHGAP31* gene (3q13) is causative.

16.3.9 Dyskeratosis Congenita (OMIM 127550)

Dyskeratosis congenita is a family of disorders, usually caused by heterozygous mutation in the gene that encodes telomerase ribonucleic acid (RNA) component (*TERC* gene; 3q). Clinical findings are variable and include bone marrow failure, pulmonary and hepatic fibrosis, predisposition to malignancy, skin pigmentation abnormalities, leukoplakia, and nail dystrophy. Retinal nonperfusion may occur. Hoyeraal–Hreidarsson syndrome (OMIM 305000) is the X-linked form of dyskeratosis congenita. It is due to mutations in *DKC1* (Xq28), and presents with cerebellar hypoplasia and aplastic anemia. Dyskeratosis congenita also presents as Revesz syndrome (OMIM 268130), with Coats-like exudative retinopathy and possible peripheral nonperfusion and retinal detachment, brain calcifications, ataxia, bone marrow failure with pancytopenia, alopecia, and failure to thrive. Revesz syndrome is due to mutations in *TINF2* (14q12).

16.3.10 Wyburn–Mason Syndrome

Also known as Bonnet–Dechaume–Blanc syndrome, this syndrome may have peripheral retinal nonperfusion in the setting of congenital arteriovenous malformations of the brain and retina or facial nevi. This multisystemic syndrome can affect the skin, bones, kidneys, muscles, and the gastrointestinal tract. Retinal vascular abnormalities can be unilateral with marked dilatation and tortuosity. Symptoms begin to appear in the second and third decades of life. There is no known genetic cause.

16.3.11 Cutis Marmorata Telangiectatica Congenita (OMIM 219250)

Individuals with this condition present with a permanent mottled appearance of the dermal vasculature, which may include telangiectasia and superficial ulceration. Also observed may be developmental delay, seizures, cerebral atrophy, and periventricular white matter calcifications. Peripheral retinal nonperfusion may present as bilateral total retinal detachment with secondary neovascular glaucoma. Congenital glaucoma or retinal hemorrhages may be seen as well. Pulmonary hypertension has also been described.

16.4 Uncommon Manifestations

Persistent fetal vasculature may be seen in IP, although recent reports describe it more frequently (up to 14%). Foveal hypoplasia or microphthalmia has also been described. Reports of cataract, nystagmus, and strabismus represent secondary phenomena in eyes that have experienced retinal detachment. Other rare finding include pulmonary hypertension.

16.5 Clinical Testing

16.5.1 Intravenous Fluorescein Angiography

Early IVFA is recommended to detect retinal nonperfusion. IVFA can reveal vascular anomalies and progression of disease is sometimes not detected by indirect ophthalmoscopy.

16.5.2 Complete Physical Examination

Complete physical examination should be performed with emphasis on the skin, hair, nails, and neurologic system.

16.5.3 Electroencephalogram and Magnetic Resonance Imaging

Electroencephalogram is necessary in case of seizures and magnetic resonance imaging (MRI) in all patients with IP to assess the extent of central nervous system involvement.

16.6 Genetic Testing

The first test could be targeted analysis to identify the common *IKBKG* 11.7-kb deletion (65–80% of females). If this test is negative, sequencing and deletion/duplication analysis can be performed (9 and 4%, respectively, in females). Skin biopsy can also be considered to support diagnosis understanding that many conditions have the same findings as IP with cells that are incontinent of pigment (e.g., nevus spilus). This is especially valuable in females with atypical findings in whom molecular testing has not revealed the mutation. Biopsy should show eosinophilic infiltration or extracellular melanin granules. In the case of males, somatic mosaicism should always be considered. Therefore, *IKBKG* should be tested on affected skin if blood testing does not reveal an explanatory chromosomal aberration.

16.7 Problems

16.7.1 Case 1

Which one of the following signs makes us consider the possibility of IP in an infant female with blistering lesions?
a) Fever.
b) History of father with isolated retinal detachment.
c) Retinal peripheral neovascularization.
d) Maternal history of vaginal herpes.

Correct answer is c.
In the initial blistering stage of IP, differential diagnosis includes herpes simplex, varicella, bullous impetigo, and epidermolysis bullosa. Retinal peripheral neovascularization is a hallmark of IP and occurs in the absence of other signs of infection.
a) **Incorrect.** Infectious conditions may be associated with fever or other systemic signs. Fever is not a sign associated with IP.
b) **Less likely.** Survival of male patients with IP is very rare, usually associated with systemic findings, and explained by somatic mosaicism or a 47,XXY karyotype. Transmission to a daughter has not been reported to our knowledge. This father's isolated retinal detachment is likely unrelated to his daughter's IP.
c) **Correct.**
d) **Incorrect.** This would be more supportive of herpes simplex infection in the infant.

16.7.2 Case 2

A 26-year-old woman comes for ocular genetic consultation. She was born prematurely at 29-weeks' gestation with normal ROP screening. She had four miscarriages, two of them in the fourth month of gestation, and all males. Family history demonstrates that her mother had two male miscarriages. Her physical examination shows hyperpigmentation on her back that does not respect the lines of Blaschko and dental abnormalities. Her vision is normal and her ocular examination shows bilateral retinal peripheral vessel straightening. IVFA confirms peripheral retinal nonperfusion. Which of the following tests would be most likely to confirm the diagnosis?
a) *NDP* sequencing.
b) *IKBKG* targeted mutation analysis.
c) *IKBKG* sequencing.
d) No genetic testing as findings due to ROP.

Correct answer is b.
The history of multiple male miscarriages and characteristic skin and dental findings makes the diagnosis of IP likely.
a) **Incorrect.** Familial exudative vitreoretinopathy (FEVR) associated with *NPD* is X-linked recessive and therefore not associated with male miscarriages. It does not present with skin or dental findings.
b) **Correct.**
c) **Less appropriate.** First test of choice should be targeted mutation analysis, which identifies the causative deletion in 65% of cases.
d) **Incorrect.** Although peripheral retina nonperfusion can result from ROP, the patient had a history of normal neonatal screening and shows no demarcation line on examination. There would also not be associated skin or dental findings.

16.7.3 Case 3

A 1-month-old boy presents with segmental erythema followed by vesicles that follow a linear distribution that evolves into a swirling pigmentation. Fundus examination reveals peripheral retinal perfusion, neovascularization, and straightening of the vessels. He has developmental delay, brain anomalies, and eosinophilia. Which from the following genetic tests is more appropriate?
a) *NDP* sequencing.
b) *IKBKG* targeted mutation analysis.
c) *IKBKG* sequencing.
d) Karyotype.

Correct answer is d.
IP is usually lethal in male patients. Survival is explained by somatic mosaicism or a 47,XXY karyotype (Klinefelter syndrome). This child has all of the clinical manifestations of IP. Karyotype should be performed to help guide the genetic evaluation. If the karyotype shows an extra X chromosome, then *IKBKG* studies can ensue. If it is normal, somatic change should be considered by skin biopsy for analysis of *IKBKG*.
a) **Less appropriate.** FEVR is not associated with these systemic signs.
b) **Less appropriate.** Karyotype would be recommended to help guide gene-specific testing strategy.

c) **Less appropriate.** *IKBKG* sequencing does not explain male survival and would only be considered after karyotype and, if indicated, failed targeted testing.

d) **Correct.**

16.7.4 Case 4

A 3-year-old girl presents with verrucous lesions that do not follow the lines of Blaschko, occurring mostly on the limbs. She also has dental anomalies and developmental delay. Which from the following tests would be most helpful in confirming IP?

a) Herpes simplex PCR (polymerase chain reaction).

b) IVFA.

c) Scrapings and cultures of the lesions.

d) C-reactive protein.

Correct answer is b.

Clinical presentation in this case is very suggestive of IP. IVFA will help confirm diagnosis, and in addition assess the possible need for treatment to lessen the risk for retinal detachment.

a) **Incorrect.** Neonatal herpes simplex is not associated with dental anomalies and developmental delay.

b) **Correct.**

c) **Incorrect.** These tests would be considered if there were signs suggestive of infection. The presence of dental anomalies and developmental delay suggest that a noninfectious process is taking place.

d) **Incorrect.** This test would be more appropriate if one were considering an inflammatory disease.

Suggested Reading

[1] Aradhya S, Woffendin H, Jakins T, et al. A recurrent deletion in the ubiquitously expressed NEMO (IKK-gamma) gene accounts for the vast majority of incontinentia pigmenti mutations. Hum Mol Genet. 2001b; 10(19):2171–2179

[2] Badgwell AL, Iglesias AD, Emmerich S, Willner JP. The natural history of incontinentia pigmenti as reported by 198 affected individuals. Abstract 38. Nashville, TN: American College of Medical Genetics Annual Meeting; 2007

[3] Chang TT, Behshad R, Brodell RT, Gilliam AC. A male infant with anhidrotic ectodermal dysplasia/immunodeficiency accompanied by incontinentia pigmenti and a mutation in the NEMO pathway. J Am Acad Dermatol. 2008; 58(2):316–320

[4] Conte MI, Pescatore A, Paciolla M, et al. Insight into IKBKG/NEMO locus: report of new mutations and complex genomic rearrangements leading to incontinentia pigmenti disease. Hum Mutat. 2014; 35(2):165–177

[5] Demirel N, Aydin M, Zenciroglu A, et al. Incontinentia pigmenti with encephalocele in a neonate: a rare association. J Child Neurol. 2009; 24(4):495–499

[6] Fiorillo L, Sinclair DB, O'Byrne ML, Krol AL. Bilateral cerebrovascular accidents in incontinentia pigmenti. Pediatr Neurol. 2003; 29(1):66–68

[7] Franco LM, Goldstein J, Prose NS, et al. Incontinentia pigmenti in a boy with XXY mosaicism detected by fluorescence in situ hybridization. J Am Acad Dermatol. 2006; 55(1):136–138

[8] Fusco F, Paciolla M, Conte MI, et al. Incontinentia pigmenti: report on data from 2000 to 2013. Orphanet J Rare Dis. 2014; 9:93

[9] Fusco F, Paciolla M, Pescatore A, et al. Microdeletion/duplication at the Xq28 IP locus causes a de novo IKBKG/NEMO/IKKgamma exon4_10 deletion in families with incontinentia pigmenti. Hum Mutat. 2009; 30 (9):1284–1291

[10] Hayes IM, Varigos G, Upjohn EJ, Orchard DC, Penny DJ, Savarirayan R. Unilateral acheiria and fatal primary pulmonary hypertension in a girl with incontinentia pigmenti. Am J Med Genet A. 2005; 135(3):302–303

[11] Holmström G, Thorén K. Ocular manifestations of incontinentia pigmenti. Acta Ophthalmol Scand. 2000; 78 (3):348–353

[12] Minić S, Trpinac D, Obradović M. Incontinentia pigmenti diagnostic criteria update. Clin Genet. 2014; 85(6): 536–542

[13] Tomotaki S, Shibasaki J, Yunoki Y, et al. Effectiveness of corticosteroid therapy for acute neurological symptoms in incontinentia pigmenti. Pediatr Neurol. 2016; 56:55–58

[14] Chen CJ, Han IC, Goldberg MF. Variable expression of retinopathy in a pedigree of patients with incontinentia pigmenti. Retina. 2015; 35(12):2627–2632

[15] Swinney CC, Han DP, Karth PA. Incontinentia pigmenti: a comprehensive review and update. Ophthalmic Surg Lasers Imaging Retina. 2015; 46(6):650–657

[16] Chen CJ, Han IC, Tian J, Muñoz B, Goldberg MF. Extended follow-up of treated and untreated retinopathy in incontinentia pigmenti: analysis of peripheral vascular changes and incidence of retinal detachment. JAMA Ophthalmol. 2015; 133(5):542–548

17 Retinitis Pigmentosa

René Moya

Abstract

Retinitis pigmentosa is a group of related hereditary disorders characterized by loss of night vision followed by progressive loss of peripheral vision while often sparing central visual acuity until later in the disease. Characteristic clinical features include "bone spicule" pigmentary clumps initially in the midperiphery of the fundus, retinal vascular attenuation, and optic disc pallor. Other common findings are posterior subcapsular cataracts and pigment in the anterior vitreous. Patients may also develop intraretinal cystoid spaces or cystoid macular edema, epiretinal gliosis, or premature vitreous detachment. It is a progressive primary retinal degeneration involving the death of rod photoreceptors followed by loss of cone photoreceptors. Retinitis pigmentosa can be classified as nonsyndromic or syndromic (association with other affected organs or tissues).

Keywords: retinitis pigmentosa, retinal degeneration, retinal dystrophy, bone spicule, cataract, cystoid macular edema

Key Points

- Retinitis pigmentosa (RP) is the most common retinal dystrophy and a major cause of incurable blindness with prevalence that ranges from 1:4,000 to 1:8,000.
- RP is characterized by a common pattern of vision loss starting with loss of night vision followed by loss of peripheral vision. Central vision is often preserved for decades.
- RP is the prototypical rod–cone dystrophy and is associated with "bone spicule" pigmentary clumping in the midperiphery, retinal vessel attenuation, "waxy pallor" of the optic nerves, and posterior subcapsular cataract. Intraretinal cystoid spaces or cystoid macular edema may also be observed and may respond to treatment with carbonic anhydrase inhibitors.
- RP is characterized by high genetic heterogeneity as well as variability in age of onset, association with systemic findings, prognosis, and inheritance patterns.

17.1 Overview

Retinitis pigmentosa (RP) is a group of related hereditary disorders characterized by loss of night vision followed by progressive loss of visual acuity. Characteristic clinical features include "bone spicule" pigmentary clumps initially in the midperiphery of the fundus, retinal vascular attenuation, and optic disc pallor (▶ Fig. 17.1). Other common findings are posterior subcapsular cataracts (PSC) and pigment in the anterior vitreous. Patients may also develop intraretinal cystoid spaces or cystoid macular edema (CME), epiretinal gliosis, or premature vitreous detachment. It is a progressive primary retinal degeneration involving the death of rod photoreceptors followed by loss of cone photoreceptors.

The estimated prevalence of RP ranges from 1:3,000 to 1:8,000 individuals. RP can be classified as nonsyndromic (not affecting other organs or tissues) or syndromic (association with other affected organs or tissues; see text box below). Major forms of syndromic

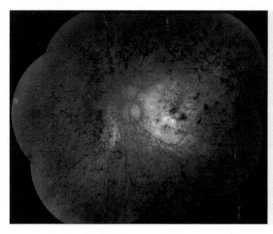

Fig. 17.1 End-stage retinitis pigmentosa, showing 360 degrees of "bone spicule" pigmentary clumping, severe vessel attenuation, pale optic disc, and macular atrophy.

RP are Usher syndrome in which there is variable sensorineural deafness with/without vestibular abnormalities and Bardet–Biedl syndrome (BBS), which includes obesity, polydactyly, renal abnormalities, and developmental delay as well as other features.

Syndromic Retinitis Pigmentosa (OMIM)

- Usher syndrome.
- Bardet-Beidl syndrome.
- Congenital disorders of glycosylation (212065).
- Mitochondrial disorders.
  - Kearns–Sayre syndrome (530000).
  - RP-deafness syndrome (500004).
  - Neuropathy, ataxia, and RP (NARP; 551500).
  - Leigh syndrome (256000).
- Mitochondrial myopathy, encephalopathy, lactic acidosis, and strokelike episodes (MELAS; 540000).
- Peroxisomal disorders.
- Rhyns syndrome (602152).
- Abetalipoproteinemia (Bassen–Kornzweig disease; 200100).
- Ataxia with vitamin E deficiency (277460).
- Short-rib thoracic dysplasia with or without polydactyly (266920; includes Ellis–van Creveld syndrome; Jeune syndrome; asphyxiating thoracic dystrophy; short-rib polydactyly syndrome; Mainzer–Saldino syndrome).
- Senior–Løken syndrome (266900).
- Epiphyseal dysplasia, microcephaly, and nystagmus (Lowry–Wood syndrome; 226960).
- Polyneuropathy, hearing loss, ataxia, retinitis pigmentosa, and cataract (PHARC; 612674).
- Posterior column ataxia with RP (609033).
- Neuronal ceroid lipofuscinoses.
- Joubert syndrome (213300).
- Oregon eye disease.

RP may be inherited as autosomal dominant (AD), autosomal recessive (AR), X-linked recessive, X-linked dominant, or mitochondrial. Rare digenic forms also occur. There are likely over 100 genes that can result in RP when mutated. RP simplex is a term applied when an individual is the only affected family member. Any of the inheritance patterns may apply. AD RP can be caused by mutations in *RDS/PRPH2*, rhodopsin, or 21 other genes currently described. Although AD RP is generally less severe with later age of onset, and X-linked recessive RP more severe with earlier onset, this is not always the case. Whereas carriers of AR RP may show mild abnormalities on electroretinogram (ERG), 50% of female carriers of X-linked RP may show ERG abnormalities, pigmentary retinopathy, and/or a tapetal reflex.

Vision loss occurs either from cataract, CME or intraretinal cystoid spaces, or the natural history of the retinal degeneration, which affects the central macula last. Approximately only 1-in-1,000 patients progress to no light perception. CME or intra-retinal cystoid spaces are seen in 15 to 50% of patients with RP. The distinction between the two is made by intravenous fluorescein angiography (IVFA), but treatment with topical and/or carbonic anhydrase inhibitors may be effective for either. Nonleaking intraretinal cystoid spaces have been reported with RP due to mutations in *NR2E3*, *XLRS*, *CRB1*, *GPR98*, *MAK*, *CNGB1*, and others, which will likely be described.

Supportive treatment for RP may include vitamin A palmitate (15,000 IU per day), which remains controversial and is likely best used for certain genotypes, a correlation that is yet to be elucidated. It should not be used in children, pregnant women, or women of child-bearing age not on birth control. It should also not be used in RP due to mutations in *ABCA4*. A high dose of vitamin E should be avoided. Increased intake of docosahexaenoic acid and lutein–zeaxanthin, especially through dietary fatty fish, may slow progression, as well as ultraviolet A (UVA) and UVB blocking sunglasses. Although cataract surgery may be useful, patients with RP have a higher rate of postoperative CME that may be irreversible and vision compromising. Even small PSC may have a large effect on vision in patients with very constricted visual fields. Other treatments, such as intravitreal triamcinolone injection, intravitreal VEGF (vascular endothelial growth factor) inhibitors, hyperbaric oxygen, acupuncture, and light deprivation lack evidence of efficacy. The Food and Drug Administration (FDA) approved the first retinal implant, the Argus II Retinal Prosthesis System, for selected patients with advanced RP aged 25 years or older. Clinical trials are under way using neurotrophic factors, stem cells, and gene therapy. Patients should also be encouraged to seek low vision services, vocational counseling, and mobility training as indicated.

17.2 Molecular Genetics

With more than 55 genes identified, many loci within which the gene has yet to be found, and over 3,000 mutations in the genes already described, RP is clearly a genetically heterogeneous disorder. Mutations in 23 genes are known to cause AD RP, 36 genes cause AR RP, and two genes cause X-linked RP. Although the proportion varies in different regions, approximately 40% of RP is sporadic (RP simplex) with no other affected family members. Of these cases, approximately 1 to 2% are X-linked, up to 10 to 15% AD, and the remainder AR. In places were consanguinity is more common, AR inheritance pattern can be higher (up to 40%). Digenic forms of RP are infrequent (e.g., heterozygous mutations in both *ROM1* and *PRPH2*).

The most frequent genes associated with AD RP include *RHO* (up to 30%), *PRPF31* (up to 10%), *PRPH2* (up to 10%), and *RP1* (up to 4%). Other genes may be frequent in specific populations (e.g., *GUCA1B* or *FSCN2* in Japan). More than 100 pathogenic variants in *RHO* have been reported. Of the *RP1* known mutations, c.2029C > T and c.2285_2289delTAAAT account for approximately half of the cases.

In patients with AR RP, the population particularly influences the estimated proportion of specific genes. For instance, *USH2A* (up to 15%), *ABCA4* (up to 5%), *PDE6A* (up to 5%), or *PDE6B* (up to 5%) are frequently found in European families, and other genes, such as *CRB1* or *EYS*, are more frequent in Hispano Americans.

X-linked RP is mostly caused by two genes. *RPGR* (also known as *RP3*) is associated with 70 to 90% of cases and *RP2* accounts for 10 to 20%. In the case of *RPGR*, the identification of exon *ORF15* increased the mutation detection rate. The *RPGR* gene has 23 exons, including the alternatively spliced exons 9a, *ORF15*, 15a, and 15b. Most pathogenic variants are located in *ORF15*, which is predominantly present in retinal transcripts.

Patients with mitochondrial DNA (deoxyribonucleic acid) mutations can get isolated RP. More commonly, affected individuals or their family members can present with other findings such as neurologic abnormalities or myopathy.

17.3 Differential Diagnosis

17.3.1 Choroideremia (OMIM 303100)

This X-linked recessive disorder can be distinguished by the early fundus appearance. The predominant finding is choroidal loss, which appears to be primary with the retina degeneration secondary. It is caused by mutations in *CHM*. End-stage choroideremia can be somewhat indistinguishable from end-stage RP. The symptoms experienced by affected individuals are also much like that seen with RP.

17.3.2 Gyrate Atrophy (OMIM 258870)

This is an AR disorder that is caused by mutations in *OAT*. It is characterized by sharply defined, scalloped defects of the retinal pigment epithelium (RPE) and choroid, which begin peripherally and progress toward the macula. Patients have elevation of plasma ornithine concentration caused by deficiency of the enzyme ornithine–ketoacid aminotransferase.

17.3.3 Cone–Rod Dystrophies

These disorders are characterized by loss of central visual acuity, photophobia, and color vision defects. In more advanced disease, the rod system becomes involved with peripheral visual loss and defective dark adaptation.

17.3.4 Leber Congenital Amaurosis

This is a group of congenital retinal dystrophies usually diagnosed in the first year of life. Most forms are AR. Although there are multiple phenotypes, the retinal appearance may be indistinguishable from classic RP.

17.3.5 Bietti's Crystalline Corneoretinal Dystrophy (OMIM 210370)

This is an AR retinal dystrophy characterized by decreased vision, nyctalopia, and paracentral scotomas with onset usually in the second to fourth decades of life. Some patients may experience photophobia. Visual field loss and visual impairment progress by the fifth decade of life. Patients exhibit yellow-white crystals in the posterior retina, associated with RPE atrophy, pigmentary clumps, and choroidal sclerosis. Many patients also have crystals at the corneoscleral limbus. Full-field ERG is affected, either with a rod–cone or cone–rod pattern. This disorder is caused by mutations in *CYP4V2* (4q35).

17.3.6 Paravenous Retinochoroidal Atrophy (OMIM 172870)

This is a slowly progressive condition characterized by bone spicule pigmentation seen in a paravenous distribution. Individuals are usually asymptomatic for many years.

17.3.7 Pericentric Retinitis Pigmentosa

In this condition, the clinical features are similar to RP except that pigmentary changes are confined to the midperiphery, in a circle immediately around the macula. Many cases are mild with satisfactory vision beyond the fifth decade of life. The inheritance pattern is considered AD, although sporadic cases have been reported. Mutations in several different genes are likely possible causes.

17.3.8 "Bear-Track" Pigmentation

This benign retinal finding is caused by hypertrophic RPE in irregularly shaped patches throughout the retina, which resemble the footprints of a bear. They are often seen in a quadrant of retina. The condition is asymptomatic.

17.3.9 Cancer-Associated Retinopathy/Melanoma-Associated Retinopathy/Autoimmune Retinopathy

This is a spectrum of conditions characterized by diffuse retinal degeneration in the context of a systemic disease that triggers an antiretinal antigen immune response, which creates antibodies that cross-react with retinal proteins. Patients usually present with severe acute or subacute vision loss, which is usually bilateral, but can present as sequential and asymmetric. The diagnosis involves the detection of antiretinal antibodies with concurrent clinical and electrophysiological evidence of retinopathy. Although rods are usually the predominant affected cells, cone-dominant retinal destruction may occur. Antirecoverin antibody is the most frequent antibody associated with cancer-associated retinopathy (CAR). Other examples of antibodies include anticarbonic anhydrase, anti-transducin B, anti-alpha enolase, anti-TULP1, anti-HSC 70 and anti-arrestin.

17.3.10 Metabolic Disorders

Metabolic disorders, such as alpha mannosidosis or some mucopolysaccharidoses, can manifest with retinal degeneration that resembles RP. These disorders must be suspected in cases of progressive developmental delay, motor dysfunction, hepatosplenomegaly, hearing loss, recurrent respiratory infections, facial dysmorphism, and skeletal anomalies.

17.3.11 Pseudo-Retinitis Pigmentosa

These disorders may present with a pigmentary retinopathy very similar to RP but without a genetic etiology. They are usually nonprogressive and without the symptoms seen in RP. Examples include diffuse unilateral subacute neuroretinitis (DUSN), acute zonal occult outer retinopathy (AZOOR), multifocal choroiditis, panuveitis, syphilis, toxoplasmosis, congenital rubella, phenothiazine/thioridazine toxicity, deferoxamine, prior ocular trauma, prior vascular obstruction, chronic retinal detachment, and cancer-/melanoma-/autoimmune-associated retinopathy.

17.4 Uncommon Manifestations

17.4.1 Unilateral Retinitis Pigmentosa

This diagnosis is made when only one eye has typical changes of RP and the other has no clinical or electrophysiological findings after a follow-up period of 5 years.

17.4.2 Retinitis Pigmentosa Sine Pigmento

This term has been used to refer to a retina that has the typical retinal vessel attenuation, pallor of the optic nerve, and other features of RP but without "bone spicule" pigmentary clumping. Abnormal ERG consistent with rod–cone dystrophy as well as typical findings of RP on other studies such as optical coherence tomography (OCT) are also present. It has been suggested that this term is a misnomer and these patients would be more accurately classified by their genotype or as an otherwise unspecified retinal dystrophy.

17.4.3 Exudative Vasculopathy (Coats-like Disease)

Telangiectatic vessels, lipid deposits in the retina, and serous retinal detachment have been associated with AR RP due to mutations in the *CRB1* gene.

17.4.4 White Dots (Retinitis Punctata Albescens)

White dots (retinitis punctata albescens) can be seen at the level of the RPE. This finding differentiates from fundus albipunctata (a flecked retina disorder) in that there is progressive loss of visual field and the presence of pigmentary changes and retinal vascular attenuation, findings that are not present in fundus albipunctata.

17.4.5 Drusen of the Optic Nerve Head

This finding may be associated with arcuate visual field loss.

17.4.6 Paravascular Pattern

A pattern of pigmented paravenous chorioretinal atrophy may be seen with *CRB1*.

17.4.7 Sector Retinitis Pigmentosa

This term describes changes in one quadrant or one half of the retina. Some of these cases develop over time into a diffuse disease. Patients with this condition may not initially have symptoms such as nyctalopia, although full-field (ff) ERG can detect abnormalities. Because sector RP is usually asymptomatic, its prevalence may be underestimated. The *RHO* mutation (c.68C > A) is one of the most frequent.

17.5 Clinical Testing

17.5.1 Optical Coherence Tomography

In RP, the OCT will show loss of photoreceptors beyond the perifovea, with subfoveal photoreceptor sparing until late in the disease. Surface gliosis may be seen and eventually there is retinal thinning, flattening of the foveal contour, and loss of normal retinal lamination. Intraretinal cystoid spaces or CME is indistinguishable by OCT. Other findings may include hyper-reflective specks in various retinal layers and "debris" at the level of the photoreceptors. Outer retinal tubulation can be seen as well. Tubulation corresponds to degenerating photoreceptors that present as round hyporeflective spaces with hyper-reflective borders with variable size. Morphologic features range from single straight or branching tubules to complex cavitations, frequently overlying areas of RPE alteration or subretinal fibrosis. These lesions generally remain stable over time. These changes are frequently seen in advanced diseases affecting the outer retina and RPE, such as RP.

17.5.2 Full-Field Electroretinogram

Rods are typically affected earlier and worse than cones, but eventually the ERG becomes isoelectric to all stimuli.

17.5.3 Multifocal Electroretinogram

This will record residual macular function in patients with advanced disease and can be used for follow-up even when the ffERG is isoelectric.

17.5.4 Goldmann Visual Field

This test will show different findings, depending on the stage of the disease. These include a progressive concentric loss of peripheral visual fields. Field loss often begins superiorly and subsequently evolves into an arcuate scotoma that may leave an isolated temporal island or a complete or incomplete midperipheral "ring scotoma." In the end stages of the disease, the field may only be a small residual central area of vision. This test is recommended for visual function follow-up and disability/legal blindness definition. It is also helpful in case of cataracts for determining the impact on the residual central field.

17.5.5 Fundus Autofluorescence

As the disease progresses, this test will show increasing patchy hypofluorescence as well as blocking by the retinal pigment clumps. A hyperautofluorescent ring in the macula represents a transition zone from relatively well preserved to abnormal retina. Some gene mutations are associated with a double hyperautofluorescent ring.

17.6 Genetic Testing

Next-generation sequencing panels are available at several centers for simultaneous testing of many genes that when mutated result in RP, including those that can result in isolated RP or syndromic disease (e.g., *USH2A*). In some cases, the phenotype may suggest a specific gene the testing of which could reduce cost, for example, the paravascular sparing or the exudative vasculopathy with *CRB1*-related RP. If panel sequencing is negative, then exome sequencing may be indicated, especially for syndromic disease.

17.7 Additional Resources

Foundation Fighting Blindness: http://www.blindness.org/.

17.8 Problems

17.8.1 Case 1

A 45-year-old woman with RP due to homozygous *MAK* gene mutation presents with a 3-year history of progressive loss of central visual acuity in both eyes. She has nyctalopia and reduced peripheral vision. She is the only affected family member and otherwise well. Best corrected visual acuities are 20/80 in the right eye and 20/100 in the left eye. Anterior segment examination shows subtle, eccentric, PSC. Fundus examination reveals the typical findings of RP including retinal vascular attenuation, midperipheral "bone spicule" pigmentary clumps, and "waxy pallor" of the optic nerves. The foveal reflex is blunted. OCT shows cystoid spaces in the macula of both eyes but preserved photoreceptors in the subfoveal regions. Visual field testing revealed marked constriction in both eyes (15 degrees). IVFA does not reveal any leakage from the macular cystoid spaces. Which of the following better explains her declining vision?

a) Intraretinal cystoid spaces.
b) Natural history of RP.
c) Posterior subcapsular cataract.
d) A different disorder.

Correct answer is a.

Intraretinal cystoid spaces (nonleaking CME) are one manifestation of RP and are seen in particular when specific genes are mutated. Vision may be improved through the use of topical and/or oral carbonic anhydrase inhibitors.

a) **Correct.**
b) **Incorrect.** Although one cannot absolutely rule out a component of natural progression, the presence of preserved subfoveal photoreceptors on OCT, a field that is still at 15 degrees, and the presence of another explanation suggest that the natural progression of the retinal dystrophy is not the cause of her vision loss.
c) **Incorrect.** Although small PSC can be a cause of vision loss, in particular in patients with RP and very constricted visual fields, the visually significant PSC should be in the visual axis.
d) **Incorrect.** As all findings are consistent with the clinical picture, there is no need to pursue another diagnosis at this time.

17.8.2 Case 2

A 35-year-old woman presents with unilateral retinal abnormalities found in her left eye on routine optometric examination. She is completely asymptomatic. Ocular history reveals a blunt trauma with paintball when she was a teenager. She was told at that time "everything was ok" and she did not see an eye doctor. Her visual acuity is 20/20 in both eyes. Ophthalmoscopy shows normal examination of the right eye. Left eye reveals diffuse, granular appearance of the retinal pigment epithelium, with "bone spicule" pigmentary clumps throughout the superior and inferior temporal quadrants. Humphrey perimetry shows peripheral nasal constriction of the visual field of the left eye. An ffERG is normal. FAF of the macula is unremarkable but shows decreased fluorescence in the affected area of retina. What is the most likely diagnosis?

a) RP.
b) X-linked RP carrier.
c) Sector RP.
d) Pseudo-RP due to trauma.

Correct answer is d.

The most likely diagnosis in this case is pseudo-RP. The patient is asymptomatic and has a normal ERG, focal findings, and no evidence of degeneration.

a) **Incorrect**. Although truly unilateral RP can very rarely occur, the normal ffERG rules out this diagnosis. The ERG is always abnormal in RP when ocular findings are apparent on examination.

b) **Incorrect**. Most carriers of X-linked RP have findings diffusely in both eyes. In many cases, obligate carriers can be identified by ERG testing or the presence of a tapetal sheen.

c) **Less appropriate**. Although this diagnosis can be consistent with the patient's history and clinical findings, one would expect an abnormal ffERG. The prior ocular trauma also makes this possibility less likely. Many patients with sector RP remain asymptomatic and some can progress into more diffuse disease.

d) **Correct**.

17.8.3 Case 3

A 10-year-old male patient is brought for assessment by his concerned parents as two maternal uncles in their 20s had a recent diagnosis of RP. The child's mother is asymptomatic although when examined she has a tapetal-like reflex and some scattered fine pigmentary clumping in her midperipheral retina. She has noted that her son has problems with his night vision and seems to bump into things more than other children. His ERG shows dramatic reduction of rod more than cone responses. OCT and FAF (autofluorescence) also show typical abnormalities for RP. Molecular analysis shows a previously reported missense mutation G576C in the *RPGR* gene compatible with the diagnosis of X-linked RP. What is the chance for this boy's younger brother to be affected?

a) 25%.
b) 8%.
c) 50%.
d) 100%.

Correct answer is c.

The mother is an obligate carrier. She also has some fundus changes compatible with a carrier state that results from inactivation of her normal X chromosome. There is a 50% chance that the younger son is affected.

17.8.4 Case 4

A 22-year-old female is diagnosed with RP due to homozygous mutation in *ABCA4* (c.1622T > C). Which of the following interventions should be avoided?
a) Increasing dietary fish.
b) Vitamin A supplementation.
c) Docosahexaenoic acid and lutein–zeaxanthin.
d) UV blocking sunglasses.

Correct answer is b.

Vitamin A should be avoided in patients with *ABCA4* mutations as it may induce lipofuscin accumulation. In addition, this treatment is relatively contraindicated in women of child-bearing age due to the risk of fetal malformation.
a) **Incorrect.** Fish intake is not contraindicated and there is some evidence that it may slow the progression of RP.
b) **Correct.**
c) **Incorrect.** Although the benefits of these supplements are controversial and unclear, they are not contraindicated in RP.
d) **Incorrect.** UV blocking sunglasses are recommended to slow disease progression.

Suggested Reading

[1] Daiger SP, Bowne SJ, Sullivan LS. Perspective on genes and mutations causing retinitis pigmentosa. Arch Ophthalmol. 2007; 125(2):151–158

[2] Haim M. Epidemiology of retinitis pigmentosa in Denmark. Acta Ophthalmol Scand Suppl. 2002; 233(233): 1–34

[3] US Food and Drug Administration. FDA approves first retinal implant for adults with rare genetic eye disease. FDA, February 14, 2013

[4] RetNet: Retinal Information Network. 2013. Available from: http://www.sph.uth.tmc.edu/Retnet/. Accessed March 2013

[5] HGMD. Human Gene Mutation Database (Biobase Biological Databases); 2013

[6] Branham K, Othman M, Brumm M, et al. Mutations in RPGR and RP2 account for 15% of males with simplex retinal degenerative disease. Invest Ophthalmol Vis Sci. 2012; 53(13):8232–8237

[7] Sohocki MM, Daiger SP, Bowne SJ, et al. Prevalence of mutations causing retinitis pigmentosa and other inherited retinopathies. Hum Mutat. 2001; 17(1):42–51

[8] Noble KG. Hereditary pigmented paravenous chorioretinal atrophy. Am J Ophthalmol. 1989; 108(4):365–369

[9] Buettner H. Congenital hypertrophy of the retinal pigment epithelium. Am J Ophthalmol. 1975; 79(2):177–189

[10] Carr RE, Siegel IM. Unilateral retinitis pigmentosa. Arch Ophthalmol. 1973; 90(1):21–26

[11] den Hollander AI, Heckenlively JR, van den Born LI, et al. Leber congenital amaurosis and retinitis pigmentosa with Coats-like exudative vasculopathy are associated with mutations in the crumbs homologue 1 (CRB1) gene. Am J Hum Genet. 2001; 69(1):198–203

[12] Kim YJ, Joe SG, Lee DH, Lee JY, Kim JG, Yoon YH. Correlations between spectral-domain OCT measurements and visual acuity in cystoid macular edema associated with retinitis pigmentosa. Invest Ophthalmol Vis Sci. 2013; 54(2):1303–1309

[13] Lenassi E, Troeger E, Wilke R, Hawlina M. Correlation between macular morphology and sensitivity in patients with retinitis pigmentosa and hyperautofluorescent ring. Invest Ophthalmol Vis Sci. 2012; 53(1): 47–52

[14] Tucker T, Marra M, Friedman JM. Massively parallel sequencing: the next big thing in genetic medicine. Am J Hum Genet. 2009; 85(2):142–154

18 Usher Syndrome

Abstract

Usher syndrome is an autosomal recessive condition involving sensorineural hearing loss and retinitis pigmentosa. It is the most frequent cause of deaf-blindness in humans. Penetrance is usually complete. Although hearing loss in children will be detected by either newborn hearing screening or later audiologic evaluation, most often due to delays or other abnormalities in speech, the diagnosis of Usher syndrome typically lags 5 to 10 years behind the identification of the hearing loss depending on the onset of its visual impairment. There are three subtypes of Usher syndrome, differentiated by the presence of vestibular involvement, age of retinitis pigmentosa onset, and pace of disease progression. Many genes are associated with this condition.

Keywords: Usher syndrome, retinitis pigmentosa, hearing loss, Usher type I, Usher type II, Usher type III

Key Points

- Usher syndrome is an autosomal recessive condition characterized by sensorineural hearing loss and retinitis pigmentosa (RP).
- There are three subtypes of Usher syndrome, differentiated by the presence or absence of vestibular involvement, age of RP onset, and pace of disease progression.

18.1 Overview

Usher syndrome is an autosomal recessive (AR) condition involving sensorineural hearing loss and retinitis pigmentosa (RP). It is the most frequent cause of deaf-blindness in humans. The approximate incidence of Usher syndrome is 1 to 6 per 100,000. It accounts for up to 6% of all childhood deafness and approximately 50% of all patient deaf-blindness. Penetrance is usually complete. Although hearing loss in children will be detected by either newborn hearing screening or later audiologic evaluation, most often due to delays or other abnormalities in speech, the diagnosis of Usher syndrome typically lags 5 to 10 years behind the identification of the hearing loss depending on the onset of its visual impairment.

There are three subtypes of Usher syndrome, differentiated by the presence of vestibular involvement, age of RP onset, and pace of disease progression. A diagnosis of Usher syndrome type I (USH1) is suspected when a patient presents with congenital profound bilateral sensorineural hearing loss, severe vestibular abnormalities (which may be clinically unapparent), and early-onset RP that typically progresses slowly. Affected patients develop abnormal speech. Vestibular areflexia is a defining feature of USH1. Because of this, children frequently walk later than usual. Older patients may experience balance issues. The remainder of the physical examination is usually normal.

Usher syndrome type II (USH2) is characterized by congenital bilateral sensorineural hearing loss that affects predominantly the higher frequencies, with normal vestibular function and adolescent-to-adult onset of RP. The most common Usher subtype is type 2, and the *USH2A* gene accounts for 75 to 80% of these cases. Usher syndrome type III (USH3) is characterized by postlingual progressive sensorineural hearing loss, later-onset RP, and variable impairment of vestibular function. In types 2 and 3, the progression of the RP is more apparent perhaps because of the later onset.

USH1 and USH2 proteins are organized into protein networks by the scaffold proteins harmonin, whirlin, and scaffold protein containing ankyrin repeats and SAM domain (SANS). USH protein networks have cytoskeletal functions as well as roles in transport processes and ciliary delivery in hair cells and photoreceptors. There are molecular links of not only USH to other ciliopathies, including nonsyndromic inner ear defects and isolated retinal dystrophies, but also to kidney diseases and syndromes like the Bardet–Biedl syndrome (BBS).

18.2 Molecular Genetics

Genes known to produce Usher syndrome when mutated are presented in ▶ Table 18.1.

Although heterozygous carriers of gene mutations causing USH1 are asymptomatic, they may show slightly subnormal audiograms.

Table 18.1 Genes associated with Usher syndrome

USH1 subtype (proportion of cases)	Gene (locus)
USH1B (up to 60%)	*MYO7A* (11q13.5)[a]
USH1C (up to 15%)	*USH1C* (11p15.1)[b]
USH1D (up to 20%)	*CDH23* (10q22.1)[c]
USH1F (up to 10%)	*PCDH15* (10q21.1)[d]
USH1G (up to 5%)	*USH1G* (17q25.1)
USH1J (Unknown)	*CIB2* (15q25.1)[e]
USH2 subtype (proportion of cases)	Gene (locus)
USH2A (up to 75%)	*USH2A* (1q41)
USH2C (up to 20%)	*ADGRV1* (5q14.3)
USH2D (up to 10%)	*DFNB31* (9q32)
USH3 subtype (proportion of cases)	Gene (locus)
USH3A (Unknown)	*CLRN1* (3q25.1)
USH3B (Unknown)	*HARS* (5q31.3)

[a]Mutations can also cause autosomal dominant nonsyndromic hearing loss (DFNA11), through a dominant negative effect.
[b]A del(11)(p14–15) that includes *USH1C* is associated with hyperinsulinism, enteropathy, and deafness. Mutations can also cause autosomal recessive (AR) nonsyndromic hearing loss (DFNB18).
[c]Missense mutations can cause AR nonsyndromic hearing loss (DFNB12). This gene can also cause digenic recessive Usher with *PCDH15*.
[d]One-third of patients have deletions or duplications. Missense mutations can cause nonsyndromic hearing loss (DFNB23).
[e]Mutations may cause AR nonsyndromic hearing loss (DFNB48).

18.3 Differential Diagnosis

18.3.1 Isolated Retinitis Pigmentosa

The main difference between Usher syndrome and RP is the absence of hearing loss. Elderly individuals may have age-related hearing loss that is unrelated to their RP.

18.3.2 Deafness, Dystonia, and Optic Neuropathy Syndrome (OMIM 304700)

These patients have prelingual or postlingual sensorineural hearing impairment, slowly progressive dystonia or ataxia in the teens, and slowly progressive decreased visual acuity from optic atrophy beginning at approximately age 20 years. In addition, individuals develop dementia in their 40s. Psychiatric changes may also be seen in the first two decades of life. Mutations of *TIMM8A* cause Dystonia and Optic Neuropathy syndrome (DDON). Inheritance is X-linked recessive.

18.3.3 Congenital Rubella

The classic triad of congenital rubella includes ocular abnormalities, heart disease, and hearing loss or deafness. Congenital rubella produces a pigmentary retinopathy without the "bone spicule" clumping or progressive changes seen in RP. Congenital cataracts and glaucoma are seen in congenital rubella but not Usher syndrome.

18.3.4 Alström Syndrome (OMIM 203800)

This condition is an AR disorder characterized by progressive cone–rod dystrophy that leads to blindness, along with sensorineural hearing loss, childhood obesity associated with hyperinsulinemia, and type 2 diabetes mellitus. Dilated cardiomyopathy is seen in approximately 70% of individuals during infancy or adolescence. Other findings include renal, pulmonary, hepatic, and urologic dysfunction. Systemic fibrosis develops with age. It is caused by *ALMS1* mutations. Although the end-stage retinopathy may be indistinguishable from RP, patients present in childhood with high-frequency small-amplitude nystagmus and photophobia with a clinical picture that is more likely confused with achromatopsia or cone dystrophy.

18.3.5 Bardet–Biedl Syndrome

The main difference of BBS from USH is the systemic findings, including obesity, kidney dysfunction, polydactyly, behavioral dysfunction, and hypogonadism.

18.3.6 PHARC (OMIM 612674)

This is an AR condition characterized by polyneuropathy, hearing loss, ataxia, RP, and cataract. It is caused by mutations in the *ABHD12* gene.

18.3.7 Mitochondrial Disorders

Patients with mitochondrial mutations can get either isolated RP or, more frequently, other concomitant findings such as deafness, early-onset diabetes, neurologic abnormalities, or myopathy.

18.3.8 CAPOS (OMIM 601338)

This syndrome includes Cerebellar ataxia, Areflexia, Pes cavus, Optic atrophy, and Sensorineural hearing loss. It is caused by heterozygous mutations in the *ATP1A3* gene.

18.3.9 Nonsyndromic Hearing Loss

Patients with nonsyndromic hearing loss have to be closely followed for the subsequent development of RP, which would lead to a diagnosis of USH. Array panel sequencing of genes associated with isolated hearing loss may relieve patients of concern about the possible development of RP. As RP (1:3,000–1:8,000) and nonsyndromic hearing loss (1:1,000) are relatively frequent conditions, the possible incidental coexistence of the two conditions should also be considered.

18.4 Uncommon Manifestations

Intraretinal cystoid spaces have been described in patients with Usher syndrome. This is more commonly seen in USH2. Rarely, bilateral Coats-like exudative retinopathy has also been described.

18.5 Clinical Testing

Patients suspected to have USH should have testing of audiology and vestibular function. Formal audiology is recommended in children with speech impairment or delay, especially in the presence of RP (see also recommended testing for RP mentioned earlier).

18.6 Genetic Testing

Multigene panels are available. Certain ethnic populations may have higher incidence of particular gene involvement, for example, *USH1F* in Ashkenazi Jews and *USH1C* and *USH2A* in people of Acadian ancestry.

A significant proportion of patients with Usher type 2 will have just one heterozygous pathogenic variant in *USH2A*, or no convincing disease-causing mutations across other Usher genes. Screening for duplications, deletions, and intronic mutations can detect up to 35% of second mutations in patients with *USH2A*. A common pathogenic deep intronic variant *USH2A*: c.7595–2144A > G should also be considered.

18.7 Additional Resources

www.usher-syndrome.org.

18.7.1 Case 1

A 16-year-old female has been experiencing progressive nyctalopia and vision acuity loss in the last year. She has been under study for hearing loss and vestibular dysfunction in the last months. Speech is normal. She has unsteady gait on physical examination. Best corrected visual acuity is 20/40 in each eye. Slit-lamp examination is normal and funduscopy reveals "bone spicule" pigmentary clumping in the midperiphery with vascular attenuation and pale optic discs in both eyes. Full-field (Ff) electroretinogram (ERG) shows severe alteration of both rod function and cone function. Which from the following is the most likely diagnosis?

a) USH1.
b) USH2.
c) USH3.
d) Rubella.

Correct answer is c.

USH3 is the most likely diagnosis based on later-onset RP, altered vestibular function, and progression of symptoms.

a) **Incorrect.** Patient has no history of early onset of the condition and hearing dysfunction is not severe or prelingual.

b) **Incorrect.** Vestibular dysfunction is not present in USH2.

c) **Correct.**

d) **is less likely.** The classic triad of congenital rubella includes congenital ocular abnormalities, heart disease, and hearing loss or deafness often with developmental delay.

18.7.2 Case 2

A 5-year-old boy comes with a previous clinical diagnosis of USH2 based on the presence of retinal degeneration associated with hearing loss and normal vestibular function. Medical history reveals type 2 diabetes mellitus and dilated cardiomyopathy. Physical examination shows obesity. He does not have polydactyly. He also has high-frequency small-amplitude nystagmus and photophobia. Full-field ERG shows cone worse than rod dysfunction. Best corrected visual acuity is 20/80 OD (oculus dextrus) and 20/70 OS (oculus sinister) wearing –1.75 sph each eye. Which is the most likely diagnosis?

a) Alström syndrome.
b) BBS.
c) USH2.
d) USH1.

Correct answer is a.

The association between cone–rod dystrophy, sensorineural hearing loss, obesity, type 2 diabetes mellitus, and dilated cardiomyopathy is highly suggestive of Alström syndrome. Nystagmus and photophobia are clinical markers that are often prominent. It is caused by *ALMS1* mutations.

a) **Correct.**

b) **Incorrect.** The patient lacks kidney dysfunction, polydactyly, and hypogonadism. Nystagmus at this age is very atypical for BBS.

c) **Incorrect.** USH2 is not associated with systemic findings other than hearing loss.

d) **Incorrect.** USH1 is not associated with systemic findings other than hearing loss.

18.7.3 Case 3

An 18-year-old female started having visual acuity decrease 2 years ago, but previously had problems with her night vision. She has congenital bilateral sensorineural hearing loss treated with cochlear implants. Directed questions do not reveal any vestibular abnormality, which is confirmed by formal testing. Medical and family history are unrevealing. She does not have nystagmus or photophobia. Best corrected visual acuity is 20/70 OD and 20/80 OS with –1.50 cylinder in each eye. Fundus examination reveals typical findings of RP. Full-field ERG confirms severe dysfunction that affects rods more than cones. An Usher gene array panel reveals a single heterozygous mutation in *USH2A*. According to these findings, which is the most correct statement?

a) Patient has an AD form of Usher syndrome.

b) Diagnosis is wrong; further workup is needed.

c) Patient has USH3.

d) Further molecular testing is necessary to reveal the second mutated allele (e.g., deletion/duplication analysis).

Correct answer is d.

Screening for duplications, deletions, and an intronic mutation can detect up to 35% of second mutations in patients with heterozygous *USH2A* mutations on initial testing.

a) **Incorrect.** Usher syndrome is an AR condition.

b) **Less appropriate.** Clinical presentation is very indicative of USH. It is possible that the deafness and RP are unrelated, but the likelihood of this event is quite low. The patients has no systemic signs to suggest another diagnosis.

c) **Incorrect.** Vestibular function is abnormal in USH3.

d) **Correct.**

Suggested Reading

[1] Astuto LM, Bork JM, Weston MD, et al. CDH23 mutation and phenotype heterogeneity: a profile of 107 diverse families with Usher syndrome and nonsyndromic deafness. Am J Hum Genet. 2002; 71(2):262–275

[2] Blaydon DC, Mueller RF, Hutchin TP, et al. The contribution of USH1C mutations to syndromic and non-syndromic deafness in the UK. Clin Genet. 2003; 63(4):303–307

[3] Bonnet C, Grati M, Marlin S, et al. Complete exon sequencing of all known Usher syndrome genes greatly improves molecular diagnosis. Orphanet J Rare Dis. 2011; 6:21

[4] Le Quesne Stabej P, Saihan Z, Rangesh N, et al. Comprehensive sequence analysis of nine Usher syndrome genes in the UK National Collaborative Usher Study. J Med Genet. 2012; 49(1):27–36

[5] Malm E, Ponjavic V, Möller C, Kimberling WJ, Stone ES, Andréasson S. Alteration of rod and cone function in children with Usher syndrome. Eur J Ophthalmol. 2011; 21(1):30–38

[6] Lingao M, Ganesh A, Karthikeyan AS, et al. Macular cysts in patients with retinal dystrophy. Ophthalmic Genet. 2016; 37(4):377–383

[7] Steele-Stallard HB, Le Quesne Stabej P, Lenassi E, et al. Screening for duplications, deletions and a common intronic mutation detects 35% of second mutations in patients with USH2A monoallelic mutations on Sanger sequencing. Orphanet J Rare Dis. 2013; 8:122

19 Bardet–Biedl Syndrome

Abstract

Bardet–Biedl syndrome is characterized by early-onset retinal dystrophy that is typically a rod–cone dystrophy but may present initially as a maculopathy. Other features include truncal obesity, postaxial polydactyly, renal abnormalities, hypogonadism, and learning difficulties. Most patients do not present with all findings. Bardet–Biedl syndrome is considered a clinically and genetically heterogeneous ciliopathy, with significant intra- and interfamilial phenotypic variability. Retinal involvement occurs in more than 90% of patients.. Most individuals present with nyctalopia and abnormal visual fields by the age of 10 years. Visual acuity progresses to legal blindness in up to 75% of patients.

Keywords: Bardet–Biedl syndrome, rod–cone dystrophy, obesity, polydactyly, renal abnormalities, hypogonadism, ciliopathy

Key Points

- Bardet–Biedl syndrome (BBS) is characterized primarily by retinal dystrophy, truncal obesity, postaxial polydactyly, cognitive impairment, hypogonadotropic hypogonadism, and renal abnormalities. Variable expression is seen and patients may have only some features.
- Full-field electroretinogram usually presents with rod–cone pattern and sometimes with cone–rod pattern.
- BBS is a ciliopathy caused by mutations in genes that are relevant to ciliary function.

19.1 Overview

Bardet–Biedl syndrome (BBS) is primarily characterized by early-onset retinal dystrophy that is typically a rod–cone dystrophy but may present initially as a maculopathy. Other features include truncal obesity, postaxial polydactyly (▶ Fig. 19.1), renal abnormalities, hypogonadism, and learning difficulties. Birth weight is typically normal in these patients, but weight gain starts within the first year. Most patients do not present with all findings. BBS is considered a clinically and genetically heterogeneous ciliopathy, with significant intra- and interfamilial phenotypic variability. Prevalence ranges from 1:100,000 to 1:160,000, although in populations with known consanguinity, frequency may be as high as 1:13,000.

Retinal involvement occurs in more than 90% of patients with BBS. Most patients present a rod–cone pattern, but sometimes have a cone–rod pattern. Initial examination may be normal, but rarely maculopathy can be seen in late childhood. Most individuals with BBS present with nyctalopia and abnormal visual fields by the age of 10 years. At the end of the second decade of life, they usually present with a central island of vision. After that, macular involvement progresses, and visual acuity falls into legal blindness, which affects up to 75% of patients with BBS. Other ophthalmic findings may include nystagmus, strabismus, refractive errors, and cataract.

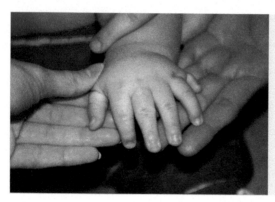

Fig. 19.1 Polydactyly in a patient with Bardet–Biedl syndrome.

Renal malformations and renal dysfunction that lead to end-stage renal disease are seen in approximately 50 to 80% of affected patients. Up to 45% of individuals with BBS have structural renal abnormalities, including cysts, scarring, agenesis, or dysplasia.

Many patients with BBS are delayed in reaching developmental milestones including speech delay, motor skills, and psychosocial skills. Approximately one-third of children with BBS also show behavioral or psychiatric disorders. Some patients may have ataxia, mild hypertonia, or anosmia. A minority of patients have severe intellectual disability. Structural brain anomalies include ventriculomegaly, cortical thinning, reduced size of the corpus striatum, and hippocampal dysgenesis. Up to 50% of individuals develop a subclinical sensorineural hearing loss.

Polydactyly is seen in up to 80% of cases. Other findings, such as brachydactyly, partial syndactyly, and clinodactyly can be found. Up to half of patients have cardiac anomalies including most commonly valvular stenosis or atrial/ventricular septal defects. BBS patients commonly show hypertension and hyperlipidemia. Liver involvement includes fibrosis, small bile ducts, biliary cirrhosis, portal hypertension, and congenital cystic dilatation of both the intrahepatic and extrahepatic biliary tract. Non–insulin-dependent diabetes mellitus is usually seen in adolescence or early adulthood. Dental crowding, hypodontia, and high-arched palate have also been described. Craniofacial defects include brachycephaly, macrocephaly, narrow forehead, frontal balding, large ears, short and narrow palpebral fissures, a long smooth philtrum, depressed nasal bridge, short nose, midface retrusion, and retrognathia.

19.2 Molecular Genetics

BBS is typically an autosomal recessive (AR) condition. At least 20 genetic subtypes have been described (▶ Table 19.1). *BBS1*, *BBS10*, and *BBS8* account for most cases (~23, 20, and 8%, respectively). *BBS6*, *BBS9*, *BBS12*, and *BBS13* each represent 5%. Other subtypes are less frequent. Although there are no clear genotype–phenotype correlations, patients with *BBS1* seem to have less severe ophthalmologic involvement than those with other genotypes (▶ Table 19.1).

CCDC28B, *MKS1*, *MKS3*, and *C2orf86* genes can modify the expression of BBS phenotypes in individuals who have pathogenic variants in other BBS genes. There are reports of unaffected individuals who carry two heterozygous mutations in the same BBS gene, which supports the notion that BBS can be more complex molecularly, requiring three mutant alleles to manifest the phenotype. This is called triallelic inheritance.

Table 19.1 Genes associated with Bardet–Biedl syndrome

Subtype	Gene (locus)
BBS1	*BBS1* (11q13)
BBS2	*BBS2* (16q13)
BBS3	*ARL6* (3q11)
BBS4	*BBS4* (15q22)
BBS5	*BBS5* (2q31)
BBS6	*MKKS* (20p12)
BBS7	*BBS7* (4q27)
BBS8	*TTC8* (14q32)
BBS9	*BBS9* (7p14)
BBS10	*BBS10* (12q)
BBS11	*TRIM32* (9q33)
BBS12	*BBS12* (4q27)
BBS13	*MKS1* (17q23)
BBS14	*CEP290* (12q21)
BBS15	*C2ORF86* (2p15)
BBS16	*SDCCAG8* (1q43)
BBS17	*LZTFL1* (3p21)
BBS18	*BBIP1* (10q25)
BBS19	*IFT27* (22q12)
BBS20	*IFT172* (2p23)
BBS21	*C8orf37* (8q22)

There is also phenotypic heterogeneity. *CEP290* mutations, which are associated with *BBS14*, can also cause Meckel syndrome, Joubert syndrome, and Senior–Løken syndrome. *SDCCAG8* (BBS16) mutations also cause Senior–Løken syndrome.

19.3 Differential Diagnosis

19.3.1 Retinitis Pigmentosa and Cone–Rod Dystrophy

Although retinal degenerations can be confused with BBS, it is the presence of systemic features that makes the diagnosis of BBS of possible. *TTC8* and *ARL6* can cause nonsyndromic RP. Mutations in *C8orf37* have been described with the BBS phenotype, as well in nonsyndromic cone–rod dystrophy (CORD) and RP.

19.3.2 Cohen Syndrome (OMIM 216550)

This is an AR multisystem condition characterized by facial dysmorphism, microcephaly, truncal obesity, intellectual disability, progressive retinopathy, high myopia, and intermittent congenital neutropenia. Cohen syndrome is caused by mutations in *COH1* (8q22).

19.3.3 McKusick–Kaufman Syndrome (OMIM 236700)

This is an AR condition characterized, in particular, by hydrometrocolpos often due to vaginal atresia. Other features include retinal dystrophy, polydactyly, and heart or gastrointestinal malformations. It is caused by *MKKS* gene mutations.

19.3.4 Meckel Syndrome 1 (OMIM 249000)

Also known as Meckel–Gruber syndrome, this is an AR ciliopathy characterized by severe developmental delay, cystic renal disease, central nervous system malformation, polydactyly, and hepatic abnormalities. It is caused by mutations in *MKS1*. There are 11 other subtypes. Mutations in *BBS2*, *BBS4*, and *BBS6* can cause occipital encephalocele, large polycystic kidneys, and postaxial polydactyly. They are usually lethal. Other anomalies include orofacial clefting, genital abnormalities, pulmonary hypoplasia, and liver fibrosis.

19.3.5 Alström Syndrome (OMIM 203800)

This AR condition is caused by mutations in *ALMS1*. It is characterized by CORD, early progression to blindness, obesity, sensorineural hearing impairment, dilated cardiomyopathy, and insulin resistance.

19.3.6 Senior–Løken Syndrome

This syndrome presents with RP and nephronophthisis. It is caused by mutations in *CEP290*, *NPHP1*, *NPHP3*, *NPHP4*, *IQCB1*, and *SDCCAG8*.

19.3.7 Joubert Syndrome (OMIM 213300)

This is a phenotypically and genetically heterogeneous disorder defined by hypoplasia of the cerebellar vermis with the neuroradiologic "molar tooth sign," and associated neurologic symptoms and developmental delay. It may include LCA (Leber congenital amaurosis) and renal abnormalities. *CEP290* mutations (*BBS14*) can also cause Joubert syndrome. Joubert syndrome is also caused by mutations in *AH1*, *TMEM67*, *NPHP1*, *RPGRIP1L*, *CC2D2A*, *ARL13B*, *INPP5E*, *OFD1*, *TMEM216*, *KIF7*, *TCTN1*, *TCTN2*, *TMEM237*, *CEP41*, *TMEM138*, *C5orf42*, and *TTC21B*.

19.3.8 MORM Syndrome (OMIM 610156)

This is a rare AR condition that includes Mental retardation, truncal Obesity, Retinal dystrophy, and Micropenis (MORM). MORM is caused by mutations in *INPP5E* (9q34).

19.3.9 Biemond Syndrome Type II (OMIM 210350)

Biemond syndrome type II (OMIM 210350) presents with intellectual disability, ocular coloboma, obesity, polydactyly, hypogonadism, hydrocephalus, and facial dysostosis. The gene associated with this disorder has not been identified.

19.4 Uncommon Manifestations

Intraretinal cystoid spaces have been described in BBS, but are not associated with a particular genotype.

Glomerular disease has been rarely reported.

19.5 Clinical Testing

19.5.1 Comprehensive Physical Examination

Comprehensive physical examination is made, especially, to evaluate genitalia, teeth, neurologic findings, weight, and cardiac system.

19.5.2 Audiology

Audiology is necessary, especially in younger children or those with speech delay.

19.5.3 Abdominal and Pelvic Ultrasound

Abdominal and pelvic ultrasound examination is performed to assess kidneys and liver in both sexes and ovaries, fallopian tubes, and uterus in affected females.

19.5.4 Renal and Liver Function Tests

Renal and liver function tests are performed to evaluate for possible kidney or liver disease.

19.5.5 Echocardiography

Echocardiography is performed to assess for heart abnormalities.

19.5.6 Magnetic Resonance Imaging

Although not obligatory, magnetic resonance imaging (MRI) may be helpful in some patients to detect structural brain abnormalities.

19.5.7 Full-Field Electroretinogram

Findings include severely reduced or extinguished responses with rod–cone or cone-rod patterns. Abnormalities are often seen after the first year of life, with most patients having significantly abnormal full-field (ff) electroretinogram (ERG) by the age of 5 years.

19.5.8 Optical Coherence Tomography

Optical coherence tomography will show loss of photoreceptors beyond the perifovea, with subfoveal photoreceptor sparing until late in the disease. Intraretinal cystoid spaces may be seen.

19.5.9 Multifocal Electroretinography

This test will often show residual macular function even in patients with advanced disease and can be used for follow-up even when the ffERG is isoelectric.

19.5.10 Goldmann Visual Field

This test will reveal progressive loss of peripheral visual fields. In the end stages of the disease, the field may only be a small residual central area of vision.

19.6 Genetic Testing

Multigene panels are the most effective approach to document pathogenic variants associated with BBS. Some laboratories may only study the most common BBS genes as an initial test. Clinical examination can guide selection of the most appropriate molecular test.

19.7 Problems

19.7.1 Case 1

A 10-year-old boy was referred for ocular examination because of polydactyly and truncal obesity. He has some learning disability. His mother thinks his night vision is poor and notes that he sometimes seems to bump into things. Speech is normal. Best corrected visual acuity is 20/60 in each eye. Cycloplegic refraction is plano. He is not dysmorphic. Slit-lamp examination is normal and funduscopy reveals rare "bone spicule" pigmentary clumping in the midperiphery with vascular attenuation in both eyes and some granular pigmentary alterations in each macula. Refraction is normal. Full-field ERG shows near isoelectric rod function, with moderate cone dysfunction. Which from the following is the most likely diagnosis?
a) BBS.
b) Alström syndrome.
c) Cohen syndrome.
d) Nonsyndromic RP.

Correct answer is a.
   BBS is the most likely diagnosis based on the systemic findings along with an ocular examination and ffERG consistent with rod–cone dystrophy.
a) **Correct.**
b) **Incorrect.** Patients with Alström syndrome usually have a CORD pattern on ffERG rather than rod–cone pattern. They do not have polydactyly.
c) **Incorrect.** Patient does not have facial dysmorphism, microcephaly, intellectual disability, or high myopia.
d) **Incorrect.** Although the systemic findings could be coincidental, a unifying diagnosis of BBS is more likely.

19.7.2 Case 2

A 12-year-old girl comes for ophthalmic evaluation. Family history reveals three cousins affected with BBS associated with a homozygous mutation in the CEP290 gene.

There are also multiple known consanguineous relationships. The girl has developmental delay, hypotonia, and ataxia. Examination shows oculomotor apraxia and retinal dystrophy. MRI shows a malformation of the midbrain–hindbrain, consisting of cerebellar vermis hypoplasia or aplasia, thick and maloriented superior cerebellar peduncles, and abnormally deep interpeduncular fossa (molar tooth sign). Renal function tests are normal. What is the best testing strategy?

a) BBS panel.

b) Retinal dystrophy panel.

c) Whole exome sequencing (WES).

d) CEP290 testing for the familial mutation.

Correct answer is d.

CEP290 mutations, which are associated with *BBS14*, can also cause allelic disorders, such as Meckel syndrome, Joubert syndrome, and Senior–Løken syndrome. The eye movement disorder, developmental delay, and molar tooth sign on brain MRI are consistent with a diagnosis of Joubert syndrome. Testing for the specific familial mutation is cost-efficient and will likely confirm the diagnosis.

a) **Incorrect.** There is already a known cause of BBS in the family. Panel testing is usually more expensive than testing for a single known mutation.

b) **Incorrect.** The diagnosis is known clinically and consistent with the family history. Expanding the testing to include more genes is not likely to be contributory and may even provide confusing information, such as variants of unknown significance in other genes on the panel.

c) **Incorrect.** See b. WES (or specific testing for other Joubert genes) may be indicated only if testing for the familial *CEP290* mutation is surprisingly negative.

d) **Correct.**

19.7.3 Case 3

A 16-year-old boy started having visual acuity decrease 2 years ago, but previously had problems with his night vision. He had surgery of his feet for an "extra toe." Family history is unrevealing. Physical examination is normal. He does not have nystagmus or photophobia. Best corrected visual acuity is 20/80 OD (oculus dextrus) and 20/100 OS (oculus sinister) with –2.00 cylinder in each eye. Fundus examination reveals typical findings of RP. Full-field ERG confirms severe rod–cone dysfunction. A retinal dystrophy panel reveals a previously reported heterozygous mutation and a novel variation of unknown significance (VOUS) in *TTC8*, inherited in trans, one from each asymptomatic parent. Which from the following seems the best alternative?

a) WES.

b) Investigate pathogenicity of the *BBS1* VOUS.

c) BBS panel.

d) Chromosomal microarray.

Correct answer is b.

There are many tools to investigate the pathogenicity of a novel VOUS, including databases, predictor algorithms, proteomics, and population frequency. For example, finding a known mutation in the same codon would support pathogenicity. Although this child does not have obesity or other frank manifestations of BBS, phenotypic heterogeneity for the disorder is well recognized and even isolated RP may occur due to

TTC8 mutation. In this child, the sequence variation was considered pathogenic by PolyPhen-2 analysis, occurred in a well-conserved codon, and was not present in 1,000 ethnically matched controls. This supports its pathogenicity and confirms the diagnosis.

a) **Incorrect.** The pathogenicity analysis of the variation confirms the diagnosis, so WES becomes unnecessary.

b) **Correct.**

c) **Incorrect.** Same answer as a.

d) **Incorrect.** Microarray may be indicated in patients with multisystem disease (in this case polydactyly plus RP), but the genotype–phenotype correlation is explanatory.

Suggested Reading

[1] Khan SA, Muhammad N, Khan MA, Kamal A, Rehman ZU, Khan S. Genetics of human Bardet-Biedl syndrome, an updates. Clin Genet. 2016; 90(1):3–15

[2] M'hamdi O, Ouertani I, Chaabouni-Bouhamed H. Update on the genetics of Bardet-Biedl syndrome. Mol Syndromol. 2014; 5(2):51–56

[3] Abu-Safieh L, Al-Anazi S, Al-Abdi L, et al. In search of triallelism in Bardet-Biedl syndrome. Eur J Hum Genet. 2012; 20(4):420–427

[4] Aldahmesh MA, Li Y, Alhashem A, et al. IFT27, encoding a small GTPase component of IFT particles, is mutated in a consanguineous family with Bardet-Biedl syndrome. Hum Mol Genet. 2014; 23(12):3307–3315

[5] Ansley SJ, Badano JL, Blacque OE, et al. Basal body dysfunction is a likely cause of pleiotropic Bardet-Biedl syndrome. Nature. 2003; 425(6958):628–633

[6] Avidor-Reiss T, Maer AM, Koundakjian E, et al. Decoding cilia function: defining specialized genes required for compartmentalized cilia biogenesis. Cell. 2004; 117(4):527–539

[7] Azari AA, Aleman TS, Cideciyan AV, et al. Retinal disease expression in Bardet-Biedl syndrome-1 (BBS1) is a spectrum from maculopathy to retina-wide degeneration. Invest Ophthalmol Vis Sci. 2006; 47(11):5004–5010

[8] Suspitsin EN, Imyanitov EN. Bardet-Biedl syndrome. Mol Syndromol. 2016; 7(2):62–71

[9] Khan AO, Decker E, Bachmann N, Bolz HJ, Bergmann C. C8orf37 is mutated in Bardet-Biedl syndrome and constitutes a locus allelic to non-syndromic retinal dystrophies. Ophthalmic Genet. 2016; 37(3):290–293

20 Cone–Rod Dystrophy

Abstract

Cone-rod dystrophy is a heterogeneous group of disorders characterized by cone degeneration that is more significant and occurs earlier than the degeneration of rods. Individuals typically complain of progressive central or paracentral visual loss associated with photophobia and color vision anomalies. Nyctalopia and peripheral visual field constriction are delayed in onset. Nystagmus can be present. Patients usually present in childhood or early adulthood. Vision ranges from 20/20 to 20/800, averaging at 20/70. Early in the onset of the disease, patients may be indistinguishable from pure cone dystrophies until the later onset of rod involvement. Examination of older affected family members may be useful to make this distinction.

Keywords: cone–rod dystrophy, retinal degeneration, photophobia, nyctalopia, bull's eye maculopathy

Key Points

- Cone–rod dystrophy (CORD) is a heterogeneous group of disorders characterized by a cone degeneration that is more significant and occurs earlier than the degeneration of rods.
- CORD has high genetic heterogeneity as well as variability in age of onset, association with systemic findings, prognosis, and inheritance patterns.

20.1 Overview

Cone-rod dystrophy (CORD) is a heterogeneous group of disorders characterized by cone degeneration that is more significant and occurs earlier than the degeneration of rods. The estimated prevalence ranges from 1:30,000 to 1:40,000. Individuals with CORD typically complain of progressive central or paracentral visual loss associated with photophobia and color vision anomalies. Nyctalopia and peripheral visual field constriction also occur but may be delayed in onset. Nystagmus can also be present.

Patients usually present in childhood or early adulthood. The average onset age is 10 years, with some patients diagnosed as early as the age of 5 years. Vision ranges from 20/20 to 20/800, averaging usually at 20/70. Night blindness often does not occur until 10 years after the first vision symptoms. Severely constricted visual field can develop on average by the age of 50 years. Early age of onset of the disease is associated with worse visual defects. Early in the onset of the disease, patients may be indistinguishable from pure cone dystrophies until the later onset of rod involvement. Examination of older affected family members may be useful to make this distinction. Although end-stage CORD may look similar to retinitis pigmentosa (RP) on full-field (ff) electroretinogram (ERG), patients with RP will tend to have better preservation of central responses on the multifocal (mf) ERG and corresponding preservation of central vision.

The majority of CORD patients present with decreased visual acuity, photophobia impaired color vision, central or paracentral scotomas, and fundus examination revealing maculopathy. With the progression of the disease, patients develop nyctalopia,

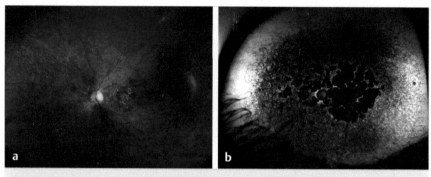

Fig. 20.1 Patient with cone–rod dystrophy caused by heterozygous mutation of the *ABCA4* gene (c.5929G > A and c.*55G > A). **(a)** Wide angle fundus picture showing pigmented macular chorioretinal atrophy associated with vessel attenuation and preretinal gliosis. **(b)** Fundus autofluorescence of same patient revealing nummular hypo-autofluorescent patches in the macula associated with a hyperfluorescent granular ring on the midperiphery.

peripheral visual field contraction, and decreasing scotopic responses on ffERG. On fundus examination, the macular appearance can be normal in the early stages or patients may have mild to moderate vessel attenuation, bull's eye maculopathy, macular atrophy, pigmentary alterations in the perifovea, and macula and/or pigmentary changes in the midperiphery (▶ Fig. 20.1). Temporal optic nerve pallor may be an early sign. Although there are no pathognomonic findings for each subtype, X-linked CORD can be associated with high myopia photophobia.

20.2 Molecular Genetics

The genetic basis of CORD is complex and highly heterogeneous (▶ Table 20.1). Inheritance can be either autosomal recessive (AR; up to 80%), autosomal dominant (AD; up to 20%), or X-linked recessive (1%). Approximately 30 genes have been implicated in CORD (https://sph.uth.edu/retnet/; March 2015). Most mutations are missense (up to 80%), but splicing defects (up to 25%) and nonsense mutations (up to 15%) also occur. Frameshift insertions or deletions have rarely been reported (▶ Table 20.1).

The most frequent genes associated with each inheritance pattern are *ABCA4* (AR), *GUCY2D* (AD), and *RPGR* (X-linked recessive). Depending on the population, mutations in *ABCA4* and *GUCY2D* can be as high as 65 and 30%, respectively. Depending on the reported clinical series, 25 to 60% of AR CORD patients have an identifiable mutation. This number is nearly 100% for AD CORD.

In approximately half of CORD3 patients, biallelic *ABCA4* mutations are found, whereas the other half show only heterozygous mutations. Deep intronic sequencing can increase the detection rate by an additional 30%. The molecular etiology of the remaining patients remains unknown and could theoretically include digenic disease, epigenetic effects, or an unknown regulator of *ABCA4*. The amount of residual *ABCA4* function appears to determine the phenotype. Whereas *ABCA4* null alleles produce RP, the combination of a null allele and a moderately affected allele may produce CORD. Sometimes this clinical continuum can be defined only on the basis of the ERG patterns.

Table 20.1 Molecular Genetics of Cone-Rod Dystrophy (CORD)

CORD (OMIM)	Locus	Gene (inheritance)[a]
CORD1 (600624)	18q21.1-q21.3	Unknown (AD)
CORD2 (120970)	19q13.3	CRX (AD)
CORD3 (604116)	1p22	ABCA4 (AR)
CORD4 (162200)	17q11.2	Associated with NF1[b]
CORD5 (600977)	17p13	PITPNM3 (AD)
CORD6 (601777)	17p13.1	GUCY2D (AD)
CORD7 (603649)	6q13	RIMS1 (AD)
CORD8 (605549)	1q12-q24	Unknown (AR)
CORD9 (612775)	8p11	ADAM9 (AR)
CORD10 (610283)	1q22	SEMA4A (AD)
CORD11 (610381)	19p13.3	RAXL1 (AR)
CORD12 (612657)	4p15	PROM1 (AD)
CORD13 (608194)	14q11	RPGRIP1 (AR)
CORD14 (602093)	6p21.1	GUCA1A (AD)
CORD15 (613660)	10q23.1	CDHR1 (AR)
CORD16 (614500)	8q22.1	C8ORF37 (AR)
CORD17 (615163)	10q26	Unknown (AD)
CORD18 (615374)	4p15	RAB28 (AR)
CORD19 (615860)	14q24	TTLL5 (AR)
CORD20 (615973)	12q21	POC1B (AR)
CORD21 (616502)	1p13	DRAM2 (AR)
CORDX1 (304020)	Xp21.1-p11.3	RPGR (X-linked)
CORDX2 (300085)	Xq27.2-28	Unknown (X-linked)
CORDX3 (300476)	Xp11.4-q13.1	CACNA1F (X-linked)

[a]Other genes described in CORD: (1) AD inheritance—AIPL1, PRPH2, and UNC119; (2) AR inheritance—ATF6, C21orf2, CACNA2D4, CERKL, CNGA3, CNGB3, CNNM4, GNAT2, KCNV2, PDE6C, PDE6H, and RDH5.
[b]One case of CORD associated with neurofibromatosis type 1.

Despite genetic heterogeneity, some phenotype–genotype correlation can be observed. CORD2, CORD8, and CORD13 frequently present with profound visual loss. CORD8 additionally can have severe photophobia and epiphora, with a high degree of fundus granularity and marked macular degeneration. In addition to childhood onset, moderate myopia and pendular nystagmus have been seen in CORD6. Patients with CORD7 may present with late-onset symptoms between the ages of 20 and 40 years, with difficulty in bright light, foveal pigmentary changes, and macular atrophy. Patients with CORD11 have electronegative b-waves. CORD15 has been associated with coexistent oculocutaneous albinism in the absence of mutations in TYR or OCA2. Adult-onset RP has been observed as an alternate phenotype in CORD15 and CORD16. High myopia and aggressive CORD have been described in CORD18, with nondetectable photopic responses and reduced scotopic responses. Recessive PROM1 mutations have been seen in CORD associated with high myopia and nystagmus.

20.3 Differential Diagnosis

20.3.1 Cone Dystrophy (OMIM 180020;602903;610478)

This group of disorders can be distinguished from CORD because the latter have eventual rod involvement or concomitant progressive loss of both cones and rods on ffERG. Symptoms can be similar to CORD, with loss of visual acuity, photophobia, and color vision alterations. Patients with CORD may also experience nyctalopia, and show retinal vascular attenuation and midperipheral pigment deposits. Inheritance patterns can be AD, AR, or X-linked recessive. *CACNA2D4, POC1B, CNGA3, CNGB3, CACNA2D4,* and *KCNV2* gene mutations have been seen in AR cone dystrophy (COD). *GUCA1A, GCAP1, RETGC-1/GUCY2D,* and *PDE6H* mutations have been associated with AD COD. X-linked recessive COD has been associated with mutations in *RPGR, GUCA1, OPN1LW, OPN1MW,* and *CACNA1F.*

20.3.2 Achromatopsia (OMIM 262300)

This condition usually presents with nystagmus from infancy and unlike CORD is nonprogressive, with normal retinal appearance and normal rod responses. CORD usually is not associated with hyperopia, which can be seen in up to 30% of patients with achromatopsia.

20.3.3 Oligocone Trichromacy (OMIM 303900)

This stationary condition presents with vision that ranges between 20/40 and 20/400. Color vision and ffERG are usually normal, and mfERG shows reduced macular responses.

20.3.4 Blue Cone Monochromatism (OMIM 303700)

Color vision is affected in the deutan/protan axis. Patients often have nystagmus.

20.3.5 Bornholm Eye Disease (OMIM 300843)

This X-linked recessive condition is characterized by high myopia, amblyopia, and deuteranopia. Other signs include optic nerve hypoplasia and nonspecific retinal pigment abnormalities. *CXORF2* is a candidate gene although mutations in *OPN1LW* have also been suggested.

20.3.6 Stargardt Disease (OMIM 248200)

Classic Stargardt disease should not have rod involvement and unlike CORD is associated with subretinal lipofuscin flecks, normal retinal vessels, and silent choroid on intravenous fluorescein angiography (IVFA).

20.3.7 Retinitis Pigmentosa

Patients with RP typically develop night blindness and progressive impairment of the peripheral visual field before a reduction in central vision. In addition, they show scotopic amplitudes more severely reduced than their photopic amplitudes.

20.3.8 Bardet–Biedl Syndrome

This AR disease is associated with retinal dystrophy along with polydactyly, obesity, hypogonadism, psychomotor delay, and renal abnormalities. It can resemble RP although a CORD-like phenotype has been described.

20.3.9 Spinocerebellar Ataxia Type 7 (OMIM 164500)

Spinocerebellar Ataxia Type 7 (OMIM 164500) is an AD spinocerebellar degeneration due to expansions of polyglutamine in the ataxin protein. The retinal degeneration usually begins with macular granularity that progressively spreads out to the rest of the retina while macular atrophy progresses.

20.3.10 Aplasia Cutis Congenital, High Myopia, and Cone–Rod Dysfunction (OMIM 601075)

This is a rare AR condition. No causative gene has been described.

20.3.11 Jalili/Heimler Syndrome (OMIM 217080)

These conditions are characterized by CORD and amelogenesis imperfecta. In Heimler syndrome, abnormal great toenails and hearing deficits may also be observed. Although the phenotypes overlap, Jalili syndrome is caused by biallelic mutations in the *CNNM4* gene and Heimler syndrome is caused by mutations in the *PEX1* or *PEX6* genes.

20.3.12 Alström Syndrome (OMIM 203800)

These patients may be confused with CORD because they present in childhood with high-frequency, small-amplitude nystagmus and photophobia with abnormalities in ffERG that can be almost indistinguishable from achromatopsia. Rod involvement and eventual blindness ensue thereafter. Associated systemic findings such as sensorineural hearing loss, obesity, hyperinsulinemia, type 2 diabetes mellitus, and dilated cardiomyopathy lead to the diagnosis. It is caused by *ALMS1* mutations.

20.3.13 Cohen Syndrome (OMIM 216550)

This is an AR disorder characterized by facial dysmorphism, microcephaly, truncal obesity, intellectual disability, intermittent neutropenia, and progressive retinopathy that may resemble CORD in the initial stages. It is caused by *COH1* gene mutations.

20.3.14 Thiamine-Responsive Megaloblastic Anemia (OMIM 249270)

Also known as Roger syndrome, this entity is characterized by megaloblastic anemia, diabetes mellitus, and sensorineural deafness. A CORD-like retinal degeneration has been occasionally described. It is caused by *SLC19A2* gene mutations.

20.3.15 Spondylometaphyseal Dysplasia with Cone–Rod Dystrophy (OMIM 608940)

This condition is characterized by postnatal growth deficiency resulting in short stature, rhizomelia with bowing of the lower extremities, platyspondyly, progressive metaphyseal irregularity, and cupping with shortened tubular bones. These patients present with early-onset visual impairment associated with progressive CORD. *PCYT1A* gene mutations are causative.

20.3.16 Cone–Rod Dystrophy Associated with *ADAMTS18*

Mutations in *ADAMTS18* have been associated with microcornea, ectopia lentis, corectopia, and early-onset CORD. These features overlap with Knobloch syndrome, caused by mutations in the same gene, which demonstrates a severely myopic fundus with geographic macular atrophy and possible retinal detachment.

CORD can also be seen in other rare conditions, such as hypotrichosis with juvenile macular dystrophy (OMIM 601553) or metabolic dysfunctions such as Refsum's disease (OMIM 266500).

20.4 Uncommon Manifestations

Childhood CORD with macular cystic degeneration from recessive *CRB1* mutations has been reported (homozygous *CRB1* mutation; c.80G > T). ERG shows CORD with an electronegative waveform. Hypogonadism and hearing impairment have been associated with CORD1. Anterior polar cataracts have been described in CORD9. Serpentine subretinal deposits can also be seen in CORD patients.

20.5 Clinical Testing

20.5.1 Full-Field Electroretinogram

Early in the disease, the photopic cone b-wave amplitude is reduced more than the scotopic rod b-wave amplitude. Initially, the scotopic responses may even be normal. Later, both rod and cone responses tend to be severely affected, resembling RP. ERG testing can also be used as a method for prediction of disease progression.

20.5.2 Multifocal Electroretinogram

Multifocal ERG depicts reduced nondetectable responses.

20.5.3 Optical Coherence Tomography

Optical coherence tomography (OCT) reveals macular thinning with loss of the central photoreceptors.

20.5.4 Fundus Autofluorescence

The usual finding is macular hypo-autofluorescence. In CORD due to *ABCA4* pathogenic variation, lipofuscin accumulation can be seen as hyper-autofluorescence.

20.5.5 Intravenous Fluorescein Angiography

Sometimes, clinical findings can orient toward a molecular etiology, such as flecks or silent choroid on IVFA (*ABCA4*). It is also helpful to differentiate true CME (cystoid macular edema) from intraretinal cystoid spaces.

20.5.6 Goldmann Visual Field

Goldmann visual field initially shows central or paracentral scotoma. It is not till later in the disease when peripheral constriction also occurs.

20.5.7 Color Vision

Color vision is mildly to moderately impaired usually without a specific color axis.

20.6 Genetic Testing

CORD multigene panels are available. Broader panels for retinal dystrophy or RP may be useful as well, especially when unusual manifestations are present. Many patients are presumed to have COD and have negative panels that are later explained by the onset of rod involvement.

20.7 Problems

20.7.1 Case 1

A 40-year-old woman comes for a second opinion. She was diagnosed with RP when she was 30 years old. Her first symptoms were when she was 10 years old, presenting with progressive decrease of visual acuity. Nyctalopia and visual field constriction started in her 20s. Family history is unremarkable. Examination reveals visual acuity of 20/400 in both eyes. Funduscopy shows macular atrophy, vascular peripheral attenuation and midperipheral pigmentary changes without clumping. ffERG shows moderate rod dysfunction, and severe cone dysfunction. Which is the best diagnostic tool to confirm this patient's condition?

a) RP panel.
b) CORD panel.
c) *ALMS1*.
d) Chromosomal microarray.

Correct answer is b.
   Based on the ERG and history of central vision loss before peripheral vision loss, the patient has CORD rather than RP. As there is no specific finding for a known gene, a CORD panel would be most appropriate.

a) **Incorrect**. Patient's history and ffERG suggest cone greater and earlier than rod involvement. RP has rod involvement greater and earlier than cones. Macular atrophy is a later finding in RP, whereas "bone spicule" pigmentary clumping in the midperiphery is seen earlier.
b) **Correct**.
c) **Incorrect**. The patient has no systemic signs of Alström syndrome.
d) **Incorrect**. In the absence of involvement of another organ system or additional malformations, a copy number variation is unlikely.

20.7.2 Case 2

A 45-year-old man comes for his annual eye examination. He has seen the same ophthalmologist for the last 15 years and was diagnosed with "possible CORD." His symptoms started at the age of 16 years, presenting with progressive decrease of visual acuity and photophobia. He has no other symptoms. Family history is unremarkable. He also brings you two ffERGs (from 10 and 5 years ago, respectively) that show progressive cone involvement, but no rod dysfunction. Examination reveals visual acuity of 20/200 in both eyes. Funduscopy shows macular atrophy, no vascular attenuation, and normal periphery. You perform a new ffERG that shows no rod dysfunction and severe cone dysfunction. Which from the following seems a better alternative to explain patient's condition?

a) Patient has COD instead of CORD.
b) Patient has CORD but needs more time to develop rod dysfunction.
c) Retinal dystrophy panel should be performed to elucidate the diagnosis.
d) CORD panel is the better alternative to differentiate from COD.

Correct answer is a.

Based on the consecutive ERG and history of central but no peripheral vision loss, the patient has COD instead of CORD. The patient has had enough follow-up to determine that rods were not part of his condition.

a) **Correct.**
b) **Incorrect.** Ten years is sufficient time for rod dysfunction to develop.
c) **Incorrect.** Phenotype clearly reveals that there is not diffuse retinal dysfunction. It won't be cost-effective to order a retinal dystrophy panel.
d) **Incorrect.** Same as c. COD panel would be sufficient to diagnose this patient.

20.7.3 Case 3

A 17-year-old female presents with retinal dystrophy. She has progressive decrease of visual acuity. She complains of mild nyctalopia. Family history reveals that her parents are first-degree cousins. Complete physical examination shows mild facial dysmorphism, microcephaly, and obesity. She also has some "developmental delay" and recurrent gingival and skin infections. Examination reveals visual acuity of 20/150 and 20/70 respectively. Fundus examination shows macular atrophy and midperipheral pigmentary granularity. Full-field ERG shows mild to moderate rod dysfunction and severe cone dysfunction. IVFA does not reveal silent choroid. Which one seems the best candidate gene?

a) BBS1.
b) PEX1.
c) ALMS1.
d) COH1.

Correct answer is d.

The combination of consanguinity, facial dysmorphism, microcephaly, obesity, intellectual disability, recurrent infections, and progressive retinopathy makes us think it is Cohen syndrome. *COH1* gene is causative.

a) **Less appropriate.** Although the patient has obesity and retinal dystrophy, she does not have polydactyly, hypogonadism, or renal abnormalities.

b) **Incorrect**. The patient does not have amelogenesis imperfecta, abnormal great toenails, or hearing deficit.

c) **Less appropriate**. She has no nystagmus, sensorineural hearing loss, type 2 diabetes mellitus, or dilated cardiomyopathy.

d) **Correct**.

20.7.4 Case 4

A 20-year-old man comes in with a history of progressive decrease of visual acuity. He has no nyctalopia or visual field constriction. Family history is noncontributory. Examination shows visual acuity of 20/200 in both eyes. Funduscopy shows beaten bronze appearance macula with some mild degree of atrophy. The patient comments to you that a colleague thought that he has CORD because of some peripheral pigmentary changes but you do not interpret them as pathologic. Further testing reveals macular involvement, with an ffERG showing normal rod function and severe cone dysfunction, a severely affected mfERG, an OCT with macular atrophy but no edema or cystoid spaces, normal Farnsworth's test and IVFA that has window defect, and silent choroid. Which from the following seems the best diagnosis for this patient?

a) Stargardt disease.

b) CORD.

c) Achromatopsia.

d) Enhanced S-cone syndrome.

Correct answer is a.

History and clinical testing make Stargardt disease the first possibility. The typical peripheral findings of CORD include pigmentary deposits that resemble bone spicules, frequently more concentrated in the macular area, accompanied by attenuation of the retinal vessels, sometimes waxy pallor of the optic disc and various degrees of retinal atrophy. Nevertheless, peripheral findings can be interpreted as pathologic or not based on the ERG that in this case shows no rod involvement. The definite sign that confirms *ABCA4* is the silent choroid.

a) **Correct**.

b) **Incorrect**. There is no rod dysfunction in the ffERG.

c) **Incorrect**. Color vision was normal.

d) **Incorrect**. OCT and scotopic ERG were normal.

Suggested Reading

[1] Maugeri A, Klevering BJ, Rohrschneider K, et al. Mutations in the ABCA4 (ABCR) gene are the major cause of autosomal recessive cone-rod dystrophy. Am J Hum Genet. 2000; 67(4):960–966

[2] Bax NM, Sangermano R, Roosing S, et al. Heterozygous deep-intronic variants and deletions in ABCA4 in persons with retinal dystrophies and one exonic ABCA4 variant. Hum Mutat. 2015; 36(1):43–47

[3] Michaelides M, Hardcastle AJ, Hunt DM, Moore AT. Progressive cone and cone-rod dystrophies: phenotypes and underlying molecular genetic basis. Surv Ophthalmol. 2006; 51(3):232–258

[4] Roosing S, Thiadens AA, Hoyng CB, Klaver CC, den Hollander AI, Cremers FP. Causes and consequences of inherited cone disorders. Prog Retin Eye Res. 2014; 42:1–26

[5] Huang L, Xiao X, Li S, et al. Molecular genetics of cone-rod dystrophy in Chinese patients: New data from 61 probands and mutation overview of 163 probands. Exp Eye Res. 2016; 146:252–258

[6] Mayer AK, Rohrschneider K, Strom TM, et al. Homozygosity mapping and whole-genome sequencing reveals a deep intronic PROM1 mutation causing cone-rod dystrophy by pseudoexon activation. Eur J Hum Genet. 2016; 24(3):459–462

[7] Rahner N, Nuernberg G, Finis D, Nuernberg P, Royer-Pokora B. A novel C8orf37 splice mutation and genotype-phenotype correlation for cone-rod dystrophy. Ophthalmic Genet. 2016; 37(3):294–300

[8] Khan AO, Bolz HJ. Pediatric cone-rod dystrophy with high myopia and nystagmus suggests recessive PROM1 mutations. Ophthalmic Genet. 2015; 36(4):349–352

[9] Khan AO, Aldahmesh MA, Abu-Safieh L, Alkuraya FS. Childhood cone-rod dystrophy with macular cystic degeneration from recessive CRB1 mutation. Ophthalmic Genet. 2014; 35(3):130–137

[10] Hamel CP. Cone rod dystrophies. Orphanet J Rare Dis. 2007; 2:7

21 Choroideremia

Abstract

Choroideremia is an X-linked recessive condition that should be suspected in male patients with nyctalopia and progressive chorioretinal degeneration. Patients also experience peripheral visual field loss that initially manifests as a ring scotoma. Fundus changes are seen generally by the second decade of life. The characteristic fundus consists of patchy areas of chorioretinal degeneration that generally begin in the midperiphery and proceed posteriorly. Female carriers have patchy chorioretinal changes that may correspond to visual field scotomas, but generally they do not have symptoms.

Keywords: choroideremia, nyctalopia, chorioretinal degeneration, lyonization, gene therapy, *CHM*

Key Points

- X-linked recessive condition characterized by progressive chorioretinal degeneration.
- Symptoms in affected males evolve from night blindness to peripheral visual field loss, with central vision preserved often for several decades.
- The diagnosis is confirmed with the identification of a mutation in the *CHM* gene.

21.1 Overview

The *CHM* gene codes Rab escort protein-1 (REP-1), which attaches to several Rab GTPases. REP-1 is a key component of Rab geranylgeranyl transferase, an enzyme complex that mediates intracellular vesicular transport. Most of the mutations in *CHM* result in a truncated product that is degraded. This results in chorioretinal degeneration. The presence of crystals in peripheral blood lymphocytes, significant plasma fatty acid abnormalities, and red blood cell membrane abnormalities suggests that choroideremia (CHM) may be a systemic condition.

CHM is an X-linked recessive condition that should be suspected in male patients with a history of nyctalopia and progressive chorioretinal degeneration. Patients also experience peripheral visual field loss that initially manifests as a ring scotoma that follows the initial changes in the fundus appearance but progresses to severe constriction. Fundus changes are seen generally by the second decade of life. The estimated prevalence is 1:50,000. Individuals present with a characteristic fundus, which consists of patchy areas of chorioretinal degeneration that generally begin in the midperiphery and proceed posteriorly (▶ Fig. 21.1). Areas of degeneration typically demonstrate marked retinal pigment epithelium (RPE) and choriocapillaris loss, but with preservation of the deep choroidal vessels. RPE loss is the primary cause of photoreceptor degeneration in CHM, with a thinner choroid from early stages, which is consistent with a developmental defect. Photoreceptors lose outer segments following loss of underlying RPE. The central macula is usually preserved until late in the disease course and appears as a preserved island of retina often with somewhat scalloped edges. Affected males may not note any symptoms until their teenage years. Visual acuity usually deteriorates after the third decade. Severe visual field constriction is present by

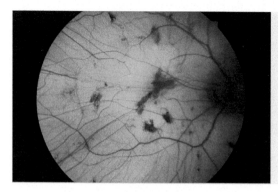

Fig. 21.1 Severe chorioretinal atrophy in a patient with choroideremia.

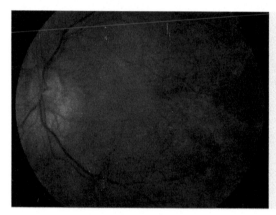

Fig. 21.2 Fundus photography of a female carrier of a mutation in the *CHM* gene showing areas of retinal pigment epithelium change and atrophy due to lyonization.

their 40s, although central visual acuity can be spared until even later. As the disease progresses, CHM may have midperipheral "bone spicule" pigmentary clumps. About 40 to 60% of CHM patients will have macular cystic spaces in at least one eye on optical coherence tomography (OCT). Posterior subcapsular cataracts can be found in one-third of affected males. Female carriers have patchy chorioretinal changes (▶ Fig. 21.2) that may correspond to visual field scotomas, but generally they do not have symptoms. Adverse lyonization can result in even more demonstrable changes. While no accepted treatment exists for CHM, promising approaches using viral vector gene therapy are entering clinical trials. Results from the first gene therapy trial revealed sustained visual improvement over 6 months post-treatment, though long-term follow-up is needed.

21.2 Molecular Genetics

CHM (Xq21.2) is the only known gene associated with CHM. The mutation detection rate is nearly 95%. Nonsense mutations are the most commonly observed, although other pathogenic variants such as missense changes, complete gene deletions, intragenic deletions, and frameshifts have been reported. There is no consistent genotype–phenotype correlation.

21.3 Differential Diagnosis

21.3.1 Retinitis Pigmentosa

The retinal appearance of CHM and end-stage RP may be almost indistinguishable due to the similar advanced chorioretinal atrophy and CHM may have midperipheral "bone spicule" pigmentary clumps. Both disorders have nyctalopia and constricted visual fields with preserved central acuity. RP may be X-linked recessive. RP is distinguished from CHM by the usual degree of pigment clumping. Peripheral scalloped degeneration is not seen in RP. Molecular genetic testing may be required to make the correct diagnosis.

21.3.2 Usher Syndrome Type 1 (OMIM 276900)

This condition can be confused with CHM in the context of an Xq21 contiguous deletion syndrome, because of retinal abnormalities and deafness (deletion of the *POU3F4* gene). Nevertheless, Usher syndrome does not present with the scalloped areas of chorioretinal degeneration and like RP, early choroidal atrophy is not seen. The inheritance pattern of Usher syndrome is autosomal recessive (AR).

21.3.3 Gyrate Atrophy (OMIM 258870)

In this AR condition, the progression of scalloped areas of chorioretinal atrophy seen in gyrate atrophy can be confused with CHM although the scalloped areas tend to be more distinct in gyrate atrophy. Patients with gyrate atrophy have elevated plasma ornithine. They do not manifest the choroidal atrophy seen in CHM until the very late stages of the disease.

21.3.4 Central Areolar Choroidal Dystrophy (OMIM 215500)

Also known as choroidal sclerosis, this AR condition predominately affects the macula, resulting in a central well-defined area of atrophy of the RPE and choriocapillaris with visual decline usually between the ages of 30 and 60 years. It has been mapped to 17p13. Genetic heterogeneity has also been described, with CACD2 (OMIM 613105) caused by mutation in the *PRPH2* gene (6p21.2-p12.3) and the CACD3 (OMIM 613144) locus yet to be identified.

21.3.5 Boucher–Neuhauser Syndrome (OMIM 215470)

This is an AR condition caused by biallelic mutation in *PNPLA6* (19p13). This syndrome is characterized by the triad of spinocerebellar ataxia, hypogonadotropic hypogonadism, and visual impairment due to chorioretinal dystrophy. Most patients develop one or more symptoms in the first decade of life, which is earlier than CHM. Chorioretinal dystrophy can be absent.

21.3.6 Leber Congenital Amaurosis

Although Leber congenital amaurosis (LCA) can be confused with CHM, earlier presentation and absence of scalloped chorioretinal degeneration characterize LCA.

21.3.7 Mitochondrial Trifunctional Protein Disorders (OMIM 609015)

Mitochondrial trifunctional protein catalyzes three steps in mitochondrial beta-oxidation of fatty acids: long-chain 3-hydroxyacyl-CoA dehydrogenase (LCHAD), long-chain enoyl-CoA hydratase, and long-chain thiolase activities. Trifunctional protein deficiency is characterized by decreased activity of all three enzymes. Clinically, mitochondrial trifunctional protein disorder (MTPD) can be classified as neonatal onset (severe, usually lethal), infantile onset with a hepatic Reye-like syndrome, and late-adolescent onset of skeletal myopathy. Some affected individuals have a progressive course associated with myopathy, rhabdomyolysis, and sensorimotor axonal neuropathy. LCHAD subtype of MTPD usually have visually disabling chorioretinopathy that may resemble CHM. MTPD is associated with *HADHA* and *HADHB* gene mutations.

21.4 Uncommon Manifestations

When CHM is due to a contiguous gene deletion, other findings may include severe cognitive deficits (caused by deletion of the *RSK4* gene), cleft lip and palate, deafness and agenesis of the corpus callosum.

21.5 Clinical Testing

21.5.1 Intravenous Fluorescein Angiography

IVFA (intravenous fluorescein angiography) demonstrates preservation of the deep choroidal vessels but marked loss of RPE and superficial choroidal vessels.

21.5.2 Visual Field

Peripheral visual field loss typically manifests as a ring scotoma early, followed by severe constriction.

21.5.3 Full-field Electroretinogram

This test reveals in affected males a pattern of rod–cone degeneration that can progress to severe alteration of scotopic and photopic function. The full-field (ff) electroretinogram (ERG) may also be abnormal in female carriers.

21.5.4 Multifocal Electroretinogram

Often the central responses are remarkably preserved even when the scotopic ffERG is isoelectric.

21.5.5 Fundus Autofluorescence

There are marked areas of hypofluorescence and this test may highlight the scalloped loss in the periphery. Female carriers show patchy areas of hypofluorescence that radiate out from the macula.

21.5.6 Optical Coherence Tomography

Central retinal thinning is associated with visual acuity loss. Outer retinal tubulation can be seen as well. Peripapillary chorioretinal atrophy, central retinal thickness, and subfoveal choroidal thickness are useful in monitoring disease progression.

Color vision is abnormal in half of the patients.

21.6 Genetic Testing

Sequencing of the *CHM* gene is usually the first test if the patient is systemically well. If no mutation is found, deletion/duplication analysis can be performed. In the presence of developmental delay, cleft lip and palate, agenesis of the corpus callosum or hearing loss, karyotype, or CMA (chromosomal microarray) should be performed.

21.7 Problems

21.7.1 Case 1

A 30-year-old man complains of nyctalopia. His symptoms started when he was 25 years old. Family history shows that his maternal grandfather died blind at his 50s. The patient's best corrected visual acuity is 20/30 in each eye. Slit-lamp examination is normal. Fundus examination shows scalloped chorioretinal degeneration in the periphery. Full-field ERG reveals severe rod and cone dysfunction. Which from the following tests seems more appropriate?

a) Retinal dystrophy panel.
b) LCA panel.
c) Audiometry.
d) *CHM* sequencing.

Correct answer is d.

This case is the typical presentation of CHM. The scalloped peripheral lesions, early preserved central vision, and family history suggestive of X-linked recessive inheritance are particularly indicative.

a) **Less appropriate.** Although many panels may include *CHM*, this strategy would not be cost-effective.
b) **Incorrect.** Symptoms started in adulthood.
c) **Incorrect.** Patient is not complaining about hearing loss and most late presentation patients with Usher syndrome are symptomatic by the age of 20 years.
d) **Correct.**

21.7.2 Case 2

A 35-year-old man presents for genetic counseling. He has three unaffected sisters, an affected brother, and their maternal grandfather and his brother died "blind." Examination shows severe diffuse chorioretinal atrophy, some pigment clumps throughout the retina and abolished ffERG. Which of the following tests is most appropriate?

a) *CHM* sequencing.
b) *RPGR/RP2* sequencing.
c) Mitochondrial panel.
d) Retinal dystrophy panel.

Correct answer is d.

End-stage CHM can resemble end-stage RP. Therefore, it is extremely difficult to suggest specific gene sequencing. Although family history suggests X-linked recessive inheritance, this could be X-linked recessive RP or CHM. In this case, testing revealed a hemizygous *CHM* mutation.

a) **Incorrect.** Clinical presentation not specific for CHM.

b) **Incorrect.** Clinical presentation not specific for RP.

c) **Incorrect.** Patients did not have any systemic signs suggestive of mitochondrial disease.

d) **Correct.**

21.7.3 Case 3

A 20-year-old man presents with nyctalopia and reduced visual acuity. Family history shows that he has an affected brother and maternal grandfather, with two unaffected sisters. His best corrected visual acuity is 20/30 in both eyes. Slit-lamp examination is normal. Fundus examination shows peripheral scalloped chorioretinal atrophy with mild pigment clumping within the affected areas. Full-field ERG reveals severe rod–cone dysfunction pattern. *CHM* sequencing was normal. Which of the following tests is most appropriate?

a) Retinal dystrophy panel.

b) Deletion/duplication analysis.

c) *RPGR/RP2* sequencing.

d) *PNPLA6* sequencing.

Correct answer is b.

This patient demonstrates a classic fundus appearance for early CHM associated with an X-linked recessive inheritance pattern. If sequencing is normal, deletion/duplication analysis can be performed.

a) **Incorrect.** Clinical presentation is strongly suggestive of CHM. Further molecular studies should be carried out to confirm this diagnosis.

b) **Correct.**

c) **Less appropriate.** Clinical presentation is not typical of RP.

d) **Incorrect.** *PNPLA6* mutations present with spinocerebellar ataxia, hypogonadotropic hypogonadism, and chorioretinal dystrophy.

21.7.4 Case 4

A 27-year-old asymptomatic woman was told that she "might have early RP," on an ophthalmic examination. Her father has "night vision problems" that started when he was 30 years old and poor day vision. She also has a brother who is unable to drive at night. Her best corrected visual acuity is 20/25 in both eyes. Slit-lamp examination is normal. Fundus examination shows scattered small areas of chorioretinal atrophy. Goldmann visual fields show several small relative scotomas. Full-field ERG reveals mild rod–cone dysfunction. Fundus autofluorescence (FAF) shows scattered areas of hypofluorescence corresponding to the clinical examination. OCT is normal. What is the most likely diagnosis?

a) Early RP.

b) Ocular histoplasmosis.

c) *CHM* carrier.

d) Normal variant.

Correct answer is c.

Female carriers of *CHM* mutations are generally asymptomatic. Signs of chorioretinal degeneration can be observed on fundus examination. These findings become more readily apparent after the second decade. Nyctalopia and field loss can also develop later in life due to expanding areas of chorioretinal atrophy. Symptomatic females who demonstrate clinical findings that mimic those of affected males likely have skewed X chromosome inactivation.

a) **Incorrect.** Early RP would have an ffERG with more predominant reduction in rod responses as the clinical features often follow the ffERG changes. Fundus findings more characteristically show "bone spicule" pigmentary clumping in the midperiphery and FAF shows a hyperfluorescent ring in the macula.

b) **Incorrect.** Patients have prominent chorioretinal scars and a normal ffERG as the disease is focal. Although the family history may be unrelated, histoplasmosis is not a genetic disorder.

c) **Correct.**

d) **Incorrect.** An abnormal ffERG is never a normal variant.

22 Enhanced S-Cone Syndrome and Other *NR2E3*-Related Retinal Dystrophies

Abstract

NR2E3 mutations are associated with three distinct phenotypes: enhanced S-cone syndrome, Goldman–Favre syndrome, and retinitis pigmentosa. Enhanced S-cone syndrome is a rare autosomal recessive inherited retinal dystrophy that has variable clinical presentation. In this condition, S-cones are the majority cone subtype, whereas in a normal adult retina S-cones represent approximately only 10% of total cones. Best corrected visual acuity ranges from 20/20 to 20/200. Fundus findings include nummular pigment clumping at the level of the retinal pigment epithelium along the vascular arcades and in the midperiphery, midperiphery and macular yellow flecks, macular cystoid spaces, macular hyperpigmentation with foveal sparing, and chorioretinal atrophic changes.

Keywords: enhanced S-cone syndrome, Goldman–Favre syndrome, retinitis pigmentosa, cystoid spaces, *NR2E3*

Key Points

- Enhanced S-cone syndrome (ESCS) is a retinal disorder, caused by *NR2E3* mutations, that is characterized by increased sensitivity to blue light, nyctalopia from an early age, and decreased vision. Electroretinogram shows extinguished scotopic responses and hypersensitivity to shorter blue wavelengths.
- Patients with *NR2E3* mutations may have optically empty liquefied vitreous, progressive foveal or peripheral retinoschisis, intraretinal cystoid spaces, chorioretinal atrophy, and/or pigmentary retinopathy.

22.1 Overview

The nuclear receptor class 2, subfamily E, member 3 protein is encoded by the *NR2E3* gene, which is uniquely expressed in the outer nuclear layer of the retina. In addition, there is some evidence that *NR2E3* suppresses cone differentiation during embryogenesis. *NR2E3* pathogenic variants are associated with three distinct phenotypes: enhanced S-cone syndrome (ESCS), Goldman–Favre syndrome, and retinitis pigmentosa (RP).

22.1.1 Enhanced S-Cone Syndrome

ESCS is a rare autosomal recessive (AR) inherited retinal dystrophy that has variable clinical presentation. In this condition, S-cones are the majority cone subtype, whereas in a normal adult retina S-cones represent approximately only 10% of total cones. Normal posterior pole retina associated with arcades is a rod-rich zone. In ESCS, cones replace these rods and affected individuals present with symptoms of nyctalopia and visual field constriction from an early age. Best corrected visual acuity ranges from 20/20 to 20/200. Fundus findings include nummular pigment clumping at the level of the

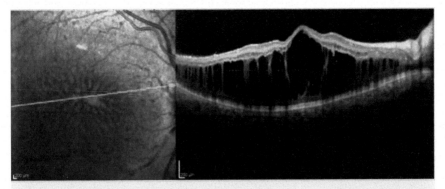

Fig. 22.1 Macular intraretinal cystoid spaces in a patient with compound heterozygous mutations in *NR2E3*. Left image shows macular spoke-wheel pattern.

retinal pigment epithelium (RPE) along the vascular arcades and in the midperiphery, midperiphery and macular yellow flecks, macular cystoid spaces (▶ Fig. 22.1), macular hyperpigmentation with foveal sparing, and chorioretinal atrophic changes. Vitreous cells, opacities, haze, and veils can be seen. Ophthalmic findings can be seen as early as 4 years of age.

22.1.2 Goldmann–Favre Syndrome

The classic Goldmann–Favre phenotype includes vitreous liquefaction with fibrillar strands and veils, nyctalopia, and severely abnormal full-field electroretinogram (ffERG) in early childhood. Patients tend to be hyperopic. As the condition progresses, patients develop chorioretinal atrophy, pigmentary retinal degeneration, marked visual field loss, peripheral and macular retinoschisis, and subcapsular cataract.

22.1.3 Retinitis Pigmentosa

NR2E3 mutations have been implicated in progressive degeneration of rods and subsequent involvement of cones, with characteristic "bone spicule" midperipheral pigmentation of RP. Disease may be AR or autosomal dominant (AD). Affected individuals show a decline of cone function relatively late, at a time when rod function is already undetectable.

22.1.4 Clumped Pigmentary Retinal Degeneration

Some patients may present with a specific pattern called clumped pigmentary retinal degeneration, which is found in less than 1% of RP cases. This pattern is characterized by abnormal nummular pigment clumping in the midperiphery or in the region of the arcades.

22.2 Molecular Genetics

These phenotypes are caused by *NR2E3* mutations although there are no clear genotype–phenotype associations. RP shows genetic heterogeneity.

22.3 Differential Diagnosis

22.3.1 Retinitis Pigmentosa

Mutations in *NR2E3* can present as RP with the presence of nummular pigmentary clumping or subretinal fibrosis is often seen as part of *NR2E3* RP.

22.3.2 Congenital Stationary Night Blindness (OMIM 310500; 300071; 257270; 613216)

Because of early nyctalopia, this condition may be confused with ESCS. Nevertheless, nystagmus is a hallmark feature of congenital stationary night blindness (CSNB), which is not present in ESCS.

22.3.3 X-Linked Juvenile Retinoschisis (OMIM 312700)

This condition, characterized by impaired vision and macular intraretinal cystoid spaces, may be difficult to distinguish from ESCS by optical coherence tomography (OCT). Juvenile X-linked retinoschisis (JXLR) occurs almost exclusively in males, making ESCS a primary differential in female patients with intraretinal cystoid spaces. Mutations in *RS1* cause JXLR. Peripheral retinoschisis is also seen in many patients although this can also be seen in Goldman–Favre syndrome.

22.3.4 Other Disorders with Intraretinal Cystoid Spaces

Other disorders with intraretinal cystoid spaces include fenestrated sheen dystrophy, pathologic myopia, *NR2E3* retinopathies, degenerative macular schisis, drug induced (niacin), vitreomacular traction, isolated foveomacular schisis, and a wide range of retinal dystrophies.

22.3.5 Cystoid Macular Edema

As opposed to the nonleaking intraretinal cystoid spaces of ESCS and other disorders, the clinical diagnosis of cystoid macular edema (CME) is made based on a pattern of late progressive hyperfluorescence (leakage) on intravenous fluorescein angiography (IVFA) often showing a perifoveal petaloid pattern. There is a wide range of causes including inflammation, diabetes, optic nerve pits, and other conditions including the genetic disorder AD CME.

22.3.6 Clumped Pigmentary Retinopathy

Some patients with this phenotype have mutations in *CRB1* or *TULP1*.

22.3.7 Torpedo Maculopathy

ESCS-associated torpedo-like lesions differ from the typical isolated torpedo lesions, which tend to be relatively large with a sharp narrowed end that points to the foveola and are usually located temporal to the fovea, with normal surrounding RPE. The isolated torpedo lesions are congenital and are thought to be produced by abnormal RPE or choroidal or ciliary vasculature maldevelopment.

22.4 Uncommon Manifestations

Torpedo-like lesions may be seen in some patients. These are variable in size and can be located through the posterior pole. They present with central depigmentation or chorioretinal atrophy with a hyperpigmented border with surrounding abnormal RPE. These lesions are nonprogressive.

Circumferential macular fibrosis (helicoid fibrosis) may also be seen in patients with ESCS, and may be associated with subretinal hemorrhages. Vasoproliferative retinal tumors have been rarely observed with Goldmann–Favre syndrome.

22.5 Clinical Testing

22.5.1 Optical Coherence Tomography

OCT reveals the characteristic intraretinal cystoid spaces. Other findings include epiretinal membrane, subretinal fibrosis, outer retinal tubulations, intraretinal lesions (in the context of yellow dots), photoreceptor loss, and patchy RPE loss.

22.5.2 Fundus Autofluorescence

Patients with ESCS may have a large macular hypo-autofluorescent ring with a hyper-autofluorescent center. The hypo-autofluorescent ring usually corresponds to areas of subretinal fibrosis. Some individuals will have blocking to clumped pigmentary changes in the RP phenotype; fundus autofluorescence (FAF) may reveal three concentric rings of hyper-autofluorescence.

22.5.3 Electroretinogram

Characteristic findings of ESCS include extinguished scotopic responses and hypersensitivity to shorter blue wavelengths. There is a disproportionately reduced 30-Hz cone flicker to the single-flash cone amplitude. Specific S-cone stimuli show supernormal responses. RP and clumped pigmentary phenotypes will show a pattern of rod–cone dystrophy.

22.6 Genetic Testing

NR2E3 full gene analysis is available.

22.7 Problems

22.7.1 Case 1

A 12-year-old girl was referred for nyctalopia and reduced visual acuity. Her family history is unrevealing. Vision acuity was 20/100 in both eyes with insignificant refractive error. Fundus examination showed some small yellow round flecks in the macula and

some patches of subretinal fibrosis. Vitreous was normal. FAF demonstrated hypo-autofluorescence corresponding to the areas of fibrosis and a ring of hyper-autofluorescence. OCT showed intraretinal cystoid spaces in the maculas that did not leak on IVFA. Her ffERG revealed extinguished scotopic responses and hypersensitivity to shorter blue wavelengths. Which from the following seems the most appropriate diagnosis?
a) X-linked retinoschisis.
b) CSNB.
c) Goldmann–Favre syndrome.
d) ESCS.

Correct answer is d.

The history of nyctalopia and decreased visual acuity is associated, and the typical clinical findings and diagnostic testing results suggest a diagnosis of ESCS. The patient was found to be a compound heterozygote for previously reported mutations in *NR2E3* (c.119–2A > C and c.767C > T).

a) **Incorrect.** The patient is female, so this is unlikely.

b) **Less appropriate.** There is no nystagmus and ERG showed hypersensitivity to shorter blue wavelengths. CSNB usually shows electronegative responses.

c) **Incorrect.** There are no vitreous abnormalities. Photopic ERG in Goldman–Favre syndrome is usually below normal.

d) **Correct.**

22.7.2 Case 2

A 20-year-old man comes for visual acuity decrease and nyctalopia that began at the age of 8 years. He has an affected sister with the same condition. His parents are second cousins. Best corrected visual acuity was counting fingers with +4.00 sph OD and +3.00 sph OS. Anterior segment examination was unremarkable. Fundus examination revealed multiple vitreous membranes, posterior vitreous detachment, macular pigment clumping, equatorial chorioretinal atrophy at one quadrant, and lamellar macular holes. OCT demonstrated intraretinal cystoid changes, in addition to the lamellar macular holes in both eyes. Full-field ERG showed markedly reduced scotopic a-wave and b-wave amplitudes. Which from the following seems the most appropriate diagnosis?
a) Juvenile X-linked retinoschisis.
b) CSNB.
c) Goldmann–Favre syndrome.
d) ESCS.

Correct answer is c.

The combination of significant vitreous abnormalities, nyctalopia, and severely affected ffERG is very indicative of Goldmann–Favre syndrome. The family history of consanguinity raises the probability of an AR condition. The patient was found to be homozygous for an *NR2E3* mutation (c.1117 A > G).

a) **Incorrect.** Although the patient is male, he has an affected sister. JXLR only affects males as it is an X-linked recessive condition. Vitreous abnormalities are more severe in Goldmann–Favre syndrome. The ERG in JXLR typically shows electronegative responses.

b) **Incorrect.** There is no nystagmus, the history reveals progressive visual loss, and the presence of vitreoretinal abnormalities rules out CSNB. Full-field ERG in CSNB often shows electronegative responses.

c) **Correct.**

d) **Incorrect.** The patient has severe vitreous abnormalities, more consistent with Goldmann–Favre syndrome rather than ESCS. The photopic ERG is supernormal to S-cone stimuli in ESCS and in this case it is not.

22.7.3 Case 3

A 30-year-old woman was referred for evaluation of nyctalopia. Her symptoms started when she was 20 years old. She has an affected brother. Her parents are consanguineous. Best corrected visual acuity is 20/60 in both eyes (–1.00 sph oculus uterque [OU]). Fundus changes reveal bone spicules, vascular attenuation, and pale optic discs. Full-field ERG was severely impaired, presenting a rod–cone pattern. Which from the following tests seem more appropriate to order?

a) *RHO* sequencing.

b) *NR2E3* sequencing.

c) CORD (cone–rod dystrophy) panel.

d) Retinal dystrophy panel.

Correct answer is d.

Clinical presentation of this RP, which is likely AR, is nonspecific, so directed *NR2E3* or other gene sequencing is not appropriate as there is no specific genotype–phenotype correlation and there is a large number of possible gene mutations that could explain the phenotype.

a) **Incorrect.** Mutations in *RHO* usually cause AD RP. The presence of consanguinity in the parents and two affected siblings suggest AR disease.

b) **Incorrect.** Although NR2E3 mutation is possible, there are no characteristic features of this patient's RP, which would suggest *NR2E3* mutations.

c) **Incorrect.** Full-field ERG has rod–cone pattern, not cone–rod pattern.

d) **Correct.**

Suggested Reading

[1] Yzer S, Barbazetto I, Allikmets R, et al. Expanded clinical spectrum of enhanced S-cone syndrome. JAMA Ophthalmol. 2013; 131(10):1324–1330

[2] Coppieters F, Leroy BP, Beysen D, et al. Recurrent mutation in the first zinc finger of the orphan nuclear receptor NR2E3 causes autosomal dominant retinitis pigmentosa. Am J Hum Genet. 2007; 81(1):147–157

[3] Jacobson SG, Marmor MF, Kemp CM, Knighton RW. SWS (blue) cone hypersensitivity in a newly identified retinal degeneration. Invest Ophthalmol Vis Sci. 1990; 31(5):827–838

[4] Marmor MF, Jacobson SG, Foerster MH, Kellner U, Weleber RG. Diagnostic clinical findings of a new syndrome with night blindness, maculopathy, and enhanced S cone sensitivity. Am J Ophthalmol. 1990; 110 (2):124–134

[5] Jacobson SG, Román AJ, Román MI, Gass JD, Parker JA. Relatively enhanced S cone function in the Goldmann-Favre syndrome. Am J Ophthalmol. 1991; 111(4):446–453

[6] Milam AH, Rose L, Cideciyan AV, et al. The nuclear receptor NR2E3 plays a role in human retinal photoreceptor differentiation and degeneration. Proc Natl Acad Sci U S A. 2002; 99(1):473–478

[7] Bonilha VL, Fishman GA, Rayborn ME, Hollyfield JG. Retinal pathology of a patient with Goldmann-Favre syndrome. Ophthalmic Genet. 2009; 30(4):172–180

[8] Khan AO, Aldahmesh MA, Al-Harthi E, Alkuraya FS. Helicoid subretinal fibrosis associated with a novel recessive NR2E3 mutation p.S44X. Arch Ophthalmol. 2010; 128(3):344–348

[9] Pachydaki SI, Klaver CC, Barbazetto IA, et al. Phenotypic features of patients with NR2E3 mutations. Arch Ophthalmol. 2009; 127(1):71–75

[10] Zweifel SA, Engelbert M, Laud K, Margolis R, Spaide RF, Freund KB. Outer retinal tubulation: a novel optical coherence tomography finding. Arch Ophthalmol. 2009; 127(12):1596–1602

[11] Cassiman C, Spileers W, De Baere E, de Ravel T, Casteels I. Peculiar fundus abnormalities and pathognomonic electrophysiological findings in a 14-month-old boy with NR2E3 mutations. Ophthalmic Genet. 2013; 34(1–2):105–108

[12] Nakamura M, Hotta Y, Piao CH, Kondo M, Terasaki H, Miyake Y. Enhanced S-cone syndrome with subfoveal neovascularization. Am J Ophthalmol. 2002; 133(4):575–577

[13] Sharon D, Sandberg MA, Caruso RC, Berson EL, Dryja TP. Shared mutations in NR2E3 in enhanced S-cone syndrome, Goldmann-Favre syndrome, and many cases of clumped pigmentary retinal degeneration. Arch Ophthalmol. 2003; 121(9):1316–1323

[14] Hull S, Arno G, Sergouniotis PI, et al. Clinical and molecular characterization of enhanced S-cone syndrome in children. JAMA Ophthalmol. 2014; 132(11):1341–1349

23 Stargardt Disease and Other *ABCA4* Retinopathies

Abstract

Stargardt disease is the most frequent childhood recessively inherited macular dystrophy. It is usually caused by *ABCA4* mutations. Patients most commonly present with bilateral or sequential central visual loss. The characteristic retinal finding is a maculopathy with "pisciform" subretinal lipofuscin deposits (flecks). Other phenotypes are associated with *ABCA4* mutations, including age-related macular degeneration, macular atrophy without flecks, bull's eye maculopathy, autosomal recessive cone–rod dystrophy, and autosomal recessive retinitis pigmentosa.

Keywords: Stargardt disease, macular dystrophy, *ABCA4*, lipofuscin, flecks

Key Points

- Stargardt disease (SGD) is the most frequent childhood recessively inherited macular dystrophy.
- Usually caused by *ABCA4* mutations.
- Patients most commonly present with bilateral or sequential central visual loss.
- The characteristic retinal finding is a maculopathy with "pisciform" subretinal lipofuscin deposits (flecks).
- *ABCA4* mutations may present phenotypes other than SGD.

23.1 Stargardt Disease Overview

Stargardt disease (SGD) is the most frequent childhood recessively inherited macular dystrophy. Most patients present with central visual loss in the early teenage years and ophthalmoscopy classically shows macular atrophy with yellowish "pisciform" subretinal flecks at the posterior pole due to lipofuscin deposition (▶ Fig. 23.1). When the flecks extend throughout the retina, the disease is called fundus flavimaculatus. The estimated prevalence is 1 per 10,000 individuals. SGD is caused by mutations in the *ABCA4* gene.

SGD results from the accumulation of lipofuscin in the retinal pigment epithelium (RPE) with secondary photoreceptor dysfunction and subsequent death. *ABCA4* encodes a transmembrane protein that is localized specifically to the retina. It is found in the disc membranes in cone and rod outer segments, where it participates in the retinoid cycle through which 11-cis-retinal recycles, and returns the photoreceptor to its dark adapted state, enabling further phototransduction. It is thought that *ABCA4* works as a "flippase" that transports N-retinylidene-phosphatidylethanolamine across the disc membranes. When *ABCA4* activity drops, there is progressive accumulation of A2E in the RPE as lipofuscin deposits. This is the histological hallmark of SGD. In SGD, lipofuscin can be accumulated up to five times above normal values. This produces a negative effect on the RPE function and survival, altering the cell membrane architecture and

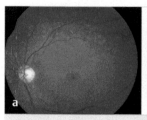 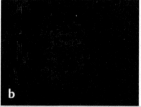 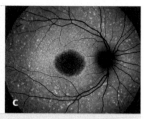

Fig. 23.1 Stargardt disease. **(a)** Fundus picture of a patient with Stargardt disease showing posterior pole subretinal yellow flecks, associated with mild macular atrophy. **(b)** Silent choroid sign on fluorescein angiography in a patient with Stargardt disease due to a mutation in *ABCA4*. **(c)** Fundus autofluorescence in a patient with Stargardt disease revealing multiple hyperfluorescent lesions (corresponding with subretinal flecks) and macular hypo-autofluorescence (corresponding with atrophy).

inducing apoptosis. Loss of RPE leads to secondary photoreceptor degeneration and, consequently, loss of vision.

SGD most commonly presents with bilateral central visual loss, color vision abnormalities, central scotomas, and slow dark adaptation with or without photophobia. Some patients may enjoy normal or only mildly reduced visual acuity despite a very abnormal retinal appearance. Eventually these patients usually experience further central vision loss. Generally, initial vision deterioration is otherwise rapidly progressive, but its age of onset is highly variable. Few patients deteriorate as far as to counting finger or hand motion. Visual prognosis is dependent on age of disease onset: patients who present with significantly compromised vision earlier have worst outcomes.

There is a particular form of SGD called childhood-onset, early-onset, or juvenile SGD. These patients tend to develop early severe visual acuity loss (usually worse than 20/40), before 10 years old, markedly compromised retinal function on electroretinogram (ERG) with generalized rod and cone system dysfunction, and rapid progression of RPE atrophy, from mild to severe findings in approximately 12 years. Approximately half of these patients have a diagnostic delay, which averages 3 years. Individuals with adult-onset SGD are more likely to retain useful visual acuity for longer and show milder retinal dysfunction at diagnosis. At presentation, 30% have flecks and 3% have a normal looking retina.

Paradoxically, fundus examination can be normal early in the course of disease, even when patients already have visual complaints. Later on, pigment mottling, a "beaten bronze" appearance of the macula, macular atrophy, fundus flecks, or even bull's eye maculopathy may arise. Flecks are typically "pisciform," round, amorphous, or dotlike yellow-white lesions. Their distribution may change with time. The number of flecks does not have a good correlation with the visual loss.

Patients with SGD can develop eccentric fixation. Furthermore, *ABCA4*-related disorders tend to spare the structure and function of the parapapillary retina, demonstrated by fundus autofluorescence and optical coherence tomography (OCT). This area can become a preferred retinal locus of fixation in up to one-third of patients.

It should be noted that SGD and fundus flavimaculatus differ in significant aspects. Individuals with fundus flavimaculatus often have a later disease onset and slower visual deterioration. Therefore, fundus flavimaculatus is often a milder condition with the macula less involved, and because of it, generally results in a better visual acuity than SGD.

Current treatment options include photoprotection and low-vision aids as needed. Patients may benefit from ultraviolet-blocking sunglasses. Vitamin A should be avoided as supplementation increases the lipofuscin accumulation in the RPE. The role of compounds that decrease lipofuscin deposits, such as deuterium-enriched vitamin A or isotretinoin, is under investigation, as are stem cell therapy and gene therapy.

23.2 *ABCA4* Retinopathies Overview

Other *ABCA4*-related phenotypes present as a spectrum that includes age-related macular degeneration (AMD), macular atrophy without flecks, bull's eye maculopathy, autosomal recessive (AR) CORD, and AR RP. Some overlap or intermediate forms can also be seen with different progression rates during the course of the conditions. In addition, different presentations may converge to the same end stage, characterized by diffuse atrophy. Symptoms may vary as well. For example, photoaversion may be seen in isolated cone dysfunction syndromes, while nyctalopia develops more frequently in patients with RP and cone–rod dystrophy (CORD). There are, however, clues that can suggest *ABCA4*. For instance, if an RP phenotype shows severe pigmentary changes in the macula or posterior pole atrophy as opposed to mild peripheral disease, *ABCA4* can be suspected. In addition, silent choroid on angiography can be seen in RP and CORD due to *ABCA4* pathogenic variants. It is estimated that 30 to 50% of CORD is due to *ABCA4* mutations.

23.3 Stargardt Disease Molecular Genetics

ABCA4 (chr 1p22.1) is a large gene that comprises 50 exons and has great allelic heterogeneity, with over 800 disease-associated variants described, most of which are missense mutations. The most frequent *ABCA4* pathogenic variations account for only approximately 10% of patients. There are ethnic group-specific *ABCA4* alleles demonstrating founder effects in different regions (e.g., T1428 M allele in Japan). The carrier frequency for *ABCA4* mutations is relatively high, usually 4 to 5% of the general population, although it can be higher in some populations. The estimated prevalence of *ABCA4* mutations in AR CORD ranges from 30 to 60%. Later-onset SGD is seen in patients with missense mutations that do not affect functional domains of *ABCA4*, resulting in milder mutant alleles and leaving some *ABCA4* activity. For early-onset SGD, the prevalence of *ABCA4* mutations can be as high as 90%. Deep intronic mutations have also been described in *ABCA4*opathies. Full sequencing of *ABCA4* coding and intronic sequences in individuals with SGD find two disease-associated alleles in 65 to 75% of patients, one mutation in 15 to 20% of individuals, and no mutations in approximately 15%. Most nonsense mutations are associated with classic SGD, whereas mutations found in patients with fundus flavimaculatus and late-onset SGD are usually missense mutations. It is not uncommon to find two or more mutations on the same *ABCA4* allele, creating a mutation number greater than 2. Familial segregation analysis is therefore crucial to determine pathogenicity and determine if the patient truly has biallelic mutations (in trans) as opposed to two mutations on the same allele (in cis).

Some phenotype–genotype correlations are noted for specific mutations. The G1961E *ABCA4* allele contributes to central macular changes rather than generalized retinal dysfunction, and is a cause of bull's eye maculopathy in either the homozygous or the compound heterozygous state. The c.2588G > C allele is associated with typical

SGD instead of "early-onset" SGD (this allele is seen in up to 4% of patients with early-onset SGD vs. 30% of individuals with classic SGD). Loss of peripapillary sparing is likely associated with the more deleterious mutations of the *ABCA4* gene.

23.4 *ABCA4* Retinopathies Molecular Genetics

Different combinations of affected *ABCA4* alleles are predicted to result in distinct phenotypes, in a spectrum of retinal manifestations of which severity is inversely proportional to the residual *ABCA4* activity. *ABCA4* has been described in the pathogenesis of AMD (*ABCA4* polymorphisms), CORD (residual *ABCA4* activity), and retinitis pigmentosa (full null alleles). Even within families, the same *ABCA4* allelic combinations can produce diverse phenotypes. It has been described that heterozygotes for the G1961E and D2177N *ABCA4* alleles have an increased risk of developing AMD. However, co-segregation studies in families with AMD have failed to establish a direct correlation between the condition and *ABCA4* variations.

23.5 Stargardt Disease Differential Diagnosis

23.5.1 Autosomal Dominant (AD) Stargardt Disease (STGD4, OMIM 603786)

Stargardt-like disease with AD inheritance pattern has been described in families with heterozygous mutations in the *PROM1* gene (4p). Patients typically have a bull's eye maculopathy. These patients may be indistinguishable from classic SGD, although central vision loss with significant outer nuclear atrophy in the context of an AD pattern of inheritance is the key factor.

23.5.2 Stargardt Like Macular Dystrophy (STGD3, OMIM 600110)

Stargardt like macular disease with AD inheritance pattern has been described in families with heterozygous mutations in the *ELOVL4* gene (6q14.1). Affected individuals have normal visual acuity in early childhood but start decreasing between the ages of 5 and 23 years. Flecks are present early in most cases. Central atrophy develops in later stages, with visual acuity decreasing to 20/200 or worse in all affected individuals by adulthood. Intravenous fluorescein angiography (IVFA) does not show a silent or dark choroid sign.

23.5.3 Malattia Leventinese and Doyne Honeycomb Retinal Dystrophy (OMIM 126600)

These two AD diseases due to mutation in *EFEMP1* (2p16.1) are characterized by yellow-white drusenoid deposits that accumulate beneath the RPE. Drusen are seen typically in the second and third decades of life, although there are reports of earlier onset (15 years old). Drusen tend to be bilateral, elongated, and with radial distribution. Drusen are more regular in shape and can extend beyond the arcade and nasal to the disc, which are uncommon in SGD. RPE and macular atrophy develop later.

23.5.4 Kandori's Flecked Retina (OMIM 228990)

This AR rare condition is characterized by irregular flecks, with variability in size and tendency to confluence, distributed in the equator or midperiphery. The macula is spared. The genetic basis remains unknown.

23.5.5 Familial Benign Fleck Retina (228980)

This is an AR condition associated with a pattern of diffuse, yellow-white, flecklike lesions extending to the far periphery of the retina but sparing the fovea. These individuals are asymptomatic and electrophysiology is normal. It is caused by biallelic mutation in the *PLA2G5* gene (1p36). Hyaline deposits occur along the cuticular layer of Bruch's membrane, looking as multiple deep yellowish white lesions of variable size and shape.

23.5.6 Sorsby's Fundus Dystrophy (OMIM 136900)

This is an AD retinal dystrophy characterized by loss of central vision as a result of macular disease by the fourth to fifth decade of life. Peripheral visual loss develops later. It is usually manifest at the age of approximately 40 years, beginning as a macular lesion showing edema, hemorrhage, and exudates; the latter may be confused with lipofuscin. Atrophy with pigmentation and extension peripherally occurs later, with sclerotic choroidal vessels. It is associated with mutations in *TIMP3* (22q12.3).

23.5.7 Pattern Macular Dystrophy (OMIM 169150)

Patterned dystrophies of RPE refer to a heterogeneous group of macular disorders, defined by an abnormal macular accumulation of lipofuscin. Three main patterns have been reported: reticular dystrophy, macroreticular ("spider-shaped") dystrophy, and butterfly dystrophy. It is caused by heterozygous mutation in the RDS–peripherin gene (*PRPH2*; 6p21). It is frequently manifest by the age of 40 years.

23.5.8 Age-Related Macular Degeneration (OMIM 603705)

Because of drusen, and geographic atrophy in the macula, ARMD can be confused with SGD. The age of onset is typically much later than classic SGD but may coincide with late-onset SGD. ARMD is the most common cause of acquired visual impairment in the elderly. Mild forms of ARMD are seen in 30% of those who are 75 years and older, and advanced stages occur in about 7% of individuals in this age group. ARMD is considered a complex phenotype and therefore, genetic testing still is not recommended. Multiple pathogenic variants have been associated with AMD (*CFH, CFB, ABCA4, TIMP3, BEST1,* and *EFEMP1* genes) and might suggest AMD is a polygenic disease, resulting from the presence of disease variants in multiple different genes.

23.5.9 Basal Laminar Drusen (OMIM 126700)

This term refers to an early adult-onset drusen phenotype that presents with a pattern of uniform small yellow subretinal nodules randomly scattered in the macula. Some authors consider it to be part of a spectrum of disease that includes ARMD. On IVFA, a typical "stars in the sky" appearance may be seen. *CFH* gene mutation may be associated with this condition.

23.5.10 Central Areolar Choroidal Atrophy (OMIM 215500)

Patients present a well-defined area of atrophy of the RPE and choriocapillaris in the center of the macula. It is usually diagnosed at the age of 40 to 60 years. It is an AR condition, associated with a mutation in the *PRPH2* gene (6p21.2-p12.3). Flecks are not present and the choroid is only affected under the geographic lesion.

23.5.11 Kjellin Syndrome (OMIM 270700)

Spastic paraplegia-15 is a neurodegenerative disorder defined by progressive spasticity primarily affecting the lower limbs, associated with mental retardation, hearing and visual defects, and thin corpus callosum. It is an AR disorder caused by biallelic mutations in the gene *ZFYVE26* (14q24.1). *SPG11* mutations (15q21.1) can also cause Kjellin syndrome. Retinal findings include macular atrophy and posterior pole flecks. The systemic associations easily differentiate it from SGD.

23.5.12 Fundus Albipunctatus (OMIM 136880)

This flecked retina disorder is characterized by discrete uniform white dots over the entire fundus with greatest density in the midperiphery and less macular involvement. It presents with nyctalopia. Scotopic full-field (ff) ERG typically improves after dark adaptation. It is associated with mutations in *RDH5* or *RLBP1* (▶ Fig. 23.2).

23.5.13 Alport Syndrome (OMIM 203780; 30105)

Alport syndrome has a frequency of 1 in 5,000 individuals, and 85% of patients have the X-linked recessive form. The characteristic findings include interstitial nephritis,

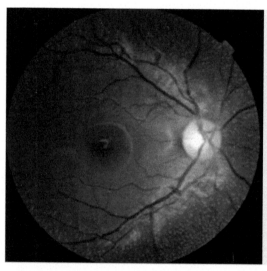

Fig. 23.2 Fundus albipunctata in a patient with discrete uniform white dots in the midperiphery and no macular involvement. (The image is provided courtesy of Sergio Zacharias, MD, and René Moya, MD.)

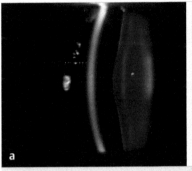
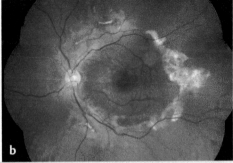

Fig. 23.3 Alport disease. (a) Anterior lenticonus. (b) Central and perimacular fleck retinopathy. The patient also has subretinal fibrosis. (These images are provided courtesy of Sergio Zacharias, MD.)

hearing loss, and ophthalmic findings including fleck maculopathy (85%), anterior lenticonus (25%; ► Fig. 23.3), and, less commonly, posterior lenticonus. Additional ophthalmic features described in X-linked Alport syndrome include microcornea, corneal arcus, iris atrophy, spontaneous lens rupture, spherophakia, posterior lenticonus, a poor macular reflex, and electro-oculogram (EOG) and ERG abnormalities. Mutations in *COL4A5* (Xq22.3) cause the X-linked recessive form, *COL4A3* the AD form, and *COL4A4* (2q36.3) the AR form. The AD form may present with solely ocular findings. An AD condition sharing the clinical findings of Alport syndrome but with the addition of macrothrombocytopenia, is known as Fechtner syndrome (OMIM 153640; *MYH9* gene, 22q11).

23.5.14 Enhanced S-Cone Syndrome (OMIM 268100)

This AR retinopathy is characterized by increased sensitivity to blue light, visual loss, nyctalopia, and retinal degeneration. Fundus findings include nummular pigment clumping at the level of the RPE along the vascular arcades and in the midperiphery, midperiphery and macular yellow flecks, macular cystoid spaces, macular hyperpigmentation with foveal sparing, and chorioretinal atrophic changes. Vitreous cells, opacities, haze, and veils can be seen. It is caused by *NR2E3* pathogenic variants.

23.5.15 Macular Dystrophy Associated with Mitochondrial DNA A3233G Mutation

The A3243G point mutation in mitochondrial deoxyribonucleic acid (mtDNA) is associated with MIDD syndromes (maternally inherited diabetes and deafness) and MELAS (mitochondrial encephalomyopathy with lactic acidosis and strokelike episodes). These two entities can have diffuse retinopathy or isolated macular alterations. Retinal findings include subretinal pale deposits and nummular perifoveal RPE atrophy. This macular dystrophy should be suspected when RPE abnormalities are found in the context of suggestive systemic findings.

23.6 *ABCA4* Retinopathies Differential Diagnosis

23.6.1 Cone–Rod Dystrophies

Patients with CORD not associated with *ABCA4* mutations usually lack flecks and do not show the dark choroid sign.

23.6.2 Retinitis pigmentosa

See RP section.

23.6.3 SGD and Its Differential Diagnosis

SGD and its differential diagnosis would also apply especially for the *ABCA4*opathies other than RP and CORD.

23.7 Stargardt Disease Uncommon Manifestations

Foveal sparing may occur in individuals with late-onset SGD with surprisingly good visual acuity. Conversely, some patients may develop large areas of geographic atrophy that are best seen on FAF.

23.8 *ABCA4* Retinopathies Uncommon Manifestations

Generalized choriocapillaris dystrophy is a progressive *ABCA4*-related phenotype defined by early-onset macular dystrophy that expands to extensive end-stage chorioretinal atrophy with profound visual loss.

23.9 Stargardt Disease Clinical Testing

23.9.1 Intravenous Fluorescein Angiography

IVFA shows the "dark-choroid" sign in up to 70% of individuals. This sign derives from a lack of early choroidal hyperfluorescence, which is blocked by high-grade lipofuscin accumulation in the RPE.

23.9.2 Fundus Autofluorescence

Hyperfluorescence on FAF represents excessive lipofuscin accumulation in the RPE. In typical SGD, multiple hyperfluorescent flecks are seen throughout the macula. Hypofluorescence relates to low-level RPE metabolic activity, which is associated with local atrophy with secondary photoreceptor loss. Large geographic areas of complete absence of fluorescence can be seen in SGD. Less frequently, macular hyperfluorescent rings can be found.

23.9.3 Full-Field Electroretinogram

SGD patients generally maintain normal or only mildly subnormal ffERG scotopic and photopic responses.

23.9.4 Multifocal Electroretinogram

Multifocal (mf) ERG is usually abnormal in patients with SGD and often shows more effect centrally with peripheral recovery of amplitudes and implicit times.

23.9.5 Optical Coherence Tomography

OCT provides significant ultrastructural information, such as early detection of lipofuscin accumulation at the RPE layer, or photoreceptor layer disorganization. When combining with FAF data, OCT can be helpful in disease staging.

23.9.6 Color Vision

SGD patients typically have a mild red–green dyschromatopsia or a tritan axis deviation.

23.9.7 Visual Field Testing

This is often normal in early disease stages, but progresses to relative to absolute central scotomas.

23.9.8 Melanin-Related Near-Infrared Fundus Autofluorescence

This can be altered earlier than FAF.

23.10 *ABCA4* Retinopathies Clinical Testing

23.10.1 Intravenous Fluorescein Angiography

IVFA may show the "dark-choroid" sign. Other findings include a central hypofluorescent spot, hyperfluorescent dots or granularity due to RPE abnormalities, or confluent hypofluorescent patches of chorioretinal atrophy.

23.10.2 Fundus Autofluorescence

FAF can reveal hyperfluorescence that corresponds with flecks, but the most frequent findings in patients with these non-SGD *ABCA4*opathies are hypofluorescent patches, diffuse hypofluorescence, or geographic atrophy.

23.10.3 Full-Field Electroretinogram

These disorders differ from SGD in that the ffERG shows abnormal scotopic and photopic responses.

23.10.4 Optical Coherence Tomography

OCT photoreceptor layer disorganization, atrophy, and inner–outer segment junction loss can be seen.

23.10.5 Visual Field Testing

Unlike SGD, these phenotypes may have peripheral field constriction in addition to central scotomas.

23.11 Stargardt Disease Genetic Testing

SGD diagnosis is typically clinical, based on history and laboratory testing. Genetic testing is used to confirm the clinical diagnosis and provide counseling. Although it may be cost efficient to consider targeted screening for common mutations, many patients require full sequencing of *ABCA4*. It is important to include deep intronic sequencing, particularly when only one mutation is found, as the frequency of this type of mutations is higher than previously thought.

23.12 *ABCA4* Retinopathies Genetic Testing

Often patients with CORD or RP will need multigene panels to make the molecular diagnosis as there may not be a specific feature that suggests *ABCA4*opathy. On occasion, the history reveals that age of onset and clinical findings are suggestive of *ABCA4*. For example, a prior IVFA revealing dark choroid, flecks on fundus photography, or macular atrophy that progressed into an RP phenotype can provide helpful hints to suggest that the workup be initiated by *ABCA4* sequencing. In some laboratories, panel testing may be more cost-effective than *ABCA4* sequencing and may even include *ABCA4* sequencing.

23.13 Problems

23.13.1 Case 1

A 14-year-old girl presents with consecutive visual loss to 20/100 in each eye over a period of 2 weeks. Family history is unremarkable. Her fundus examination shows a "beaten bronze" area of macular atrophy and yellowish subretinal scattered flecks of varying size throughout the macula bilaterally. Full-field ERG is normal, but there is mild reduction of responses centrally on mfERG. FAF demonstrates hyperfluorescent flecks throughout the posterior pole. Macular thinning with some photoreceptor loss and subretinal deposits are seen on OCT. IVFA shows a silent choroid. What is your clinical diagnosis?
a) Pattern macular dystrophy.
b) CORD.
c) SGD.
d) Doyne's honeycomb macular dystrophy.

Correct answer is c.
　The combination of age of onset, macular atrophy with "beaten bronze" appearance, subretinal lipofuscin flecks, and her testing results are consistent with a clinical diagnosis of SGD.

a) **Incorrect.** Fleck distribution is not patterned. Adolescence is not the typical age of onset. Silent choroid not seen with pattern dystrophy.

b) **Incorrect.** Full-field ERG showed normal rod function and only mildly reduced scotopic responses.

c) **Correct.**

d) **Incorrect.** Fleck distribution is not typical of Doyne's honeycomb macular dystrophy. Age of onset for vision loss is usually older and slower onset. Silent choroid is not seen in Doyne's dystrophy.

23.13.2 Case 2

A 14-year-old girl was referred for possible SGD. Her main complaint was reduced vision over the preceding year. Visual acuity is 20/80 OD (oculus dextrus) and 20/100 OS (oculus sinister) with no significant refractive error. Her ocular examination shows "bull's eye" maculopathy and some flecks in the posterior pole. Further testing revealed an abnormal mfERG, borderline abnormal cone function but normal rod function on ffERG, double hyperfluorescent ring, and hyperfluorescent flecks in the macula on FAF and foveal thinning with photoreceptor loss on OCT. IVFA was suggestive of a silent choroid. Family history is negative. A cone dystrophy DNA array panel, including "hot spot" exonic sites, showed a previously reported pathogenic mutation associated with SGD in her *ABCA4* gene (c.4539 + 2028C > T), which she inherited from her clinically normal father. What would be the next step?

a) Retinal dystrophy panel.

b) Whole exome sequencing (WES).

c) No further testing.

d) *ABCA4* full sequencing.

Correct answer is d.

In up to 15% of patients with *ABCA4*opathy, just one affected allele is found in the usual exonic *ABCA4* testing. This technique, although an effective screen, may miss novel mutations or deep intronic changes. Deep intronic sequencing can find the second mutation in approximately 30% of these patients. In this case, c.4539 + 2001G > A (V4) was found.

a) **Incorrect.** The possibility of finding a digenic condition is lower than the chance of finding a second *ABCA4* affected allele with deep intronic sequencing. In addition, silent choroid on IVFA and flecks were suggestive of *ABCA4* mutation as the cause.

b) **Incorrect.** In this case, WES is not cost-effective and can provide information that is not related with the phenotype, which may be difficult to interpret and carry unnecessary risk.

c) **Incorrect.** Full sequencing should be done.

d) **Correct.**

23.13.3 Case 3

A 22-year-old man was referred for reduced vision. He has no systemic findings. Family history is unrevealing. Visual acuity was 20/200 OU (oculus uterque) with insignificant refractive error. His ocular examination showed macular internal limiting membrane irregularity, loss of foveal reflex, and some scattered subretinal yellowish lesions

throughout the macula. Further testing revealed an abnormal mfERG, abnormal cone function but normal rod function on ffERG, macular hyperfluorescent ring and hypo-fluorescence in the foveal area on FAF with hyperfluorescent subretinal lesions, foveal thinning with photoreceptor loss on OCT, and IVFA with no silent choroid. *ABCA4* gene sequencing found a known polymorphism (c.5682G > C) in one allele. Which one of the following alternatives would be your next step?
a) Retinal dystrophy panel.
b) Macular dystrophy panel.
c) *PRPH2* sequencing.
d) *ABCA4* deep intronic sequencing.

Correct answer is b.
What is clear from this case is that the condition is confined to the macula. Clinical and laboratory findings were not specific for other conditions, so macular dystrophy panel seems to be the most appropriate test of choice.
a) **Incorrect.** Rods are not affected on ERG and examination beyond the macula was normal.
b) **Correct.**
c) **Incorrect.** There are no specific findings that suggest *PRPH2* mutation and the patient is younger than might be expected for a phenotype related to this gene.
d) **Incorrect.** This test is unlikely to be helpful in a scenario where there are no other *ABCA4* affected alleles.

23.13.4 Case 4

A 42-year-old woman comes for evaluation of SGD. She was diagnosed when she was 18 years old, but in the last few years, vision has decreased and she started having nyctalopia. She has an affected brother. Best corrected visual acuity is 20/200 OD and 20/400 OS. Her ocular examination revealed macular atrophy, yellowish subretinal flecks in the posterior pole, and RPE granularity in the midperiphery. On diagnostic testing, ffERG shows moderate dysfunction in both the cone and rod systems, FAF shows hypofluorescence in the macula and midperiphery, OCT shows diffuse retinal and macular thinning with photoreceptor loss, and IVFA shows a silent choroid. *ABCA4* gene full sequencing (including introns) found a reported mutation (c.5929G > A, inherited maternally and a novel variant [c.5461–1389C > A], inherited paternally). Parental examination and testing was normal. What would be your next step?
a) Examine her brother and test him for her mutations.
b) CORD panel.
c) No further testing required. Perform counseling based on this report.
d) Suspect RP and perform a retinal dystrophy panel.

Most appropriate answer is a.
History and examination is concordant with CORD caused by *ABCA4*. Genetic testing revealed an *ABCA4* mutation and one novel variant. Based on segregation, the variation is likely pathogenic, but testing the affected brother would further support the pathogenicity of the novel variant.
a) **Correct.**
b) **Incorrect.** *ABCA4* mutation is concordant with clinical and laboratory findings. There is no need to search for another etiology.

c) **Less appropriate**. Although we might assume the novel variation is likely pathogenic based on segregation, confirming with the affected brother will improve the counseling accuracy.

d) **Incorrect**. ERG is moderately affected, there is no pigmentary clumping, and IVFA shows a silent choroid. These findings support the diagnosis of *ABCA4*-related CORD.

23.13.5 Case 5

A 44-year-old man comes for evaluation of SGD. He was diagnosed when he was 35 years old. Besides low visual acuity, he has no other complaints. His deceased father was legally blind when he was 40 years old. Best corrected visual acuity is 20/100 OU. His ocular examination shows macular atrophy, patterned flecklike lesions in the posterior pole in a butterfly-shaped pattern, with normal midperiphery and periphery. Full-field ERG shows a moderate dysfunction of cones, and mfERG is also altered. EOG is normal. FAF shows a patterned hyperfluorescence in the macula, without abnormalities in the periphery. OCT reveals macular thinning, photoreceptor loss, and deposits above the RPE. The choroid is normal on IVFA. Which from the following seems the most appropriate test?

a) *ABCA4* sequencing.
b) *BEST1* sequencing.
c) *PRPH2* sequencing.
d) Macular dystrophy panel.

Correct answer is c.

Pattern dystrophies are a heterogeneous group of macular disorders, defined by an abnormal macular accumulation of lipofuscin. They are most often caused by heterozygous mutation in the RDS–peripherin gene (*PRPH2*). It is frequently manifest by the age of 40 years. The presence of a likely affected parent increases the chance of AD disorder. Testing and clinical findings are consistent with this diagnosis. *PRPH2* sequencing showed a heterozygous mutation (c.422A > G).

a) **Incorrect**. Based on age of onset, patterned appearance of the flecks, and IVFA without silent choroid, this option is less likely to yield positive results.

b) **Incorrect**. EOG was normal and the typical macular lesion is absent.

c) **Correct.**

d) **Less appropriate**. Although most macular dystrophy panels will include *PRPH2*, clinical and laboratory findings in this patient are highly consistent with a *PHPR2* pattern dystrophy.

Suggested Reading

[1] Parodi MB, Iacono P, Triolo G, et al. Morpho-functional correlation of fundus autofluorescence in Stargardt disease. Br J Ophthalmol. 2015; 99(10):1354–1359

[2] Zernant J, Xie YA, Ayuso C, et al. Analysis of the ABCA4 genomic locus in Stargardt disease. Hum Mol Genet. 2014; 23(25):6797–6806

[3] Fujinami K, Zernant J, Chana RK, et al. Clinical and molecular characteristics of childhood-onset Stargardt disease. Ophthalmology. 2015; 122(2):326–334

[4] Lambertus S, van Huet RA, Bax NM, et al. Early-onset Stargardt disease: phenotypic and genotypic characteristics. Ophthalmology. 2015; 122(2):335–344

[5] Rozet JM, Gerber S, Souied E, et al. Spectrum of ABCR gene mutations in autosomal recessive macular dystrophies. Eur J Hum Genet. 1998; 6(3):291–295

[6] Jiang F, Pan Z, Xu K, et al. Screening of ABCA4 gene in a Chinese cohort with Stargardt disease or cone-rod dystrophy with a report on 85 novel mutations. Invest Ophthalmol Vis Sci. 2016; 57(1):145–152

[7] Ścieżyńska A, Oziębło D, Ambroziak AM, et al. Next-generation sequencing of ABCA4: high frequency of complex alleles and novel mutations in patients with retinal dystrophies from Central Europe. Exp Eye Res. 2016; 145(145):93–99

[8] Bax NM, Sangermano R, Roosing S, et al. Heterozygous deep-intronic variants and deletions in ABCA4 in persons with retinal dystrophies and one exonic ABCA4 variant. Hum Mutat. 2015; 36(1):43–47

[9] Bauwens M, De Zaeytijd J, Weisschuh N, et al. An augmented ABCA4 screen targeting noncoding regions reveals a deep intronic founder variant in Belgian Stargardt patients. Hum Mutat. 2015; 36(1):39–42

[10] Burke TR, Tsang SH. Allelic and phenotypic heterogeneity in ABCA4 mutations. Ophthalmic Genet. 2011; 32 (3):165–174

24 Best Vitelliform Macular Dystrophy (Best Disease)

Abstract

Best vitelliform macular dystrophy (Best disease) is an autosomal dominant macular dystrophy defined by an early central macular egg yolk–like (vitelliform) lesion, which then progresses over time. Lesions are typically bilateral, but can be unilateral. The lesions may be initially asymptomatic with remarkably preserved vision despite the obvious macular lesion. Peripheral vision and dark adaptation should be normal. There are defined clinical stages, but the condition does not necessarily progress through each of these stages in every patient. Best disease may show incomplete penetrance. Variable expression is a hallmark of the disease and given that patients may be asymptomatic, examination and testing of family members who may report themselves as unaffected is essential. Affected patients are at risk for subretinal neovascularization, especially in later stages.

Keywords: Best disease, macular dystrophy, vitelliform lesions, electro-oculogram, *BEST1, gene*

Key Points

- Best vitelliform macular dystrophy is a macular dystrophy that slowly affects central vision, with typical onset in childhood.
- Affected patients initially have a classic yellow yolklike (vitelliform) macular lesion on posterior pole. Lesions are usually bilateral, but can be asymmetric, multifocal, and/or unilateral.

24.1 Overview

Best vitelliform macular dystrophy (VMD) is an autosomal dominant (AD) macular dystrophy defined by the early central macular egg yolk–like (vitelliform) lesions, which then progress over time (▶ Fig. 24.1). Lesions are typically bilateral, but can be unilateral. Deposits outside the macula may also occur. It typically progresses slowly. Generally, VMD has an onset in childhood, but occasionally can appear in later teenage years. The lesions may be initially asymptomatic with remarkably preserved vision despite the obvious macular lesion. Initial symptoms may include decreased visual acuity or metamorphopsias. Peripheral vision and dark adaptation should be normal. Clinical stages are listed in ▶ Table 24.1, but the condition does not necessarily progress through each of these stages in every patient. Up to 75% of patients retain a visual acuity of 20/40 or better in their better eye.

There is also an AD adult-onset form of the disease in which symptoms and retinal changes begin later, usually after the age of 40 years, and causes vision loss that tends to worsen over time. This condition is also characterized by subretinal yellowish flecks in the posterior pole. Electro-oculogram (EOG) is normal or mildly reduced, but Arden's ratio is always above 1.5.

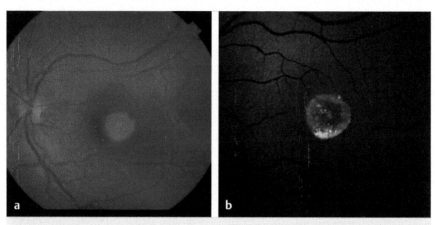

Fig. 24.1 Best vitelliform macular dystrophy. **(a)** Central macular egg yolk–like lesion. **(b)** Autofluorescence reveals some hyper-autofluorescence within the lesion and pooling inferiorly.

Because of the distinctive presentation, the diagnosis of VMD is clinical, based on macular appearance, EOG, and, when present, AD family history. VMD may show incomplete penetrance although those with the gene mutation almost invariably have an abnormal EOG even when the clinical examination is normal. Variable expression is a hallmark of the disease and given that patients may be asymptomatic, examination and testing of family members who may report themselves as unaffected is essential. The prevalence is unknown.

Table 24.1 Best vitelliform macular dystrophy clinical stages

Stage	Clinical appearance	Testing
0	Normal macula	Abnormal EOG
1	Previtelliform stage. Macular RPE disruption	Window defect on FA
2 2a	Circular, well-circumscribed, yellow-opaque, homogeneous yolklike macular lesion Vitelliform lesion contents become less homogeneous ("scrambled-egg" appearance)	FA shows marked hypofluorescence in the lesion FA shows partial blockage of fluorescence with a nonhomogeneous hyperfluorescence
3	Pseudo-hypopyon phase (fluid level of a yellow-colored vitelline content)	FA shows in macular lesions inferior hypofluorescence from the blockage by the vitelline material, along with superior hyperfluorescent defect
4a 4b 4c	Orange-red lesion with atrophic RPE and choroid visibility Fibrous scarring of the macula Choroidal neovascularization or subretinal hemorrhage	FA shows hyperfluorescence without leakage FA reveals hyperfluorescence and late staining

Abbreviations: EOG, electro-oculogram; this is abnormal at every stage, although there are reports of mutations in *BEST1* that have a normal EOG; FA, fluorescein angiogram; RPE, retinal pigment epithelium.

Individuals with VMD are at risk for subretinal neovascularization, especially for those in stage 4. Either laser or anti-VEGF (vascular endothelial growth factor) agents may be helpful. Smoking should be discouraged.

24.2 Molecular Genetics

BEST1 (formerly known as VMD2; 11q12.3) is the gene that when mutated is most commonly the cause of Best disease. Its protein product is bestrophin-1, and it is expressed in the basolateral membrane of the retinal pigment epithelium (RPE) cells. Disruption of bestrophin-1 function may produce an abnormal ion and fluid transport by the RPE, disrupting the interaction with photoreceptors. Patients with VMD have lipofuscin deposits within the RPE, predominantly in the macula. This explains the characteristic electrophysiologic finding of an abnormal EOG. The BEST1 gene has 11 exons. The majority of pathogenic variants are in the first five exons, whereas most of the polymorphisms occur in noncoding regions.

Pathogenic mutations in the PRPH2 gene can also cause the adult-onset form of VMD; however, it has been classically said that less than 25% of all affected patients have mutations in BEST1 or PRPH2 genes. In patients with adult-onset vitelliform dystrophy, IMPG1 and IMPG2 genes are causal genes in 8% of patients who were negative for BEST1 and PRPH2 mutations. These individuals usually have moderate visual impairment, drusen like lesions, and, on optical coherence tomography (OCT), normal reflectivity of the RPE line and vitelliform deposits located between ellipsoid and interdigitation lines.

Individuals with VMD may have no pathogenic variants in BEST1 due to incomplete exon sequencing, deep intronic mutations, or genetic heterogeneity (e.g., pathogenic variants in PRPH2 for adult-onset VMD). In VMD, the proportion of patients who present as a de novo mutation is unknown. If a proband has an apparent de novo pathogenic variant, and fundus examination of parents is normal, EOG on the parents is still recommended for ruling out variable expressivity.

Sequence analysis of BEST1 exons and intron–exon boundaries has approximately a 95% detection rate. To the best of our knowledge, there are no reported pathogenic deletions or duplications of the BEST1 gene. There is a specific Swedish mutation (c.383G > C); targeted analysis could be tried first with proper counseling in that group as a cost-saving measure. Evidence of genotype–phenotype correlation is scarce. p.Val89Ala is associated with late-onset VMD. p.Tyr227Asn has been seen with late-onset small vitelliform lesions.

24.3 Differential Diagnosis

The differential diagnosis of Stargardt disease (SGD) applies to VMD. In addition, the following disorders also deserve consideration.

24.3.1 Central Serous Retinopathy

Central serous retinopathy (CSR) is characterized by leakage of fluid under the neurosensory retina. It is typically seen in young males, and it is exacerbated by stress or corticosteroid use. It causes a circular macular elevated lesion similar to that seen in VMD but without lipofuscin, although exudates may be seen. Intravenous fluorescein angiography (IVFA) will usually show a typical "smoke stack" focus of leakage CSR that is usually unilateral. EOG is normal.

24.3.2 Toxoplasmosis Retinochoroiditis

White focal retinitis with overlying vitritis ("headlight in the fog"), accompanied by adjacent pigmented retinochoroidal scars, can help distinguish from VMD. Lipofuscin accumulation is not seen.

24.3.3 Solar Retinopathy

This condition is caused by photochemical toxicity, usually occurring at the fovea. It is associated with sun-gazing or eclipse viewing, and results in visual acuity deficit or paracentral scotomas. At examination, a very small foveal yellowish spot is seen in the fovea without elevation. EOG would be normal.

24.3.4 Autosomal Recessive Bestrophinopathy (OMIM 611809)

Autosomal Recessive Bestrophinopathy (ARB) is an AR disorder that differs from VMD in that it is multifocal and involves the retina more widely. Patients have multiple yellowish subretinal lesions (▶ Fig. 24.2), which show hyperfluorescence on fundus autofluorescence (FAF) as well as subretinal fluid or fibrosis. EOG is characterized by significant reduction or absence of light rise. Patients have patchy deep hyperfluorescent areas on IVFA, which usually extend beyond the retinal arcades. Intraretinal cystoid spaces or subretinal neovascularization may also be seen. Although the full-field electroretinogram (ffERG) is usually normal in the early stages of the condition, it has been reported that some ARB patients have severe photoreceptor dysfunction, characterized by prolonged latencies of the photopic responses. The multifocal ERG shows mild to markedly abnormal responses throughout the macula. OCT can reveal subretinal yellowish lesions and scars corresponding to hyper-reflective accumulations within or just above the RPE layer. Serous subretinal fluid or intraretinal cystoid spaces can also be observed. Color vision tests are usually normal.

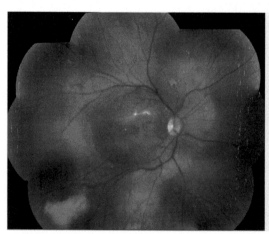

Fig. 24.2 Autosomal recessive bestrophinopathy showing subretinal yellowish deposits in the posterior pole and retinal pigment epithelium disturbances. The patient has a compound heterozygous mutation in the *BEST1* gene (c.388C > A and c.37 + 5G > A). (This image is provided courtesy of Sergio Zacharias, MD.)

ARB is usually diagnosed in the first two decades of life. Other associated abnormalities include hyperopia, amblyopia, narrow angles, and/or short axial length. In individuals with biallelic mutations in the *BEST1* gene, subretinal neovascular lesions with hemorrhage may occur. Up to 50% of patients with ARB may develop angle closure glaucoma. Carbonic anhydrase inhibitors have been used to reduce intraretinal cystoid spaces in this condition.

The main differential diagnoses for ARB are SGD, drusen disorders, chronic CSR, North Carolina macular dystrophy (caused by dysregulation of the retinal transcription factor PRDM13) and age-related macular degeneration. These were described in the SGD and VMD sections earlier. Subretinal lipofuscin in SGD is not associated with subretinal fluid, a finding that can be seen in ARB. Factors that help differentiate atypical multifocal VMD from ARB include AD rather than AR inheritance, degree of EOG abnormality being worse in ARB, and larger clumps of lipofuscin in ARB. Some ARB patients have been misdiagnosed as having posterior uveitis (e.g., birdshot chorioretinitis), and treated mistakenly with systemic immunosuppressants. Patients with chorioretinitis often have vitreous cells, contrary to ARB patients.

ARB is due to biallelic mutation in the *BEST1* gene. Both mutations are found in nearly 85% of patients. The c.422G > A mutation is one of the most frequent pathogenic variants in ARB. *BEST1* full sequencing is crucial to diagnose ARB, especially in challenging cases in which clinical findings are atypical. Depending on cost and availability, for some cases the best strategy will be a macular dystrophy panel.

24.3.5 Autosomal Dominant Vitreoretinochoroidopathy (OMIM 193220)

Autosomal dominant vitreoretinochoroidopathy (ADVIRC) is an AD condition characterized by a discreet band of chorioretinal hypo- and hyperpigmentation, usually from the midperiphery to the ora serrata for 360 degrees (▶ Fig. 24.3). In addition, posterior to this ring, preretinal punctate white opacities, retinal arteriolar narrowing and occlusion, and choroidal atrophy can be seen. ADVIRC patients may have cystoid macular edema, vitreous changes (fibrillar degeneration, liquefaction, peripheral vitreal condensations), and cataract. Generally, patients present with only mild visual impairment, and rarely develop severe visual loss. In some cases, progressive central macular atrophy and cone dysfunction lead to visual impairment. Other rare manifestations

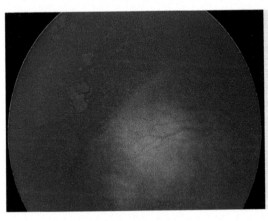

Fig. 24.3 Autosomal dominant vitreoretinochoroidopathy showing sharply demarcated peripheral hyperpigmented band (which extends 360 degrees).

include microcornea, retinal dystrophy, cataract, and posterior staphyloma, which can be seen together as a syndrome in patients who have ADVIRC. Nanophthalmos and microphthalmia have also been described. Characteristically, EOG is abnormal. Patients with ADVIRC may also have glaucoma, neovascularization, retinal detachment, vitreous hemorrhage, dyschromatopsia, or nystagmus. Progressive foveal atrophy may be seen as well.

EOG in patients with ADVIRC is typically abnormal. Full-field ERG is usually normal in young affected patients and only moderately abnormal in older ones. ERG findings are variable, ranging from mild to severe alterations in scotopic and photopic responses. Multifocal ERG can reveal reduced macular responses. In areas that are apparently normal, FAF can reveal hypofluorescent zones, which suggest retinal degeneration. IVFA may show leakage from neovascularization. IVFA also helps highlight the symmetric peripheral band of pigmentary changes. It also may reveal the abrupt cessation of vessels that go into the hyperpigmented zone. Visual fields tend to constrict concentrically with age.

Retinitis pigmentosa (RP) is the main diagnosis to consider. Full-field ERG is a critical test to differentiate ADVIRC from RP. Clinically, the abrupt cessation of vessels in the peripheral pigmented zone helps identify ADVIRC. "Bone spicule" pigmentary clumping in the midperiphery, a hallmark of RP, is not seen in ADVIRC.

ADVIRC has been associated with heterozygous missense *BEST1* mutations that result in alternative splicing. When suspecting ADVIRC, *BEST1* full sequencing is the test of choice.

24.4 Uncommon Manifestations

Bull's eye maculopathy has been seen in patients with pathogenic variants in *BEST1*. Vitelliform lesions can uncommonly be unilateral, multifocal, or present outside the macula.

24.5 Clinical Testing

24.5.1 Electro-oculogram

In VMD, the EOG is abnormal with a reduced light peak/dark trough ratio, typically less than 1.5 (normal > 1.8). Arden's ratio normally decreases with age after the fourth decade, a factor that should be considered in interpretation. There are reports of pathogenic variant in *BEST1* that have a normal EOG.

24.5.2 Intravenous Fluorescein Angiography

This test shows hyperfluorescence of typical vitelliform lesions. As the condition progresses, there is a mixed pattern of hyperfluorescence and hypofluorescence. Blocking of fluorescence can be seen because of fibrosis. Late staining and leakage will indicate a subretinal neovascular net.

24.5.3 Full-Field Electroretinogram

This is usually normal, but in some cases there can be reduced amplitudes and delayed implicit time in photopic responses.

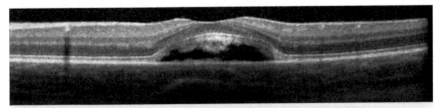

Fig. 24.4 Optical coherence tomography of the lesion showing neurosensorial retinal detachment with accumulated lipofuscin within the lesion.

24.5.4 Multifocal Electroretinogram

Multifocal ERG shows reduced central amplitudes.

24.5.5 Optical Coherence Tomography

In previtelliform stages, splitting and/or elevation at the outer retina and RPE are seen (► Fig. 24.4). For vitelliform stages, OCT defines the size/number of the deposits, in addition to the ellipsoid disruption. In the atrophic stages, thinning of the retina and RPE may be seen. OCT can also be used to detect subretinal neovascularization.

24.5.6 Fundus Autofluorescence

Hyper-autofluorescence corresponds to the lesions seen in the posterior pole during the earlier vitelliform stages. This hyperfluorescence endures with the pseudo-hypopyon stage, and becomes mottled with areas of hypo-autofluorescence during the initial atrophic stage, and eventually progresses to hypofluorescence.

24.5.7 Color Vision Tests

Many patients have anomalous color discrimination, particularly in the protan axis. This is not a routine test.

24.6 Genetic Testing

VMD diagnosis is typically made on the basis of clinical examination, history, and diagnostic testing. Genetic testing, usually by full sequencing, is used to confirm the clinical diagnosis, identify individuals who may be nonpenetrant or low expressing, and provide counseling. There are cases in which molecular testing is especially useful, particularly when vitelliform lesions are atypical (multiple throughout the posterior pole or unilateral) or when the EOG is borderline. If clinical findings are not suggestive of any macular condition or clinical presentation is atypical, macular dystrophy panels may be more cost-effective.

24.7 Problems

24.7.1 Case 1

A 33-year-old man comes for genetic counseling. He has had low vision since he was 16 years old. His 12-year-old daughter is complaining about difficulty reading. On their examination, he has bilateral macular scarring with a relatively normal retinal periphery and retinal vessels. She has subtle RPE disruption in the macular region with a small single focus of subretinal lipofuscin in one eye as suggested by OCT and FAF. Her fluorescein angiogram shows normal choroidal fluorescence with some hyperfluorescence corresponding to the lipofuscin in one eye. Both patients have an abnormal EOG. Which genetic test would you choose?
a) Sequence *ABCA4*.
b) Sequence *BEST1*.
c) Macular dystrophy panel.
d) Whole exome sequencing.

Correct answer is b.

Family history suggests an AD pattern of a condition that primarily affects the macula. Based on examination, the father has a presentation of VMD compatible with stage 4b (macular scarring) and his daughter stage 1 (RPE disruption) and early stage 2 in the other eye. The key for diagnosis is the abnormal EOG.
a) **Incorrect.** There are no suggestive clinical findings of SDG or another *ABCA4*-associated condition.
b) **Correct.**
c) **Incorrect.** Findings are very specific to a *BEST1* mutation. This approach would not likely be cost-effective.
d) **Incorrect.** Same as c.

24.7.2 Case 2

A healthy 15-year-old girl was diagnosed with retinal dystrophy when she was 5 years old. When she was 9 years old, her vision was 20/40 in both eyes with no significant refractive error. She does not have nyctalopia or other symptoms. Her physical examination was normal. Currently, she has 20/200 in both eyes. Ocular examination shows macular cystoid spaces in both eyes, with a few yellowish subretinal deposits in the left eye. Family history is unremarkable. Consecutive OCTs show cystoid spaces that are stable, with no leakage at IVFA. FAF reveals hyperautofluorescent subretinal deposits. Full-field ERG has a normal scotopic response, and a photopic altered b-wave, with prolonged implicit time and diminished amplitude. Multifocal ERG is severely affected. EOG revealed Arden's ratio of 14. Which would be the most appropriate genetic test?
a) *ABCA4* sequencing.
b) *NR2E3* sequencing.
c) *BEST1* sequencing.
d) *RS1* sequencing.

Correct answer is c.

Although EOG is abnormal in this patient, clinical presentation is atypical for VMD and family history is unrevealing. Electrophysiology confines the condition to the macula. From the listed genes, *BEST1* would be the most appropriate. In this case, sequencing showed two novel variations in the *BEST1* gene (p.Asp58His:c.172G > C; probably damaging by PolyPhen-2 with score of 1.0) and c.599delC (novel frameshift mutation). Intraretinal cystoid spaces can be caused by other genes such as *CRB1*, *NR2E3*, *MAK*, and others, but these disorders have other characteristic features, in particular widespread retinal dystrophy. As the patient is female, juvenile X-linked retinoschisis need not be considered.

a) **Incorrect.** *ABCA4* mutations are not associated with macular edema or intraretinal cystoid spaces.

b) **Incorrect.** Rod response was normal. It is unlikely that *NR2E3* is the causative gene as one would expect more severe cone involvement, or supranormal cone responses (see enhanced S-cone disorder).

c) **Correct.**

d) **Incorrect.** Patient is female and skewed X inactivation to this degree is unlikely. ERG does not show the electronegative b-wave that is characteristic of JXLR (juvenile X-linked retinoschisis).

24.7.3 Case 3

A 51-year-old man was told that he has atypical AD RP. He has an affected son and his deceased mother is believed to have had the same retinal problem. His vision is 20/40 OD (oculus dextrus) and 20/30 OS (oculus sinister). Slit-lamp examination shows bilateral subtle posterior subcapsular cataract and fibrillar vitreous degeneration. Fundus examination reveals a 360-degree well-demarcated peripheral hyperpigmented zone that extended to the ora serrata in both eyes. In addition, there is retinal arteriolar narrowing and abrupt vessel cessation into the hyperpigmented zone. There are no "bone spicule" pigment clumps. EOG is abnormal. Full-field ERG shows mild abnormalities of both rod and cone responses. FAF shows mild hypofluorescence just posterior to the 360-degree band of pigment alteration. Which from the following seems the most likely diagnosis?

a) ADVIRC.

b) AR bestrophinopathy.

c) Atypical vitelliform macular dystrophy.

d) RP.

Correct answer is a.

Clinical picture is very typical of ADVIRC, showing the peripheral band of hyperpigmentation and vessel alteration at the periphery. EOG and ERG are abnormal. This patient was found to have a heterozygous mutation in *BEST1* (c.256G > A).

a) **Correct.**

b) **Incorrect.** The absence of subretinal lipofuscin deposition in the macular region and the AD pattern of inheritance are not compatible with ARB.

c) **Incorrect.** Same as b. In addition, FAF showed a normal macula.

d) **Incorrect.** The absence of "bone spicule" pigment clumps and the mildly affected ERG rule out RP.

24.7.4 Case 4

A 22-year-old male comes for a second opinion. He was diagnosed with "atypical SGD" when he was 16 years old. His main complaint is affected central vision with normal night vision. He recently had further acute vision loss in his right eye. Best corrected vision is 20/400 OD and 20/40 OS. Anterior segment examination is normal. Fundus examination reveals bilateral, yellowish, multiple subretinal deposits of different sizes, confined mostly in the posterior pole, but some outside the arcades. His right eye has subfoveal blood. OCT shows ellipsoid preservation and hyperautofluorescent lesions corresponding to the deposits, and Arden's ratio is 1.4 OU (oculus uterque) on EOG. Full-field ERG is normal. There are mildly reduced amplitudes on multifocal ERG and leakage in the right eye on IVFA. Which from the following is the most likely diagnosis?

a) SGD.
b) Pattern macular dystrophy.
c) Multifocal Best disease.
d) Doyne's honeycomb macular dystrophy.

Correct answer is c.

This patient most likely has multifocal VMD, based on clinical findings and compatible laboratory findings.

a) **Incorrect.** Lesions are not flecks and IVFA does not show silent choroid.
b) **Incorrect.** The patient is too young for pattern macular dystrophy and EOG is less than 1.5 (pattern macular dystrophy is always above 1.8).
c) **Correct.**
d) **Incorrect.** Clinical findings do not suggest malattia leventinese or Doyne's honeycomb retinal dystrophy. In these conditions, drusen tend to be bilateral, elongated, and radially distributed.

Suggested Reading

[1] Bakall B, Marknell T, Ingvast S, et al. The mutation spectrum of the bestrophin protein–functional implications. Hum Genet. 1999; 104(5):383–389

[2] Bitner H, Mizrahi-Meissonnier L, Griefner G, Erdinest I, Sharon D, Banin E. A homozygous frameshift mutation in BEST1 causes the classical form of Best disease in an autosomal recessive mode. Invest Ophthalmol Vis Sci. 2011; 52(8):5332–5338

[3] Boon CJ, Klevering BJ, den Hollander AI, et al. Clinical and genetic heterogeneity in multifocal vitelliform dystrophy. Arch Ophthalmol. 2007; 125(8):1100–1106

[4] Burgess R, MacLaren RE, Davidson AE, et al. ADVIRC is caused by distinct mutations in BEST1 that alter pre-mRNA splicing. J Med Genet. 2009; 46(9):620–625

[5] Boon CJ, van den Born LI, Visser L, et al. Autosomal recessive bestrophinopathy: differential diagnosis and treatment options. Ophthalmology. 2013; 120(4):809–820

[6] Burgess R, Millar ID, Leroy BP, et al. Biallelic mutation of BEST1 causes a distinct retinopathy in humans. Am J Hum Genet. 2008; 82(1):19–31

[7] Krämer F, White K, Pauleikhoff D, et al. Mutations in the VMD2 gene are associated with juvenile-onset vitelliform macular dystrophy (Best disease) and adult vitelliform macular dystrophy but not age-related macular degeneration. Eur J Hum Genet. 2000; 8(4):286–292

[8] Leu J, Schrage NF, Degenring RF. Choroidal neovascularisation secondary to Best's disease in a 13-year-old boy treated by intravitreal bevacizumab. Graefes Arch Clin Exp Ophthalmol. 2007; 245(11):1723–1725

[9] MacDonald IM, Gudiseva HV, Villanueva A, Greve M, Caruso R, Ayyagari R. Phenotype and genotype of patients with autosomal recessive bestrophinopathy. Ophthalmic Genet. 2012; 33(3):123–129

[10] Querques G, Zerbib J, Santacroce R, et al. Functional and clinical data of Best vitelliform macular dystrophy patients with mutations in the BEST1 gene. Mol Vis. 2009; 15:2960–2972

[11] Testa F, Rossi S, Passerini I, et al. A normal electro-oculography in a family affected by best disease with a novel spontaneous mutation of the BEST1 gene. Br J Ophthalmol. 2008; 92(11):1467–1470

[12] Yardley J, Leroy BP, Hart-Holden N, et al. Mutations of VMD2 splicing regulators cause nanophthalmos and autosomal dominant vitreoretinochoroidopathy (ADVIRC). Invest Ophthalmol Vis Sci. 2004; 45(10):3683–3689

[13] Zhuk SA, Edwards AO. Peripherin/RDS and VMD2 mutations in macular dystrophies with adult-onset vitelliform lesion. Mol Vis. 2006; 12:811–815

[14] Boon CJ, Klevering BJ, Leroy BP, Hoyng CB, Keunen JE, den Hollander AI. The spectrum of ocular phenotypes caused by mutations in the BEST1 gene. Prog Retin Eye Res. 2009; 28(3):187–205

[15] Meunier I, Manes G, Bocquet B, et al. Frequency and clinical pattern of vitelliform macular dystrophy caused by mutations of interphotoreceptor matrix IMPG1 and IMPG2 genes. Ophthalmology. 2014; 121(12):2406–2414

[16] Chen CJ, Kaufman S, Packo K, Stöhr H, Weber BH, Goldberg MF. Long-term macular changes in the first proband of autosomal dominant vitreoretinochoroidopathy (ADVIRC) due to a newly identified mutation in BEST1. Ophthalmic Genet. 2016; 37(1):102–108

25 Leber Congenital Amaurosis

Abstract

The diagnosis of Leber congenital amaurosis typically involves two major criteria: severe visual impairment in early infancy and severely affected electroretinogram. Other clinical findings that may be seen are oculo-digital sign, near-absent pupillary reactions (or paradoxical pupils), nystagmus, high hyperopia, and photophobia. It is usually autosomal recessive. The retina may appear normal initially, but other findings may include macular geographic chorioretinal atrophy (macular "coloboma"), bone-spicule pigmentary clumping in the "midperiphery," subretinal flecks, or pigmented nummular lesions.

Keywords: Leber congenital amaurosis, childhood blindness, nystagmus, *RPE65*, gene therapy

> ### Key Points
>
> - Leber congenital amaurosis (LCA) is a severe retinal dystrophy that becomes clinically evident in the first year of life.
> - Patients present with poor visual function, frequently accompanied by nystagmus, sluggish pupillary responses (or paradoxical pupils), photophobia, and high hyperopia.
> - The appearance of the fundus is extremely variable, ranging from normal to severe pigmentary retinopathy. Mutations in 22 genes are known to cause LCA.
> - The electroretinogram is typically "nondetectable" or severely subnormal.

25.1 Overview

The diagnosis of Leber congenital amaurosis (LCA) typically involves two major criteria: severe visual impairment in early infancy and severely affected electroretinogram (ERG). Other clinical findings that may be seen are oculo-digital sign, near-absent pupillary reactions (or paradoxical pupils), nystagmus, high hyperopia, and photophobia. The prevalence is 1 in 30,000 to 50,000 births. This condition is the most frequent cause of inherited blindness of childhood. Because it is usually autosomal recessive, LCA is more prevalent if consanguinity or community constriction is present.

The retina may appear normal initially, but other findings may include macular geographic chorioretinal atrophy (macular "coloboma"), bone spicule pigmentary clumping in the "mid periphery," subretinal flecks, or pigmented nummular lesions at the retinal pigment epithelium (RPE) level (▶ Fig. 25.1). Optic nerve anomalies such as drusen may be seen. Some patients with LCA do not develop obvious fundus anomalies until later in life, but in early years have only subtle findings, including mild RPE changes, initial vessel attenuation, or internal limiting membrane irregularity. Franceschetti's oculo-digital sign (eye poking and rubbing) may be repetitive and severe. Patients often have an enophthalmic appearance. There is an association between LCA and keratoconus, which may in part be related to eye rubbing, although it has also been described in patients with LCA without eye poking.

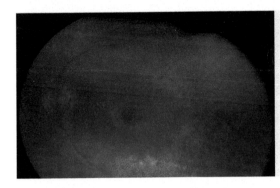

Fig. 25.1 Patient with Leber congenital amaurosis, showing attenuated vessels, early macular atrophy, surface gliosis, and pigmentary changes.

Although retinal gene therapy for LCA2 was initially shown to have positive benefit for patients with *RPE65* mutations, long-term follow-up of treated patients indicates some progressive diminution of the areas of improved vision. Perhaps additional repeat injection will be needed.

25.2 Molecular Genetics

LCA is associated to mutations in 22 genes, including *AIPL1, CEP290, CRB1, CRX, DTHD1, GDF6, GUCY2D, IFT140, IMPDH1, IQCB1, KCNJ13, LCA5, LRAT, NMNAT1, OTX2, RD3, RDH12, RPE65, RPGRIP1, SPATA7,* and *TULP1.* The most common are summarized in ▶ Table 25.1.

Pathogenic variants in these genes typically produce nonfunctional or absent protein product. Deletions or duplications are rarely reported. Heterozygotes are typically asymptomatic although symptoms and ERG findings may be seen in carriers of mutation in *GUCY2D* and *RPGR1P1*. Nonpenetrance has been reported with mutations in *NMNAT1*. Autosomal dominant LCA has been reported with mutations in cone–rod homeobox (CRX). Variable expression may occur.

Although there is no pathognomonic genotype–phenotype correlation, there is some evidence to establish common associations. Patients with *CRB1* pathogenic variants may have preserved para-arteriolar RPE, often seen best on intravenous fluorescein angiography. Some individuals with *RPE65* mutations present with star-shaped maculopathy associated with hypopigmented RPE white dots. In addition, "macular

Table 25.1 Most common genetic causes of Leber congenital amaurosis

Gene	Locus	Estimated percent of patients[a] (%)
GUCY2D	17p13.1	Up to 20
RPE65	1p31.3	Up to 15
AIPL1	17p13.2	Up to 8
CRX	19q13.33	Up to 3
CEP290	12q21.32	Up to 20
CRB1	1q31.3	Up to 15
RDH12	14q24.1	Up to 4

[a]Frequency is variable according to specific populations. Proportion of other genes is usually lower than presented in this table.

coloboma" or progressive macular atrophic lesion with sharp borders has been seen with mutations in *AIPL1*, *CRB1*, and *NMNAT1*. The phenotype of LCA in patients with *AIPL1* mutations can be relatively severe, with maculopathy and marked bonespicule pigmentary changes, with a large proportion of individuals having keratoconus and cataract. Patients with *RPGRIP1* mutations frequently progress to light perception or no light perception. These individuals are characterized by early photophobia. Other gene mutations associated with photophobia include *GUCY2D*, *RPGRIP1*, and *AIPL1*. Affected individuals with predominant night blindness may have mutations in *CRB1*, *RPE65*, *TULP1*, and *CRX*. Patients have mild hyperopia, transient improvement of visual acuity, macular atrophy with later severe progression, and may either have *RDH12* or *RPE65* mutations. Nevertheless, loss of visual acuity usually happens at an earlier age in those with *RDH12* mutations. Patients with *IQCB1* mutations usually have greater loss of rods rather than cones. In addition, these individuals may also present with renal dysfunction. Keratoconus has been associated with *CRB1* and *AIPL1* mutations.

Occasionally, LCA is associated with neurodevelopmental delay and intellectual disability, although some reports establish that these findings occur in up to 15% of patients. This is particularly true for *CEP290* mutations. Other genes that when mutated cause LCA with developmental delay include *GUCY2D* and *RPGR1P1*.

Patients with LCA usually do not have visual acuity better than 20/400. *AIPL1*, *GUCY2D*, *CRX*, and *RPGRIP1* mutations have been associated with severely decreased visual acuities in the first year of life, whereas *RPE65*, *RDH12*, and *CRB1* mutations present variable visual acuities. Patients who have better visual acuity may have a delayed onset of visual symptoms until after the first year of life.

25.3 Differential Diagnosis

Many of the genes associated with LCA phenotype have phenotypic heterogeneity. Alternative phenotypes are summarized in ▶ Table 25.2.

25.3.1 Early-Onset Retinitis Pigmentosa (Juvenile Retinitis Pigmentosa)

This condition has a later age of onset than LCA (night blindness before 10 years), presents with no nystagmus, and has a better preservation of central visual acuity than in LCA. The photopic component of ERG in early-onset RP is usually spared or mildly abnormal.

25.3.2 Achromatopsia (OMIM 216900)

Like LCA, the retinal appearance can be normal, with low vision and nystagmus. ERG shows no involvement of rod system.

25.3.3 Congenital Stationary Night Blindness (OMIM 310500)

Uncommonly, patients with complete congenital stationary night blindness (CSNB) may present with low vision. These patients (usually associated with *NYX* mutations) present nonprogressive findings, and the ERG rules out LCA.

Table 25.2 Summary of alternative phenotypes

Gene	Alternative phenotype
GUCY2D	AD CORD Early-onset RP (p.His1079GlnfsTer54)
RPE65	AR RP
AIPL1	AD CORD AD RP
RPGRIP1	CORD (p.Arg827Leu and p.Ala547Ser)
CRX	AD CORD AD RP
CRB1	AD paravascular chorioretinal atrophy AR RP CORD Coats-like RP
CEP290	BBS14 Joubert syndrome Meckel syndrome Senior–Løken syndrome
IMPDH1	AD RP
RDH12	Progressive CORD
TULP1	AR RP
KCNJ13	Snowflake vitreoretinal degeneration
IQCB1	Senior–Løken syndrome

Abbreviations: AD, autosomal dominant; AR, autosomal recessive; BBS, Bardet–Biedl syndrome; CORD, cone–rod dystrophy; RP, retinitis pigmentosa.

25.3.4 Conorenal Syndrome (OMIM 266920)

Conorenal syndrome (OMIM 266920) comprises cone-shaped digital epiphyses, cerebellar hypoplasia, and early-onset retinal dystrophy.

25.3.5 Senior–Løken Syndrome (OMIM 266900)

This is an autosomal recessive condition comprising nephronophthisis and LCA. It can be caused by mutation in the NPHP4 gene (1p36), NPHP5 gene (IQCB1,3q21), NPHP6 gene (CEP290, 12q21), SDCCAG8 gene (1q44), WDR19 gene (4p14), or TRAF3IP1 gene (2q37). Nephronophthisis manifests as normal-size or small kidneys with increased echogenicity and usually progresses to renal failure. Approximately 15% of patients with nephronophthisis associated with CEP290 mutations also have central nervous system and/or ophthalmic involvement, overlapping Joubert syndrome, and Senior–Løken syndrome.

25.3.6 Joubert Syndrome (OMIM 213300)

This is a phenotypically and genetically heterogeneous group of disorders defined by hypoplasia of the cerebellar vermis with the neuroradiologic "molar tooth sign" (▶ Fig. 25.2), and associated neurologic symptoms and developmental delay. It may

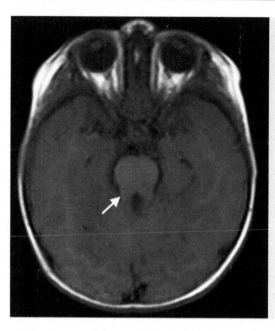

Fig. 25.2 Patient with Joubert syndrome and molar tooth sign on magnetic resonance imaging.

include LCA and renal abnormalities. More than 17 genes have been associated with Joubert syndrome.

25.3.7 Meckel–Gruber Syndrome (OMIM 249000)

This is an autosomal recessive developmental disorder caused by ciliary dysfunction during embryogenesis. The diagnostic criteria include cystic renal disease, central neurological system malformation, and hepatic anomalies. Patients have significant developmental delay. It can overlap with Joubert syndrome. Meckel–Gruber syndrome has genetic heterogeneity. It can be caused by mutations in *TMEM216* (11q13), *TMEM67* (8q), *CEP290* (12q), *RPGRIP1L* (16q12.2), *CC2D2A* (4p15), *NPHP3* (3q22), *TCTN2* (12q24.31), *B9D1* (17p11.2), *B9D2* (19q13), *TMEM231* (16q23), and *KIF14* gene (1q31).

25.3.8 SECORD (Severe Early Childhood Onset Retinal Dystrophy)

This condition is distinguished from LCA by the age of onset, usually after the first year of life. It is associated most commonly with *RPE65* mutations.

25.3.9 *OTX2* Gene Mutation with Leber Congenital Amaurosis

OTX2 gene mutation with LCA is a rare association. In a large group of LCA or early-onset retinal dystrophy, only one patient, a 7-year-old male, was described having an infantile-onset retinal dystrophy. He was reported to have an *OTX2* variant (novel heterozygous p.S138X). He had a history of failure to thrive in infancy, poor feeding, and growth hormone deficiency.

25.3.10 Boucher–Neuhauser Syndrome (OMIM 215470)

This is an autosomal recessive disorder characterized by spinocerebellar ataxia, hypogonadotropic hypogonadism, and chorioretinal dystrophy. The age at onset is variable, but most patients present in the first decade of life, sometimes in infancy. It is associated with *PNPLA6* gene mutation, which is also seen in spastic paraplegia.

25.3.11 Peroxisomal Disorders

These patients present with variable degrees of retinal dystrophy, sensorineural hearing loss, developmental delay with hypotonia, and liver dysfunction. The survival is poor: usually they die during the first year of life. Clinically, peroxisomal disorders include Zellweger syndrome (OMIM 214100), neonatal adrenoleukodystrophy (OMIM 202370), and Refsum's disease (OMIM 266510).

25.3.12 Others

Early retinal dystrophy or retinal degeneration has been documented in patients with abetalipoproteinemia (OMIM 200100), metabolic conditions such as methylmalonic aciduria, and homocystinuria cobalamin C type (OMIM 277400), hyperthreoninemia (OMIM 2737700), and mitochondrial disorders.

25.4 Uncommon Manifestations

CRB1 mutations can present with keratoconus or Coats-like RP. *CEP290* pathogenic variants may have microphthalmia and ectopia lentis.

Infrequently, optic disc swelling (*CRB1*), drusen like deposits of the optic nerve (*CRB1*), or peripapillary neovascularization have been reported. Spasmus nutans–like eye movements can also be seen (*CRB1*).

25.5 Clinical Testing

25.5.1 Electroretinogram

ERG shows severely affected photopic and scotopic components. Normal ERG responses rule out a diagnosis of LCA. In patients with *NMNAT1* mutations, electronegative b-wave may be seen.

25.5.2 Optical Coherence Tomography

In patients with LCA, three OCT patterns have been described: patients with near normal outer nuclear layer across the central retina, preserved fovea with reduced outer nuclear layers, or early macular disease (foveal maldevelopment). OCT would be particularly useful in patients with macular pseudocoloboma (▶ Fig. 25.3).

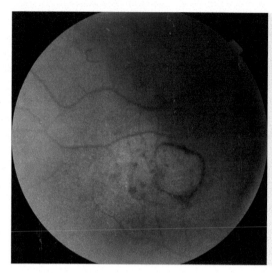

Fig. 25.3 Right eye of patient with Leber congenital amaurosis and *CRB1* gene mutations, showing macular "coloboma" (well-demarcated chorioretinal geographic atrophic lesion). Also note vessel attenuation, and grayish gliosis on retinal surface. (This image is provided courtesy of Hernán Iturriaga, MD.)

25.6 Genetic Testing

25.6.1 Leber Congenital Amaurosis Panel

Multigene testing panels are available and may vary from one laboratory to another. It is important to have a good phenotype and identify what one is looking for in order to select the best test that can provide a diagnosis. In addition to the number of genes included on a panel, laboratories may differ in their methodology, which will also make a difference in how the results are interpreted. For example, some laboratories will perform targeted mutation analysis prior to full sequencing only looking at commonly occurring mutations, while other laboratories may only perform full-sequence analysis of the genes on their panel.

25.7 Problems

25.7.1 Case 1

A 9-month-old female infant is brought for evaluation of nystagmus. Vision is subnormal but present in both eyes. Pupillary responses are sluggish. Fundus examination reveals macular "coloboma," vascular attenuation with preserved para-arteriolar RPE in the midperiphery. Family history is unremarkable. There is no developmental delay. The ERG is nearly isoelectric. Which from the following genes seems to be the most probable candidate?

a) *AIPL1*.

b) *RPE65*.

c) *GUCY2D*.

d) *CRB1*.

Correct answer is d.

The patient was found to be homozygous for a reported mutation in the *CRB1* gene: p.Cys948Tyr:c.2843G > A. Although there is no pathognomonic genotype–phenotype correlation, there is some evidence to establish common associations. Patients with *CRB1* mutations may have preserved para-arteriolar RPE, often seen best on intravenous fluorescein angiography. In addition, macular pseudocoloboma has been reported with pathogenic variants of *AIPL1*, *CRB1*, and *NMNAT1*. LCA due to mutations in *CRB1* is not associated with systemic findings or developmental delay.

a) **Less appropriate.** The phenotype of patients with *AIPL1* mutations can be relatively severe, with maculopathy and marked bone spicule pigmentary changes, but no paravascular RPE preservation.

b) **Incorrect.** Some patients with *RPE65* mutations present star-shaped maculopathy associated with hypopigmented RPE white dots.

c) **Incorrect.** These patients commonly present photophobia and retina with "normal" appearance.

d) **Correct.**

25.7.2 Case 2

A 6-month-old female infant comes for nystagmus evaluation. Her workup reveals a nearly isoelectric full field ERG. Retinal examination shows vascular attenuation, disrupted internal limiting membrane reflexes in each macula, and some midperipheral pigmentary alterations. An array LCA gene panel shows a homozygous mutation in the *CEP290* gene (c.2991 + 1655A > G). Which of the following studies seem more appropriate to order?

a) Brain magnetic resonance imaging (MRI)/renal function.
b) Echocardiogram/chest computed tomography (CT).
c) Brain MRI/echocardiogram.
d) Renal function/skeletal survey.

Correct answer is a.

CEP290 mutations may be associated with Senior–Løken and Joubert syndrome. Nephronophthisis and brain anomalies should be considered. Around 15% of patients with nephronophthisis associated with *CEP290* pathogenic variations may overlap with Joubert and Senior–Løken syndromes.

a) **Correct.**
b) **Incorrect.** These tests are not indicated.
c) **Incorrect.** Cardiac anomalies are not associated with mutations in this gene.
d) **Incorrect.** Skeletal anomalies are not associated with mutations in this gene

25.7.3 Case 3

A 9-year-old girl is referred with a clinical diagnosis of foveal hypoplasia. Clinical examination shows multidirectional nystagmus, sluggish pupillary responses, absence of foveal reflex, vascular attenuation, and midperipheral pigmentary "bone spicule" clumping. Vision has been very poor since infancy. ERG isoelectric rod and cone responses are consistent with LCA. The parents are asymptomatic and their ocular examination is normal. An array LCA gene panel shows a previously reported mutation and a novel missense variation in the *CRB1* gene (paternal p.Cys948Tyr:c.2843G > A and maternal p.Leu755Ser:c.2264T > C [PolyPhen-2 score of 0.996 out of 1.0]). The parents want to know if their daughter can be treated with gene therapy. Which is the most appropriate response currently?

a) *RPE65* treatment can be used for other types of LCA.
b) There are no current *CRB1* human clinical trials.
c) Testing should be ordered to rule out a deletion of *RPE65*.
d) Vitamin A treatment should be started.

Correct answer is b.

Although retinal gene therapy for LCA2 was initially shown to have positive benefit for patients with *RPE65* mutations, there are no current human clinical trials for *CRB1*, and therefore, gene therapy treatment cannot be recommended.

a) **Incorrect.** Each gene therapy trial is very specific to a particular gene, and in some cases, to particular mutations.
b) **Correct.**
c) **Incorrect.** Although it is certainly possible that an *RPE65* deletion could be present, the child has convincing evidence that her disease is caused by *CRB1* mutations. Digenic disease with both *CRB1* and *RPE65* involvement has not been reported.
d) **Incorrect.** Vitamin A treatment has never been tested in the treatment of children or in any patient with LCA.

25.7.4 Case 4

An 8-year-old boy comes for poor vision evaluation. Clinical examination confirmed that the patient does not fixate nor follow objects, and has at best light perception vision. Additionally, the child has horizontal symmetric nystagmus, paradoxical pupillary responses, and apparently normal fundus examination. Systemic physical examination is normal. Pedigree reveals that paternal and maternal families come from the same small region. Which would be the following step?

a) Follow-up every 3 months.
b) Three-lead VEP (visual evoked potential).
c) Full-field ERG.
d) Brain MRI.

Correct answer is c.

ERG would be the test that provides most important information as the findings are highly suggestive of LCA.

a) **Incorrect.** Obtaining a clear diagnosis will guide the follow-up and best inform the family.
b) **Incorrect.** The three-lead VEP is most useful in the setting of albinism, for which there are no clinical findings in this patient and the vision is far worse than generally expected in albinism.
c) **Correct.**
d) **Incorrect.** The paradoxical pupils point to pathology in the eye. With this visual acuity and a normal retina, LCA becomes a leading diagnosis and brain pathology much less likely.

Suggested Reading

[1] Acland GM, Aguirre GD, Bennett J, et al. Long-term restoration of rod and cone vision by single dose rAAV-mediated gene transfer to the retina in a canine model of childhood blindness. Mol Ther. 2005; 12(6):1072–1082

[2] Bainbridge JW, Smith AJ, Barker SS, et al. Effect of gene therapy on visual function in Leber's congenital amaurosis. N Engl J Med. 2008; 358(21):2231–2239

[3] Cremers FP, van den Hurk JA, den Hollander AI. Molecular genetics of Leber congenital amaurosis. Hum Mol Genet. 2002; 11(10):1169–1176

[4] den Hollander AI, Koenekoop RK, Yzer S, et al. Mutations in the CEP290 (NPHP6) gene are a frequent cause of Leber congenital amaurosis. Am J Hum Genet. 2006; 79(3):556–561

[5] Dharmaraj S, Leroy BP, Sohocki MM, et al. The phenotype of Leber congenital amaurosis in patients with AIPL1 mutations. Arch Ophthalmol. 2004; 122(7):1029–1037

[6] Galvin JA, Fishman GA, Stone EM, Koenekoop RK. Evaluation of genotype-phenotype associations in Leber congenital amaurosis. Retina. 2005; 25(7):919–929

[7] Hanein S, Perrault I, Gerber S, et al. Leber congenital amaurosis: comprehensive survey of the genetic heterogeneity, refinement of the clinical definition, and genotype-phenotype correlations as a strategy for molecular diagnosis. Hum Mutat. 2004; 23(4):306–317

[8] Koenekoop RK, Fishman GA, Iannaccone A, et al. Electroretinographic abnormalities in parents of patients with Leber congenital amaurosis who have heterozygous GUCY2D mutations. Arch Ophthalmol. 2002a; 120 (10):1325–1330

[9] Lotery AJ, Jacobson SG, Fishman GA, et al. Mutations in the CRB1 gene cause Leber congenital amaurosis. Arch Ophthalmol. 2001; 119(3):415–420

[10] Maguire AM, Simonelli F, Pierce EA, et al. Safety and efficacy of gene transfer for Leber's congenital amaurosis. N Engl J Med. 2008; 358(21):2240–2248

[11] Perrault I, Delphin N, Hanein S, et al. Spectrum of NPHP6/CEP290 mutations in Leber's congenital amaurosis and delineation of the associated phenotype. Hum Mutat. 2007; 28(4):416

[12] Bainbridge JW, Mehat MS, Sundaram V, et al. Long-term effect of gene therapy on Leber congenital amaurosis. N Engl J Med. 2015; 372(20):1887–1897

26 Achromatopsia

Abstract

Achromatopsia is a rare cause of infantile nystagmus primarily characterized by reduced or complete loss of color discrimination, reduced visual acuity, and photophobia. Visual acuity is variable, ranging from 20/70 to legal blindness. The disorder is often divided into complete and incomplete forms, the latter being less severe. The fundus is usually normal. The disorder is due to incomplete and maldevelopment of cone cells.

Keywords: achromatopsia, nystagmus, *CNGB3*, *CNGA3*, *GNAT2*, *PDE6C*, *PDE6H*

Key Points

- Achromatopsia is an autosomal recessive disorder with genetic heterogeneity that results in maldevelopment of cone cells.
- Characteristic findings include nonprogressive visual impairment, significant photophobia, nystagmus, and almost absent color discrimination.

26.1 Overview

Achromatopsia is a rare cause of infantile nystagmus primarily characterized by reduced or complete loss of color discrimination, reduced visual acuity, and photophobia. Estimated prevalence is 1 in 30,000 individuals. The nystagmus is usually horizontal, symmetric, high frequency, and small amplitude. Hyperopia may be present. Visual acuity is variable, ranging from 20/70 to legal blindness. The disorder is often divided into complete and incomplete forms, the latter being less severe. The fundus is usually normal, but macular changes and vessel narrowing may be present in some individuals. Patients may also have paradoxical pupillary constriction when transitioned from photopic to scotopic conditions. The disorder is due to incomplete and maldevelopment of cone cells.

26.2 Molecular Genetics

Five genes have been associated with achromatopsia: *CNGB3* (8q21.3), *CNGA3* (2q11.2), *GNAT2* (1p13.1), *PDE6C* (10q24), and *PDE6H* (12p13). Their protein products are expressed in cone cells and all are involved in phototransduction, involving the guanosine binding site of the transducin alpha subunit (*GNAT2*), the alpha subunit of the cone phosphodiesterase (*PDE6C*), the inhibitory gamma subunit (*PDE6H*), and the cGMP-gated cation channels (*CNGA3*/*CNGB3*). *CNGB3* and *CNGA3* are associated with up to 50 and 25% of cases, respectively. In *CNGB3*, the most typical mutation found is c.1148delC (70%). Most patients who present with mutations in *CNGA3*, *CNGB3*, *GNAT2*, and *PDE6C* have complete achromatopsia as compared to those with *PDE6H* mutations who usually present with the incomplete form.

Among Israeli and Palestinian patients who reside in Jerusalem, *CNGA3* mutations are the leading cause of achromatopsia. Two *CNGA3* founder mutations are found in approximately 50% of cases. These pathogenic variants lead to a high achromatopsia prevalence (1:5,000).

26.3 Differential Diagnosis

26.3.1 S (Blue) Cone Monochromacy

This X-linked condition is distinguished from achromatopsia with electrophysiology testing and color vision testing.

26.3.2 Cone Dystrophies

Cone function is normal at birth with a delayed onset of nystagmus as cones degenerate. Symptoms are progressive, including reduced visual acuity, photophobia, and abnormal color vision. Progressive macular pigmentary and atrophic changes may be seen. Color vision is initially normal and then declines.

26.3.3 Alström Syndrome

Although Alström syndrome may present with features indistinguishable from achromatopsia clinically or by electroretinogram (ERG), the disorder is progressive and rod involvement is inevitable with blindness often by the second or third decade of life. Patients may also have obesity, diabetes, hearing loss, and cardiomyopathy.

26.4 Uncommon Manifestations

Progressive retinal degeneration, with an evolving cone dystrophy picture, may occur, especially later in life.

26.5 Clinical Testing

26.5.1 Electrophysiology

Photopic responses are absent or markedly diminished, while the scotopic response is usually normal.

26.5.2 Color Vision Tests

Patients may learn to recognize patterns and differences in brightness, but individuals with achromatopsia have altered color discrimination in all three axes of color vision testing.

26.5.3 Optical Coherence Tomography

Optical coherence tomography (OCT) is often normal, distinguishing this condition from cone dystrophy. Rarely, patients may exhibit variable degrees of foveal hypoplasia, inner/outer segment junction disruption, or macular retinal pigment epithelium (RPE) attenuation.

26.5.4 Systemic Evaluation

It is important to ensure that patients do not have features of Alström syndrome, in particular because the cardiomyopathy can be life-threatening.

26.6 Genetic Testing

One approach is to first perform *CNGB3* sequencing or targeted mutation analysis for the common c.1148delC. *CNGA3* is the second most frequent gene involved, and can also be sequenced to establish the diagnosis. Knowing the frequency of specific gene involvement in the patient's ethnic group may also be helpful in guiding testing strategy. A different approach would be an achromatopsia panel, particularly when the phenotype and history do not suggest a specific gene, which is available in many clinical laboratories.

26.7 Problems

26.7.1 Case 1

An 8-year-old girl presents with symmetric, horizontal, low-amplitude, and high-frequency nystagmus. Which of the following would most suggest a diagnosis of achromatopsia?
a) Normal-appearing posterior pole.
b) Three-lead visual evoked potential (VEP) showing asymmetric decussations.
c) ERG showing normal scotopic responses and isoelectric photopic responses and flicker.
d) Foveal hypoplasia on OCT.

Correct answer is c.
Although the differential diagnosis list for infantile nystagmus narrows in the presence of a normal fundus examination, some subtypes of retinal or cone dystrophies could have a similar appearance early in the disease. The described ERG findings are almost pathognomonic for achromatopsia in this situation.
a) **Incorrect.** Idiopathic infantile nystagmus, Leber congenital amaurosis, blue cone monochromacy, or cone dystrophy can present with description of fairly normal clinical retinal examination.
b) **Incorrect.** The three-lead VEP shows normal decussations in achromatopsia. Asymmetric decussations would be more consistent with albinism, in which case iris transillumination is almost always present.
c) **Correct.**
d) **Incorrect.** In rare cases, patients with achromatopsia have variable degrees of foveal hypoplasia, photoreceptor disruption, or macular RPE attenuation, but in general, true foveal hypoplasia is not often seen

26.7.2 Case 2

A 5-year-old female patient comes to your clinic with her parents; they had recently immigrated from Israel. She presents with photophobia and reduced visual acuity. She has never been examined by an ophthalmologist. Best corrected visual acuity is 20/100. She has high-frequency, low-amplitude, symmetric, and horizontal nystagmus. Fundus examination is normal. Cycloplegic refraction is + 1.50 sph in both eyes. Further study reveals cone dysfunction on ERG, normal OCT, and abnormal color vision. Her pedigree reveals Arab-Muslim ancestry on both sides of the family. Which from the following genes is a good candidate for sequencing?

a) *PDE6C*.
b) *PDE6H*.
c) *CNGB3*.
d) *CNGA3*.

Correct answer is d.

Among Israeli and Palestinian patients, *CNGA3* mutations are the leading cause of achromatopsia. Two *CNGA3* founder mutations are found in approximately 50% of cases.

a) **Incorrect**. *PDE6C* is associated with the complete form, but is not frequent in this population.
b) **Incorrect**. *PDE6H* is associated with incomplete achromatopsia, and is not frequent in this specific population.
c) **Incorrect**. Although *CNGB3* is present in many cases, and is typically associated with the complete form, *CNGA3* mutations are more frequent in this population.
d) **Correct**.

26.7.3 Case 3

A 4-month-old obese boy comes with nystagmus and otherwise normal anterior pole and fundus examination. Cycloplegic refraction is + 3.00 sph in each eye. He does not have polydactyly. ERG under anesthesia shows absent photic responses with normal scotopic responses. Which of the following tests will help most in the clinical diagnosis?

a) Multifocal ERG.
b) OCT.
c) Color vision testing.
d) Audiometry and cardiologic evaluation.

Correct answer is d.

In the early stages, Alström syndrome can be indistinguishable from achromatopsia both clinically and by ERG, although this syndrome is always progressive. Screening for hearing loss and cardiomyopathy are essential to determine whether the cause for this child's subnormal vision is also the same cause for obesity. In this case, detection of associated cardiomyopathy would be life-saving.

a) **Incorrect**. Multifocal ERG requires cooperation of an awake individual. This would not be obtainable in an infant.
b) **Incorrect**. Both achromatopsia and Alström syndrome have normal OCT architecture in the beginning of the disease.
c) **Incorrect**. There is no reliable color vision assessment at this age.
d) **Correct**.

26.7.4 Case 4

A 12-year-old girl diagnosed with achromatopsia has been followed clinically every year since she was 7 years old, when she had abnormal photopic responses and unaltered scotopic responses, stable 20/200 visual acuity, typical nystagmus, and normal OCT. At that time, she had a negative *CNGB3* sequencing, but no further testing was performed because of insurance issues. She comes to see you for a second opinion because of progressive visual loss. After your examination and workup, you find 20/400 visual acuity, loss of internal limiting membrane reflex, blunted foveal reflex, and loss of foveal photoreceptors in the OCT. Which from the following should be your main concern?

a) Functional vision loss.

b) Sequence other genes that when mutated cause achromatopsia.

c) A rare form of progressive achromatopsia.

d) Diagnosis of achromatopsia may be wrong.

Correct answer is d.

Typically, achromatopsia is considered a stable condition. When a patient presents with progressive visual loss, cone or cone–rod dystrophy should be suspected. Next steps would include a repeat ERG and appropriate genetic testing.

a) **Incorrect**. This patient has subtle findings of retinal degeneration on fundus examination and OCT, which are not compatible with functional visual loss, which would have all normal testing.

b) **Incorrect**. The progressive nature of the disease suggests an alternate diagnosis.

c) **Incorrect**. The frequency of progressive achromatopsia is much less than cone dystrophy and would likely not progress this early in life.

d) **Correct**.

Suggested Reading

[1] Johnson S, Michaelides M, Aligianis IA, et al. Achromatopsia caused by novel mutations in both CNGA3 and CNGB3. J Med Genet. 2004; 41(2):e20

[2] Kohl S, Varsanyi B, Antunes GA, et al. CNGB3 mutations account for 50% of all cases with autosomal recessive achromatopsia. Eur J Hum Genet. 2005; 13(3):302–308

[3] Nishiguchi KM, Sandberg MA, Gorji N, Berson EL, Dryja TP. Cone cGMP-gated channel mutations and clinical findings in patients with achromatopsia, macular degeneration, and other hereditary cone diseases. Hum Mutat. 2005; 25(3):248–258

[4] Thiadens AA, Roosing S, Collin RW, et al. Comprehensive analysis of the achromatopsia genes CNGA3 and CNGB3 in progressive cone dystrophy. Ophthalmology. 2010; 117(4):825–30.e1

[5] Thiadens AA, Slingerland NW, Roosing S, et al. Genetic etiology and clinical consequences of complete and incomplete achromatopsia. Ophthalmology. 2009; 116(10):1984–9.e1

[6] Tränkner D, Jägle H, Kohl S, et al. Molecular basis of an inherited form of incomplete achromatopsia. J Neurosci. 2004; 24(1):138–147

[7] Wissinger B, Gamer D, Jägle H, et al. CNGA3 mutations in hereditary cone photoreceptor disorders. Am J Hum Genet. 2001; 69(4):722–737

[8] Zelinger L, Cideciyan AV, Kohl S, et al. Genetics and disease expression in the CNGA3 form of achromatopsia: steps on the path to gene therapy. Ophthalmology. 2015; 122(5):997–1007

27 Congenital Stationary Night Blindness

Abstract

Congenital stationary night blindness is a condition that is suspected in young patients with nonprogressive reduced vision, and nyctalopia with a normal appearing fundus. Visual acuity is variable, but usually ranges from 20/30 to 20/200, although worse vision can be found. Refraction is usually myopic, although in some cases can be hyperopic, with some genotype–phenotype correlation. Other findings include nystagmus and strabismus. The condition has complete penetrance with variable expressivity. It can be classified as complete or incomplete. Clinically, the most striking feature is the constant finding of severe nyctalopia in the complete form, as compared to the incomplete form, where night blindness might not always be present.

Keywords: Congenital stationary night blindness, nyctalopia, nystagmus, color blindness, electroretinogram

---

Key Points

- This condition is characterized by nonprogressive reduced visual acuity, nyctalopia, and variable myopia. Fundus examination is usually normal.
- Congenital stationary night blindness can be X-linked, autosomal dominant, or autosomal recessive, with mutations in more than 14 genes associated with this condition.

27.1 Overview

Congenital stationary night blindness (CSNB) is a condition that is suspected in young patients with nonprogressive reduced vision, and nyctalopia with a normal appearing fundus. Visual acuity is variable, but usually ranges from 20/30 to 20/200, although worse vision can be found. Refraction is usually myopic, although in some cases it can be hyperopic, with some genotype–phenotype correlation. For example, *NYX* mutations are usually associated with high myopia. Other findings include nystagmus and strabismus. Color vision is usually normal though some genetic forms may have mild color defects. Slit-lamp and fundus examination are within normal limits, although there can be tigroid fundus or myopic degeneration in the presence of high myopia. The condition has complete penetrance with variable expressivity.

CSNB can be classified as complete or incomplete. Clinically, the most striking feature is the constant finding of severe nyctalopia in the complete form, as compared to the incomplete form, where night blindness might not always be present. CSNB can also be classified based on full-field electroretinogram (ff ERG) features. The Schubert–Bornschein pattern is characterized by a b-wave that is smaller than the a-wave (electronegative ERG), whereas the Riggs subtype shows proportionally reduced a- and b-waves.

Table 27.1 Molecular causes of congenital stationary night blindness (CSNB)

Subtype (OMIM)	Gene (locus)	CSNB phenotype	Inheritance pattern
CSNB1A (310500)	NYX (Xp11.4)	Complete	X-linked recessive
CSNB1B (257270)	GRM6 (5q35.3)	Complete	AR
CSNB1C (613216)	TRPM1 (15q13.3)	Complete	AR
CSNB1D (613830)	SLC4A1 (15q22.31)	Complete	AR
CSNB1E (614565)	GPR179 (17q12)	Complete	AR
CSNB1F (615058)	LRIT3 (4q25)	Complete	AR
CSNB1G (139330)	GNAT1 (3p21.31)	Complete	AR
CSNB1 H (617024)	GNB3 (12p13.31)	Complete	AR
CSNBAD1 (610445)	RHO (3q22.1)	Complete	AD
CSNBAD2 (163500)	PDE6B (4p16.3)	Complete	AD
CSNBAD3 (610444)	GNAT1 (3p21.31)	Complete	AD
CSNB2A (300071)	CACNA1F (Xp11.23)	Incomplete	X-linked recessive
Congenital nonprogressive cone–rod synaptic disorder (CRSD)	CABP4 (11q13.1)	Incomplete	AR
Oguchi type 1 (258100)	SAG (2q37.1)	Incomplete	AR
Oguchi type 2 (613411)	RHOK/GRK1 (13q34)	Incomplete	AR

Abbreviations: AD, autosomal dominant; AR, autosomal recessive.

27.2 Molecular Genetics

The molecular causes of CSNB are described in ▶ Table 27.1. Approximately 55% of patients with typical X-linked CSNB have mutations in *CACNA1F*, whereas the other 45% have mutations in *NYX*.

There are allelic disorders associated with some of these genes. For example, *CACNA1F* mutations may also result in Åland Island eye disease (AIED), an X-linked recessive (XLr) condition characterized by decreased vision, nystagmus, red–green color deficiency, fundus hypopigmentation, progressive myopia, iris transillumination, and abnormal dark adaptation with abnormal photopic and scotopic responses on ERG. *CACNA1F* mutations have also been associated with CORD (cone–rod dystrophy) and optic atrophy.

27.3 Differential Diagnosis

27.3.1 Blue Cone Monochromacy (OMIM 303700)

This is an XLr disorder characterized by poor vision and nystagmus. It can be distinguished from CSNB because of abnormal color vision, a severely affected photopic ERG with minimally altered rod function, and, in some cases, macular atrophy. It is associated with mutations in *OPN1LW* and *OPN1MW*, the red–green photopigment genes.

27.3.2 Idiopathic Congenital Motor Nystagmus

Patients have a normal ERG and no nyctalopia.

27.3.3 Ocular and Oculocutaneous Albinism (OMIM 300500)

Although these individuals have nystagmus, clinical findings of iris transillumination, foveal hypoplasia, fundus hypopigmentation, and small gray optic nerves as well as the cutaneous and hair hypopigmentation when present allow for distinction from CSNB although there may be some confusion with AIED. The ff ERG in albinism is supranormal.

27.3.4 Oguchi Disease

Oguchi disease is a rare disorder, sometimes classified as a form of CSNB. It is more common in the Japanese population. It is caused by mutations in either the *SAG* or the *GRK1* gene. These patients characteristically show the Mizuo phenomenon, which is a golden-brown fundus with a yellow–gray metallic sheen in the light-adapted state that normalizes after prolonged dark adaptation.

27.4 Uncommon Manifestations

Rarely, individuals with CSNB may have paradoxical pupillary response, which is a miotic effect when lights are turned off or dilations response to light.

27.5 Clinical Testing

27.5.1 Full-Field Electroretinogram

Patients with CSNB have reduced scotopic b-wave amplitudes in response to bright flashes after dark adaptation, resulting in a larger amplitude a-wave compared to b-wave (electronegative b-wave; ► Fig. 27.1). In cases of complete CSNB, the b-wave is

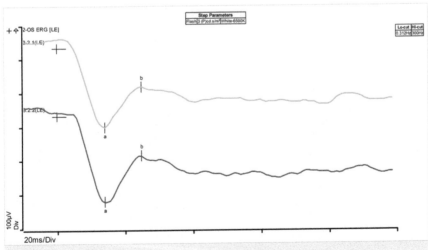

Fig. 27.1 Electronegative b-wave in a patient with congenital stationary night blindness.

severely affected or absent. Incomplete CSNB shows a b-wave that is reduced but it can be measured. Obligate female carriers of XLr CSNB usually have normal ff ERG, although reduced oscillatory potentials or reduced photopic b-wave have been described. Mild cases of CSNB may be missed if ERG is not performed.

27.5.2 Optical Coherence Tomography

Optical coherence tomography (OCT) is typically normal, but some cases can show thinner internal layers.

27.5.3 Fundus Autofluorescence

Fundus autofluorescence (FAF) is typically normal and helps in differentiating CSNB from degenerative disorders.

27.6 Genetic Testing

CSNB multigene panels are available as well as single gene tests. In the absence of family history or an identified family mutation, and when the pedigree may be compatible with more than one inheritance pattern, the multigene panel is likely more cost- and time-efficient. Again, it is important to know the methodology used by a laboratory offering a selected test when interpreting the results. The difference in methodology from one laboratory to another may also impact the choice in selecting a test.

27.7 Problems

27.7.1 Case 1

A 10-year-old boy presents with a history of nonprogressive reduced visual acuity. He does not complain of nyctalopia or other symptom. He has an affected brother and maternal grandfather. Best corrected vision is 20/40 (−2.25 sph OU [oculus uterque]). Clinical examination reveals a subtle horizontal nystagmus of low amplitude and moderate frequency. Slitlamp and funduscopy are normal. Full-field ERG reveals reduced scotopic b-wave amplitudes in response to bright flash after dark adaptation. OCT and FAF are normal. Which seems the most appropriate next step?
a) Sequence *TRPM1* gene.
b) Sequence *CACNA1F* gene.
c) Sequence *RHO* gene.
d) Sequence *SAG* gene.

Correct answer is b.
Family history strongly suggests an XLr pattern. *CACNA1F* is a good candidate gene. In this case, the patient had a hemizygous reported mutation in the *CACNA1F* gene (c.244C > T).
a) **Incorrect.** Mutations in this gene cause autosomal recessive (AR) CSNB. Pedigree strongly suggests XLr inheritance.
b) **Correct.**
c) **Incorrect.** Inheritance pattern is unlikely autosomal dominant as CSNB is fully penetrant.
d) **Incorrect.** Fundus is normal.

27.7.2 Case 2

A 3-year-old boy presents with history of nystagmus since 1 month old. The parents are concerned because he sometimes "bumps into things." He has a 7-year-old healthy sister. Best corrected vision is 20/50 (plano + 2.25 axis 80 OU). Clinical examination shows symmetric horizontal nystagmus of low amplitude and moderate frequency. Slit-lamp reveals subtle iris transillumination. Retinal examination shows macular hypoplasia, gray optic nerves, and fundus hypopigmentation. Full-field ERG is supra-normal and three-lead visual evoked potential responses showed pattern reversal. OCT confirmed macular hypoplasia. Which from the following seem the most appropriate diagnosis?

a) CSNB.
b) Albinism.
c) Blue cone monochromacy (BCM).
d) Congenital idiopathic nystagmus.

Correct answer is b.

Iris transillumination, macular hypoplasia, gray optic nerves, fundus hypopigmentation, and abnormal decussations by three-lead VEP are consistent with a diagnosis of albinism.

a) **Incorrect.** ERG is normal. Iris transillumination and macular hypoplasia are not found in CSNB. Three-lead VEP is normal in CSNB.
b) **Correct.**
c) **Incorrect.** This condition usually has severely affected photopic ERG with minimally altered rod function. Iris transillumination is not seen in BCM and three-lead VEP would be expected to be normal.
d) **Incorrect.** This is a diagnosis of exclusion. In this case, slit-lamp, funduscopy, VEP, and OCT were abnormal.

27.7.3 Case 3

Two affected siblings (a 4-year-old boy and an 11-year-old girl) with a clinical and electrophysiologic diagnosis of complete CSNB, but a negative CSNB gene panel were referred to you for a second opinion. The panel included all known CSNB genes. Deletion and duplication analysis was also performed. There is known consanguinity of the parents. Both patients have visual acuity 20/80 OU, moderate myopia, nystagmus, normal anterior segment, and normal fundus examination. Full-field ERG reveals an electronegative b-wave. Which from the following alternatives seems the best course of action?

a) Retinal dystrophy gene panel.
b) Sequencing of genes for AR OCA (oculocutaneous albinism).
c) Order a new CSNB panel from a different laboratory.
d) Whole exome sequencing (WES).

Correct answer is d.

It is certain that not all genes responsible for CSNB have been discovered. Although WES is an expensive alternative, it can be a helpful mode of testing for well-defined phenotypes in which genetic heterogeneity is suspected and the family is highly motivated to confirm the diagnosis.

a) **Incorrect**. The patient clearly has CSNB rather than another retinal dystrophy.
b) **Incorrect**. There is no transillumination, fundus examination does not suggest albinism, and ffERG is inconsistent.
c) **Less appropriate**. Most likely, it will be redundant and inefficient.
d) **Correct**.

Suggested Reading

[1] Allen LE, Zito I, Bradshaw K, et al. Genotype-phenotype correlation in British families with X linked congenital stationary night blindness. Br J Ophthalmol. 2003; 87(11):1413–1420

[2] Boycott KM, Pearce WG, Bech-Hansen NT. Clinical variability among patients with incomplete X-linked congenital stationary night blindness and a founder mutation in CACNA1F. Can J Ophthalmol. 2000; 35(4): 204–213

[3] Boycott KM, Pearce WG, Musarella MA, et al. Evidence for genetic heterogeneity in X-linked congenital stationary night blindness. Am J Hum Genet. 1998; 62(4):865–875

[4] Dryja TP. Molecular genetics of Oguchi disease, fundus albipunctatus, and other forms of stationary night blindness: LVII Edward Jackson Memorial Lecture. Am J Ophthalmol. 2000; 130(5):547–563

[5] Hemara-Wahanui A, Berjukow S, Hope CI, et al. A CACNA1F mutation identified in an X-linked retinal disorder shifts the voltage dependence of Cav1.4 channel activation. Proc Natl Acad Sci U S A. 2005; 102(21): 7553–7558

[6] Jalkanen R, Bech-Hansen NT, Tobias R, et al. A novel CACNA1F gene mutation causes Aland Island eye disease. Invest Ophthalmol Vis Sci. 2007; 48(6):2498–2502

[7] Jalkanen R, Mäntyjärvi M, Tobias R, et al. X linked cone-rod dystrophy, CORDX3, is caused by a mutation in the CACNA1F gene. J Med Genet. 2006; 43(8):699–704

[8] Miyake Y, Yagasaki K, Horiguchi M, Kawase Y, Kanda T. Congenital stationary night blindness with negative electroretinogram. A new classification. Arch Ophthalmol. 1986; 104(7):1013–1020

[9] Nakamura M, Ito S, Piao CH, Terasaki H, Miyake Y. Retinal and optic disc atrophy associated with a CACNA1F mutation in a Japanese family. Arch Ophthalmol. 2003; 121(7):1028–1033

[10] Rigaudière F, Roux C, Lachapelle P, et al. ERGs in female carriers of incomplete congenital stationary night blindness (I-CSNB). A family report. Doc Ophthalmol. 2003; 107(2):203–212

[11] Tarpey P, Thomas S, Sarvananthan N, et al. Mutations in FRMD7, a newly identified member of the FERM family, cause X-linked idiopathic congenital nystagmus. Nat Genet. 2006; 38(11):1242–1244

[12] Zeitz C, Minotti R, Feil S, et al. Novel mutations in CACNA1F and NYX in Dutch families with X-linked congenital stationary night blindness. Mol Vis. 2005; 11:179–183

[13] Zhang Q, Xiao X, Li S, et al. Mutations in NYX of individuals with high myopia, but without night blindness. Mol Vis. 2007; 13:330–336

28 Juvenile X-Linked Retinoschisis

Abstract

Juvenile X-linked retinoschisis is an X-linked recessive disorder. It has complete penetrance and variable expressivity. Affected individuals are usually diagnosed in the first decade of life. The schisis can affect many layers of the retina, mainly including the inner nuclear, outer nuclear, ganglion cell, and nerve fiber layers. Foveal lesions can present as large radial striations, microcystic spaces, honeycomb-like cysts, foveal pigment mottling, loss of the foveal reflex, or foveal atrophy. Carbonic anhydrase inhibitors can be effective in improving visual acuity and reducing foveal schisis. Approximately half of affected individuals also present with vitreous veils and peripheral schisis. Peripheral schisis may also be accompanied by inner or full-thickness retinal holes and subsequent retinal detachment in up to 20% of affected patients. Vitreous hemorrhage is seen in up to 40% of individuals. The *RS1* gene is the only known gene in which mutations cause this condition.

Keywords: Juvenile X-linked retinoschisis, macular schisis, retinal detachment, vitreous hemorrhage, *RS1*

Key Points

- This condition may be characterized by bilateral symmetric areas of schisis in the macular area with onset in the first decade of life.
- Schisis of the peripheral retina occurs in approximately half of affected patients.
- Visual acuity usually decreases until the second decade of life but then tends to remain stable provided that retinal detachment does not occur.
- Mutation in *RS1* is the only known cause of this X-linked condition.
- Patients are at risk of retinal detachment or vitreous hemorrhage.

28.1 Overview

Juvenile X-linked retinoschisis (JXLR) is an X-linked recessive (XLr) disorder with an estimated prevalence from 1:5,000 to 1:25,000. JXLR has complete penetrance and variable expressivity. JXLR is variable among family members. While carrier females show no clinical signs, affected females with biallelic mutations can present with a wide clinical spectrum, including macular schisis or macular atrophy, associated with markedly reduced autofluorescence signal and a surrounding ring of enhanced autofluorescence. On rare occasions, peripheral examination may reveal white flecks or schisis or macular dysfunction by multifactor electroretinogram (mFERG). This can be explained by skewed X-inactivation.

Affected individuals are usually diagnosed in the first decade of life. The schisis can affect many layers of the retina, mainly including the inner nuclear, outer nuclear, ganglion cell, and nerve fiber layers. Fundus examination often reveals a macular spoke-wheel pattern (▶ Fig. 28.1). Foveal lesions can present as large radial striations, microcystic spaces, honeycomb-like cysts, foveal pigment mottling, loss of the foveal reflex, or foveal atrophy. Carbonic anhydrase inhibitors can be effective in improving

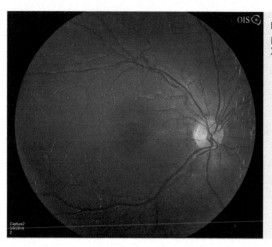

Fig. 28.1 Macular spoke-wheel pattern in a male with juvenile X-linked retinoschisis.

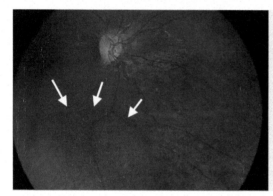

Fig. 28.2 Peripheral retina of a patient with juvenile X-linked retinoschisis, revealing peripheral schisis as marked by the arrows.

visual acuity and reducing foveal schisis. Approximately half of affected individuals also present with vitreous veils and peripheral schisis (▶ Fig. 28.2). Peripheral schisis may also be accompanied by inner or full-thickness retinal holes and subsequent retinal detachment. Retinal detachment can be seen in up to 20% of affected patients. Vitreous hemorrhage is seen in up to 40% of individuals with severe JXLR. Vitreous hemorrhage may be the presenting sign even in infancy. It is due to rupture of vessels that bridge an inner retinal hole. Surgical repair of retinal detachment is difficult. In patients older than 50 years, posterior pole pigmentary changes and retinal pigment epithelium (RPE) atrophy are common.

28.2 Molecular Genetics

The *RS1* gene (Xp22.13) is the only known gene in which pathogenic variants cause JXLR. The product is retinoschisin, which is predominantly expressed in the inner segments of the photoreceptors. Retinoschisin is an extracellular protein, although the specific function is still unknown. Nonsense mutations are usually associated with severe phenotypes. Missense, splice site, or frameshift mutations or intragenic deletion result in JXLR phenotype.

28.3 Differential Diagnosis

28.3.1 Goldmann–Favre Vitreoretinal Degeneration and Enhanced S-Cone Syndrome (OMIM 268100)

These conditions are caused by autosomal recessive (AR) *NR2E3* mutations. Unlike JXLR, females may be affected. Patients generally present with severely impaired visual acuity, visual field loss, and night blindness. Intraretinal cystoid spaces can be seen with peripheral retinoschisis. ERG shows markedly reduced a- and b-waves.

28.3.2 Retinitis Pigmentosa

Patients with RP (retinitis pigmentosa), as opposed to JXLR, present with optic nerve pallor, narrowing of retinal vessels, and "bone spicule" pigmentary clumping with a severely affected full-field (ff) ERG. They may have cystoid macular edema (CME) or intraretinal cystoid spaces that resemble JXLR.

28.3.3 *VCAN* Vitreoretinopathies

VCAN vitreoretinopathies can be confused with JXLR because of vitreous abnormalities. *VCAN*-related vitreoretinopathies can be distinguished from JXLR because of autosomal dominant (AD) inheritance (females can be affected), optically empty vitreous on slit-lamp examination, presenile cataract, night blindness, progressive chorioretinal atrophy, and moderately to severely affected scotopic, and photopic ERG without electronegative waveforms.

28.3.4 Cystoid Macular Edema

There are many causes for CME, such as inflammation, diabetes mellitus, uveitis, intraocular surgery, optic nerve pits, or AD CME. Diagnosis is based on a leakage on intravenous fluorescein angiography (IVFA; perifoveal petaloid pattern), which is not seen in JXLR.

28.3.5 Other Disorders with Intraretinal Cystoid Spaces

Other disorders with intraretinal cystoid spaces, including fenestrated sheen dystrophy, pathologic myopia, degenerative macular schisis, drug-induced (niacin), vitreomacular traction, isolated foveomacular schisis, and a wide range of retinal dystrophies.

28.3.6 Traumatic Macular Retinoschisis of Abusive Head Trauma

Traumatic macular retinoschisis of abusive head trauma should not be confused with JXLR as its appearance is completely different and may be a misnomer. Hemorrhage is seen to accumulate most often under the internal limiting membrane (ILM). There may be circumlinear hemorrhagic or hypopigmented folds at the edge of the schisis cavity. Retinal hemorrhages are usually present. The lesion can be unilateral.

28.3.7 Proliferative Vitreoretinopathy

This condition most commonly develops as a complication of rhegmatogenous retinal detachment. Advanced stages of JXLR can be confused with proliferative vitreoretinopathy.

28.4 Uncommon Manifestations

Severe and atypical findings in young patients include macular atrophy and pigmentary changes. The Mizuo phenomenon, which is characteristic of Oguchi disease, can also be seen in JXLR. It presents as a golden-brown fundus with a yellow-gray metallic sheen in the light-adapted state. After 3 to 12 hours of complete dark adaptation, the fundus appears normal. The disappearance of the shiny, yellow, fundus reflex is known as the Mizuo–Nakamura phenomenon.

Gunn's dots are tiny white dots sometimes visible overlying the nerve fiber layer that correspond to visible reflections of the ILM, created by the footplate of the Muller cells, and rarely can be seen in patients with JXLR.

28.5 Clinical Testing

28.5.1 Optical Coherence Tomography

JXLR affects primarily the inner retinal layers. This test reveals the typical intraretinal cystoid spaces (▶ Fig. 28.3). With age, some cystic spaces may flatten and atrophy may appear, especially in patients beyond the first two decades of life.

28.5.2 Fundus Autofluorescence

Fundus autofluorescence (FAF) can show increased foveal autofluorescence, sometimes in a radiating pattern consistent with the inner retinal cystoid spaces.

28.5.3 Full-Field Electroretinogram

Although ERG findings could be variable, the electronegative b-wave is a classic finding in JXLR.

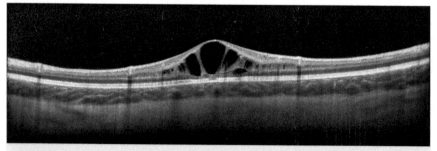

Fig. 28.3 Retinal optical coherence tomography showing macular schisis in juvenile X-linked retinoschisis.

28.5.4 Intravenous Fluorescein Angiography

This test is useful in detecting nonleaking schisis from leaking cystoid macular edema. The latter is not associated with JXLR..

28.6 Genetic Testing

Gene testing is clinically available for *RS1*. Approximately 90% of patients can be found to have a pathogenic change in *RS1*. If there is a known mutation or a population-specific mutation based on a person's ethnicity, targeted mutation analysis has an even higher yield. If sequencing is uninformative, deletion/duplication analysis should be performed.

28.7 Problems

28.7.1 Case 1

A 10-year-old boy was referred for nyctalopia and reduced visual acuity. His family history shows that his maternal grandfather and one of his brothers have "something similar." Visual acuity is 20/100 in both eyes (−0.50 sph OU [oculus uterque]). There is no nystagmus. Fundus examination reveals a macular spoke-wheel pattern of the nerve fiber layer. Vitreous is normal. FAF shows small foci of mild foveal hyper-autofluorescence. Optical coherence tomography (OCT) showed intraretinal cystoid spaces in each macula that do not leak on IVFA. His scotopic ffERG reveals reduction of the dark-adapted b-wave amplitude with relative preservation of the a-wave amplitude. Photopic ERG is normal. Which from the following is the most appropriate diagnosis?

a) X-linked juvenile retinoschisis.
b) Congenital stationary night blindness (CSNB).
c) Goldmann–Favre syndrome.
d) Enhanced S-cone syndrome.

Correct answer is a.

The history of nyctalopia and decreased visual acuity associated with the finding of a nerve fiber layer macular spoke-wheel pattern, typical ERG, and intraretinal cystoid spaces on OCT all suggest a diagnosis of JXLR. The patient was found to be hemizygous for a previously reported mutation in *RS1* (c.3G > A).

a) **Correct.**
b) **Incorrect.** Fundus in CSNB is normal, OCT is normal, and nystagmus is often present.
c) **Incorrect.** There are no vitreous abnormalities. Photopic ERG in Goldman–Favre is usually abnormal and electronegative b wave would be atypical at this age.
d) **Incorrect.** Although a macular spoke-wheel pattern due to intraretinal cystoid spaces can be seen in ESCS, the ffERG would not show the electronegative b-wave and would instead show typical abnormalities in the cone responses.

28.7.2 Case 2

A 22-year-old man comes for decreasing visual acuity that began when he was 12 years old. He has an affected brother with the same condition. Family history reveals that his maternal grandfather had bilateral retinal detachment in his youth. Best corrected visual acuity of the patient is 20/40 with correction of –2.00 sph OD (oculus dextrus) and hand movements with –1.50 sph OS (oculus sinister). Anterior segment examination is unremarkable. Fundus examination reveals some vitreous veils, posterior vitreous detachment, intraretinal cystoid spaces confirmed by OCT, and peripheral retinal schisis. The left eye examination shows a complete retinal detachment. Full-field ERG shows moderately reduced b-wave amplitudes in the OD, with normal photopic ERG and no recordable signal in OS. Which from the following seems the most appropriate diagnosis?

a) Wagner syndrome.
b) JXLR.
c) Goldmann–Favre syndrome.
d) Erosive vitreoretinopathy.

Correct answer is b.

This is a case very suggestive of JXLR, with compatible ERG and vitreous findings. Family history is suggestive of XLr inheritance pattern.

a) **Incorrect.** There is no chorioretinal atrophy and the pedigree does not show an AD pattern. Intraretinal cystoid spaces and superficial peripheral schisis are unusual for Wagner syndrome.

b) **Correct.**

c) **Incorrect.** Full-field ERG in Goldmann–Favre is usually severely affected to both cone and rod stimuli. In addition, family history does not suggest an AR pattern.

d) **Incorrect.** The family history is not consistent with erosive vitreoretinopathy. This condition usually shows a progressive pigmentary retinopathy, in particular with thinning and progressive "erosion" in the equatorial periphery. Full-field ERG is usually severely affected.

28.7.3 Case 3

A 12-year-old boy was referred for reduced visual acuity. His family history shows that his maternal grandfather is affected with "low vision since childhood" in one eye and retinal detachment in the fellow eye. Vision acuity of the proband is 20/200 in both eyes (–0.75 sph OU). There is no nystagmus. Fundus examination reveals a macular superficial spoke-wheel pattern and an inferior superficial retinoschisis with an inner retinal hole that is spanned by a retinal vessel. Vitreous is normal. OCT confirms intraretinal cystoid spaces in each macula that do not leak on IVFA. His scotopic ffERG reveals reduction of the amplitude of the dark-adapted b-wave amplitude with relative preservation of the a-wave amplitude. Photopic ERG is normal. *RS1* sequencing was negative. Which from the following is the most appropriate next step?

a) *NR2E3* sequencing.
b) Whole-exome sequencing.
c) Retinal dystrophy panel.
d) *RS1* deletion/duplication analysis.

Correct answer is d.

History and examination is very suggestive of JXLR. When *RS1* sequencing is negative in the context of a clinical presentation strongly suggestive of JXLR, deletion/duplication analysis is a good option as these abnormalities cannot be detected by sequencing. In this case, testing revealed *RS1* c.53–78del.

a) **Incorrect.** Mutations in *NR2E3* do not cause superficial retinal schisis with holes. ERG is usually more severely abnormal including photopic responses.

b) **Incorrect.** Does not detect deletions or duplications, and phenotype and history are compatible with JXLR.

c) **Incorrect.** Clinical diagnosis is JXLR.

d) **Correct.**

Suggested Reading

[1] Apushkin MA, Fishman GA, Rajagopalan AS. Fundus findings and longitudinal study of visual acuity loss in patients with X-linked retinoschisis. Retina. 2005; 25(5):612–618

[2] Bowles K, Cukras C, Turriff A, et al. X-linked retinoschisis: RS1 mutation severity and age affect the ERG phenotype in a cohort of 68 affected male subjects. Invest Ophthalmol Vis Sci. 2011; 52(12):9250–9256

[3] Eksandh L, Andréasson S, Abrahamson M. Juvenile X-linked retinoschisis with normal scotopic b-wave in the electroretinogram at an early stage of the disease. Ophthalmic Genet. 2005; 26(3):111–117

[4] Eksandh LC, Ponjavic V, Ayyagari R, et al. Phenotypic expression of juvenile X-linked retinoschisis in Swedish families with different mutations in the XLRS1 gene. Arch Ophthalmol. 2000; 118(8):1098–1104

[5] Gehrig A, Weber BH, Lorenz B, Andrassi M. First molecular evidence for a de novo mutation in RS1 (XLRS1) associated with X linked juvenile retinoschisis. J Med Genet. 1999; 36(12):932–934

[6] Grayson C, Reid SN, Ellis JA, et al. Retinoschisin, the X-linked retinoschisis protein, is a secreted photoreceptor protein, and is expressed and released by Weri-Rb1 cells. Hum Mol Genet. 2000; 9(12):1873–1879

[7] Kim DY, Mukai S. X-linked juvenile retinoschisis (XLRS): a review of genotype-phenotype relationships. Semin Ophthalmol. 2013; 28(5–6):392–396

[8] Kim LS, Seiple W, Fishman GA, Szlyk JP. Multifocal ERG findings in carriers of X-linked retinoschisis. Doc Ophthalmol. 2007; 114(1):21–26

[9] Molday RS, Kellner U, Weber BH. X-linked juvenile retinoschisis: clinical diagnosis, genetic analysis, and molecular mechanisms. Prog Retin Eye Res. 2012; 31(3):195–212

[10] The Retinoschisis Consortium. Functional implications of the spectrum of mutations found in 234 cases with X-linked juvenile retinoschisis. Hum Mol Genet. 1998; 7(7):1185–1192

29 Retinoblastoma

Vikas Khetan, Jagadeesan Madhavan, Diego Ossandón Villaseca, and Carol L. Shields

Abstract

Retinoblastoma (RB) is a childhood intraocular malignancy that most commonly presents as leukocoria. Early diagnosis can lead to excellent outcomes. Otherwise, the disease progresses to a massive tumor, with invasion of surrounding structures via the optic nerve or sclera, with risk of metastasis and subsequent mortality. Survival is therefore variable: approximately 30% in underdeveloped countries but 97% in developed countries. Inactivation of both alleles of the RB gene (*RB1*) predispose an individual to develop RB. The disease can be categorized as hereditary (25–35%) or nonhereditary (65–75%). Hereditary RB develops from a predisposition due to a de novo or inherited germline *RB1* mutation with subsequent loss of the function of the second allele (loss of heterozygosity) due to a somatic mutation. Familial RB accounts for approximately 6% of newly diagnosed RB. In the hereditary RB, 85% of tumors are early onset, bilateral, and multifocal with a cumulative average of five tumors, the distribution being random between the eyes. In nonhereditary RB, tumors are solitary and unilateral with later onset. Management of a patient with RB aims primarily to preserve life, and secondarily the globe and, ultimately, visual potential. Treatment alternatives include enucleation, radiotherapy, systemic and intra-arterial chemotherapy, and focal treatments.

Keywords: retinoblastoma, childhood ocular tumor, enucleation, intra-arterial chemotherapy, *RB1*

Key Points

- Retinoblastoma (RB) is a childhood retinal malignancy that can be hereditary or sporadic.
- RB demonstrates the two-hit hypothesis, whereby its heritable form is characterized by autosomal dominant heterozygous germline mutation with subsequent somatic loss of the other allele's function (loss of heterozygosity). A nonheritable form occurs when the function of both alleles is lost through somatic mutations in situ for each.

29.1 Overview

Retinoblastoma (RB) is a childhood ocular malignancy that most commonly presents as leukocoria. Early diagnosis can lead to excellent outcomes. Otherwise, the disease progresses to a massive tumor, with invasion of surrounding structures via he optic nerve or sclera, with risk of metastasis and subsequent mortality. Survival is therefore variable: approximately 30% in underdeveloped countries but 97% in developed countries.

Inactivation of both alleles of the RB gene (*RB1*) predisposes an individual to develop RB. The disease can be categorized as hereditary (25–35%) or nonhereditary (65–75%). Hereditary RB develops from a predisposition due to a de novo or inherited germline *RB1* mutation with subsequent loss of the function of the second allele (loss of heterozygosity [LOH]) due to a somatic mutation. Familial RB accounts for approximately 6% of newly diagnosed RB. De novo hereditary RB occurs due to the inactivation of the first *RB1* allele at the time of conception. This is uncommon. In nonhereditary RB, each allele is mutated in situ as a somatic change after conception. All cases of nonhereditary RB are sporadic.

In the hereditary RB, 85% of tumors are early onset, bilateral, and multifocal with a cumulative average of five tumors, the distribution being random between the two eyes. In nonhereditary RB, tumors are solitary and unilateral with later onset.

Management of a patient with RB aims primarily to preserve life, and secondarily the globe and, ultimately, visual potential. Treatment alternatives include enucleation, radiotherapy, systemic and intra-arterial chemotherapy, and focal treatments (cryotherapy, transpupillary thermotherapy, and laser photocoagulation).

29.2 Molecular Genetics

The *RB1* gene is located at 13q14.2. *RB1* is a tumor suppressor gene, the product of which plays a role in cell cycle regulation. Tumor development requires mutations in both copies of the gene. The first allele to be mutated may be found in the germline (hereditary RB) or in a somatic cell (nonhereditary RB). Approximately 10% of *RB1* germline mutations are due to germline mosaicism. Mosaicism is suggested when a parent with more than one affected child does not show the same mutant allele present in their children. In all forms of RB, the second allele is inactivated somatically due to mitotic nondisjunction, duplication, mitotic recombination between the *RB1* locus and the centromere, or gene conversion and deletion. LOH is the most frequent mechanism of second hit in RB. In unilateral RB, silencing of the *RB1* gene due to methylation of the promoter region is also a known mechanism by which the function of at least one allele is lost.

More recent studies also show that RB tumors may demonstrate different mutagenic pathways from normal to malignant cell. A small subset of RB is caused by amplification of the *MYCN* gene in tumor cells. It is unknown whether *MYCN* amplification is the only genomic event driving malignancy of these tumors. Further investigation is needed to examine if these tumors are different than those caused by *RB1* pathogenic variants.

In addition, *RB1* gene inactivation alone is insufficient to induce tumorigenesis. Additional genetic and stochastic events lead to uncontrolled retinal precursor cell proliferation. Comparative genomic hybridization and gene expression studies have facilitated the probing of genes controlling basic events in cellular development, proliferation, differentiation, and apoptosis. The minimal regions most frequently gained in chromosomes of RB are 1q31 (52%), 6p22 (44%), 2p24–25 (30%), and 13q32–34 (12%), and the most commonly lost is 16p22 (14%). Proposed candidate genes responsible for some of these chromosomal imbalances include the leukemic oncogene *DEK* and the transcriptional factor *E2F3*. *MYCN* or *KIF14* amplification, or overexpression, and *CDH11* (cadherin II) loss of expression are other candidates proposed to affect RB development and progression.

A small subset of hereditary RB are due to germline de novo chromosomal deletion of various sizes of the *RB1* locus chr 13q. The phenotype in del13q syndrome with RB includes prominent eyebrows, broad nasal bridge, anteverted ear lobes, a high and broad forehead, bulbous tip of the nose, large mouth, thin upper lip, thick lower lip, and long philtrum, hypertelorism, proptosis, cleft palate, macroglossia, hypotonia with severe developmental delay, and/or motor impairment (▶ Fig. 29.1). Approximately 5 to

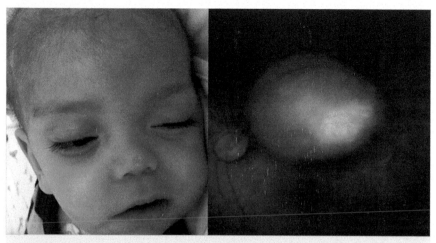

Fig. 29.1 Patient with 13q deletion syndrome demonstrating facial dysmorphism and retinoblastoma.

15% of patients with RB are heterozygous for a deletion that includes 13q14.2. The frequency of unilateral RB in these patients is likely higher than patients with intragenic mutations. Deletion of 13q has variable phenotype, depending on the location and size of the deletion: deletions proximal to 13q32 (group 1) have mild to moderate developmental delay, variable dysmorphic features, and growth retardation; deletions affecting 13q32 (group 2) have one or more major malformations including brain, genitourinary or gastrointestinal, or severe microcephaly; distal deletions involving 13q33q34 (group 3) have variable presentation.

Patients with an interstitial 13q deletion involving *RB1* can show less aggressive phenotypic expression of RB with deletions larger than 1 Mb, which contains the *MED4* gene. Other genes affected, such as *NUFIP1* and *PCDH8*, may contribute to psychomotor delay, *MTLR1* to microcephaly, and loss of *EDNRB* to feeding difficulties and deafness.

Small *RB1* mutations that produce premature termination codons almost always cause bilateral RB. It has been suggested that the tendency for total deletions to cause fewer tumors is due to contiguous deletion of an adjacent unknown gene that is essential for cell survival. Therefore, fewer and less aggressive tumors would develop in larger deletions.

29.3 Differential Diagnosis

29.3.1 Astrocytic Hamartoma

These are glial tumors of the retinal nerve fiber layer that arise from retinal astrocytes. They appear as a cream-white, well-circumscribed, elevated lesion that may present as multiple or solitary sites. A lesion is commonly seen with a multilobulated appearance, but can also be seen as flat and semitranslucent. It is most frequently associated with tuberous sclerosis but may also be seen in affected individuals with neurofibromatosis. It can also be found as an isolated presentation.

29.3.2 Ocular Toxocariasis

Ocular toxocariasis can cause a peripheral retinal mass that resembles RB, but it is usually unilateral and associated with inflammation. History of contact with puppies or dirt eating, fever, eosinophilia, pneumonitis, or hepatosplenomegaly would be helpful. Positive serum titers for toxocara canis would confirm the diagnosis.

29.3.3 Coats' Disease

Can be considered as differential in case of retinal detachment. This condition presents with abnormally dilated, tortuous vessels, associated with exudation that causes a masslike lesion of lipid with associated telangiectatic neovascularization. The exudate tends to be more yellow than white because of the presence of cholesterol. This condition is typically unilateral and predominantly affects older boys.

29.3.4 Other Differential for White Mass

Other differential for white mass include benign vasoproliferative tumors, choroidal coloboma, and myelinated retinal nerve fibers. Norrie disease and retinopathy of prematurity can be considered as RB differential when facing retinal detachment.

29.4 Uncommon Manifestations

Some children with the hereditary form of RB develop pinealoblastoma (trilateral RB). The pinealoblastoma has embryological, pathological, and immunological similarities to RB. The other clinical variants, retinoma and retinocytoma, are uncommon benign forms of RB, occurring in less than 3% of cases. This form of RB is also termed "spontaneously arrested" or "spontaneously regressed" RB.

Clinical evidence strongly suggests that the rare retinoma that remains stable and unchanging under observation can sometimes later progress to an active, malignant RB, perhaps by failure of senescence. Higher expression of *p16* in retinoma arrests its proliferative capability that results in cellular senescence.

Rarely, Hirschsprung's disease can be associated with 13q deletion syndrome.

29.5 Clinical Testing

29.5.1 Ultrasound

This test is crucial for RB diagnosis. Advantages are that it can be performed without sedation and can be repeated multiple times without exposing the patient to radiation. RB lesions appear as echogenic soft tissue masses with variable shadowing due to calcifications and heterogeneity due to necrosis or hemorrhages. Doppler may show vascularization. Vitreous may have multiple areas of echogenicity that can represent vitreous seeding, necrotic debris, or hemorrhage. Ultrasound can also reveal areas of retinal detachment.

29.5.2 Computed Tomography and Magnetic Resonance Imaging

CT (computed tomography) reveals a contrast-enhancing retrolental mass that is usually calcified. Nevertheless, MRI (magnetic resonance imaging) is the test of choice for staging, which can help in diagnosing choroidal involvement, optic nerve involvement, or extra-ocular extension.

29.5.3 Fundus Photography

This test is useful to document RB progression or tumor regression after treatment.

29.6 Genetic Testing

Although the *RB1* gene is the causative gene of RB, the *MYCN* gene has started to be studied by specialized diagnostic laboratories. *RB1* testing includes copy number changes (quantitative multiplex PCR (polymerase chain reaction) to look for exonic deletions and duplications), sequence analysis of exonic regions and flanking intronic regions, and splice site analysis. Other specific tests are for methylation of the *RB1* promoter and amino acid conservation analysis.

Fluorescence in situ hybridization (FISH) and chromosomal microarray (CMA) can be requested as well when suspecting contiguous gene deletion syndrome (deletion of chromosome 13). CMA has benefits over FISH as it can better determine the breakpoints and provide a more accurate size of the particular deletion.

29.7 Problems

29.7.1 Case 1

An 8-month-old child is presented with bilateral RB. The father of the child had enucleation performed during childhood for RB. What would be the first molecular diagnostic test to be performed?
a) Methylation status of the *RB1* gene in the peripheral blood.
b) Methylation status of the *RB1* gene in the tumor.
c) Deletion/insertion and point mutation screening of *RB1* in peripheral blood.
d) Deletion/insertion and point mutation screening of *RB1* in the tumor.

Correct answer is c.
As it is a case of familial RB, peripheral venous blood screening for insertion/deletion and point mutation will likely help in identifying the first hit in the *RB1* gene, which is responsible for disease transmission. This will help confirm familial RB and prevent the transmission of the disease to the next offspring.
a) **Incorrect.** Hyper-methylation of the promoter region of the *RB1* gene happens only in tumor and not in the peripheral blood.
b) **Incorrect.** Identifying methylation status of tumor in familial RB does not add value in the management of the disease. The first priority of the molecular diagnosis of familial RB will be to identify the first hit responsible for disease transmission in the family.
c) **Correct.**
d) **Incorrect.** It would be appropriate to screen the peripheral blood for first hit in familial RB. The identified mutation in the peripheral blood may be confirmed in the tumor if it is available.

29.7.2 Case 2

Which one of the following statements on the genetic defect of retinoma is true?
a) Presence of gene defect in *KIF14*.
b) Absence of mutation in *RB1*.
c) Absence of any genetic defect.
d) High gene expression of *p16*.

Correct answer is d.
   Higher expression of *p16* in retinoma arrests its proliferative capability that results in cellular senescence.
a) **Incorrect.** Profound expression of the *KIF14* gene has been associated with higher proliferation rate in RB. Retinoma is a spontaneously arrested tumor with very little proliferative capability.
b) **Incorrect.** The initiating mutation in *RB1* has been identified in retinoma similar to RB. With the absence of additional events for proliferation, retinoma does not progress to RB.
c) **Incorrect.** Retinoma carries an *RB1* gene defect.
d) **Correct.**

29.7.3 Case 3

A 5-month-old male infant presented with unilateral RB with invasion of optic nerve. Molecular screening of the tumor lacked *RB1* defect. Which one of the following statements would be correct with respect to the molecular profile of this tumor?
a) The peripheral blood may have *MYCN* amplification.
b) *MYCN* amplification in the tumor.
c) Very high copy numbers of *KIF14*, *DEK*, and *E2F3* in the tumor.
d) Loss of *CDH11* (cadherin 11) in the tumor.

Correct answer is b.
   MYCN amplification is the driving mutation in this tumor in the absence of *RB1* defect.
a) **Incorrect.** *MYCN* amplification is a sporadic event and happens only in tumor.
b) **Correct.**
c) **Incorrect.** Only *RBI* defect causes genomic instability that would result in amplification of various oncogenes.
d) **Incorrect.** *MYCN* amplification does not cause gross genomic instability that would result in loss of tumor suppressor gene.

29.7.4 Case 4

A 6-month-old infant was referred to the molecular diagnostic lab for RB screening. The child had bilateral RB, dysmorphic face, and delayed milestones. Which one of the following investigation is preferred?
a) Peripheral blood screening for *RB1* point mutations.
b) LOH assessment.
c) FISH in peripheral blood or CMA.
d) Peripheral blood methylation studies.

Correct answer is c.

The child most likely has 13q14 deletion syndrome. FISH technique is useful to detect large deletions. Large deletions can also sometimes be detected by conventional karyotyping if the deletion is large enough. Large deletion in 13q14 region results in loss of the *RB1* gene and other genes around *RB1* that result in bilateral RB, facial dysmorphism, and mental retardation.

a) **Incorrect.** Point mutation in *RB1* leads to isolated RB without any other systemic features.

b) **Incorrect.** LOH assessment is performed to identify the second hit in the tumor sample.

c) **Correct.**

d) **Incorrect.** Methylation studies of the promoter region of the *RB1* gene are requested for tumor samples and not in the peripheral blood.

Suggested Reading

[1] Knudson AG, Jr. Mutation and cancer: statistical study of retinoblastoma. Proc Natl Acad Sci U S A. 1971; 68 (4):820–823

[2] Shields JA, Shields CL. Intraocular tumors – A text and Atlas. Philadelphia, PA: WB Saunders Company; 1992

[3] Zimmerman LE, Burns RP, Wankum G, Tully R, Esterly JA. Trilateral retinoblastoma: ectopic intracranial retinoblastoma associated with bilateral retinoblastoma. J Pediatr Ophthalmol Strabismus. 1982; 19(6):320–325

[4] Munier FL, Thonney F, Girardet A, et al. Evidence of somatic and germinal mosaicism in pseudo-low-penetrant hereditary retinoblastoma, by constitutional and single-sperm mutation analysis. Am J Hum Genet. 1998; 63(6):1903–1908

[5] Cavenee WK, Dryja TP, Phillips RA, et al. Expression of recessive alleles by chromosomal mechanisms in retinoblastoma. Nature. 1983; 305(5937):779–784

[6] Ramprasad VL, Madhavan J, Murugan S, et al. Retinoblastoma in India : microsatellite analysis and its application in genetic counseling. Mol Diagn Ther. 2007; 11(1):63–70

[7] Rushlow DE, Mol BM, Kennett JY, et al. Characterisation of retinoblastomas without RB1 mutations: genomic, gene expression, and clinical studies. Lancet Oncol. 2013; 14(4):327–334

[8] DiCiommo D, Gallie BL, Bremner R. Retinoblastoma: the disease, gene and protein provide critical leads to understand cancer. Semin Cancer Biol. 2000; 10(4):255–269

[9] Chen D, Gallie BL, Squire JA. Minimal regions of chromosomal imbalance in retinoblastoma detected by comparative genomic hybridization. Cancer Genet Cytogenet. 2001; 129(1):57–63

[10] Bowles E, Corson TW, Bayani J, et al. Profiling genomic copy number changes in retinoblastoma beyond loss of RB1. Genes Chromosomes Cancer. 2007; 46(2):118–129

[11] Corson TW, Huang A, Tsao MS, Gallie BL. KIF14 is a candidate oncogene in the 1q minimal region of genomic gain in multiple cancers. Oncogene. 2005; 24(30):4741–4753

[12] Dimaras H, Khetan V, Halliday W, et al. Loss of RB1 induces non-proliferative retinoma: increasing genomic instability correlates with progression to retinoblastoma. Hum Mol Genet. 2008; 17(10):1363–1372

[13] Friend SH, Bernards R, Rogelj S, et al. A human DNA segment with properties of the gene that predisposes to retinoblastoma and osteosarcoma. Nature. 1986; 323(6089):643–646

[14] Cooper GM. The Cell: A Molecular Approach. 2nd ed. Sunderland, MA: Sinauer Associates; 2000

[15] Albrecht P, Ansperger-Rescher B, Schüler A, Zeschnigk M, Gallie B, Lohmann DR. Spectrum of gross deletions and insertions in the RB1 gene in patients with retinoblastoma and association with phenotypic expression. Hum Mutat. 2005; 26(5):437–445

[16] Bunin GR, Emanuel BS, Meadows AT, Buckley JD, Woods WG, Hammond GD. Frequency of 13q abnormalities among 203 patients with retinoblastoma. J Natl Cancer Inst. 1989; 81(5):370–374

[17] Mitter D, Ullmann R, Muradyan A, et al. Genotype-phenotype correlations in patients with retinoblastoma and interstitial 13q deletions. Eur J Hum Genet. 2011; 19(9):947–958

[18] Richter S, Vandezande K, Chen N, et al. Sensitive and efficient detection of RB1 gene mutations enhances care for families with retinoblastoma. Am J Hum Genet. 2003; 72(2):253–269

30 Optic Nerve Hypoplasia

Abstract

Optic nerve hypoplasia is the most frequent optic nerve head anomaly. It is a unilateral or bilateral congenital, nonprogressive developmental abnormality. The clinical presentation is extremely variable. A "double-ring sign," which is the outline of the circle formed by the lamina cribrosa unfilled by optic nerve fibers around the small optic nerve, is not always present. Patients usually present with reduced vision with or without nystagmus or strabismus. Visual acuity in affected individuals does not necessarily correlate with the size of the optic nerve head. Optic nerve hypoplasia may be associated with other ocular disorders such as microphthalmia, aniridia, and albinism, as well as systemic associations such as neurologic and endocrine anomalies (septo-optic dysplasia). Most patients with optic nerve hypoplasia do not have an identifiable molecular cause, though many may likely have an underlying genetic cause.

Keywords: optic nerve hypoplasia, double-ring sign, childhood blindness, coloboma, microphthalmia

Key Points

- Optic nerve hypoplasia (ONH) is a congenital, nonprogressive developmental abnormality characterized by small optic disc, with or without a peripapillary "double-ring sign."
- Most patients with ONH do not have an identifiable molecular cause, though many may likely have an underlying genetic cause.

30.1 Overview

Optic nerve hypoplasia (ONH) is the most frequent optic nerve head anomaly. It is a unilateral or bilateral congenital, nonprogressive developmental abnormality. The clinical presentation is extremely variable. A "double-ring sign," which is the outline of the circle formed by the lamina cribrosa unfilled by optic nerve fibers around the small optic nerve, is not always present (▶ Fig. 30.1). Retinal vascular tortuosity and a failure of the normal arcade pattern to develop are also important but inconsistent signs. Patients usually present with reduced vision with or without nystagmus or strabismus. Visual acuity in affected individuals does not necessarily correlate with the size of the optic nerve head. In mild cases, increased disc-to-macula distance/disc diameter ratio can be used to determine if ONH is present. Other visual functions such as color vision may remain unaffected. An afferent pupillary defect can be seen. ONH may be associated with other ocular disorders such as microphthalmia, aniridia, and albinism.

ONH accounts for up to one-quarter of children with significant congenital visual loss. Depending on the population, 5 to 15% of blind children have ONH. The estimated

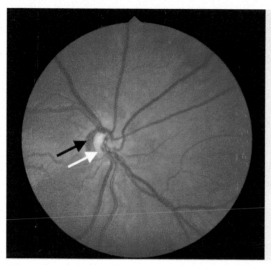

Fig. 30.1 Severe optic nerve hypoplasia. The white arrow indicates the optic nerve. The black arrow indicates the double-ring sign.

prevalence is 1.5:10,000. It is thought that fetal exposure to teratogenic agents such as alcohol or illicit drugs has increased the incidence of ONH. Carbamazepine, isotretinoin, phenytoin, quinine, and valproic acid have also been suggested as predisposing factors. Segmental inferior hemi-ONH has been associated with maternal gestational insulin-dependent diabetes.

Individuals with ONH should be evaluated for systemic associations such as neurologic and endocrine anomalies. Many syndromes have been reported with ONH (see text box below). Approximately half of patients with ONH have hypopituitarism, while neuroimaging anomalies are detected in 60% of bilaterally affected individuals, and approximately one-third of those with unilateral ONH, and include hypoplastic optic nerves with a hypoplastic chiasm, cortical heterotopia, other neuronal migration anomalies, hydrocephalus, and absent or hypoplastic corpus callosum and/or absent septum pellucidum. Less common findings include cerebral atrophy, encephalocele, cerebellar vermis hypoplasia, and other posterior fossa anomalies. The pituitary may be absent (empty sella) or, more commonly, the posterior pituitary bright spot seen on magnetic resonance imaging (MRI) is found ectopically in the pituitary stalk (▶ Fig. 30.2). The stalk itself may be hypoplastic. When pituitary abnormalities are found along with other midline brain anomalies, the term septo-optic dysplasia (SOD) is sometimes used. Although sometimes labelled de Morsier syndrome, historically it is notable that de Morsier never actually described this disorder. Patients with SOD may also show facial dysmorphism, macrocrania, and a large anterior fontanelle. Patients may have developmental delay, seizures, or cerebral palsy. Hormonal alterations include thyroid, growth, adrenal (corticosteroid), and antidiuretic hormone deficiencies. The risk of developing such hormonal abnormalities is increased in bilateral cases or if there are midline brain defects, although milder hormonal alterations may occur in unilateral cases. Testing for thyroid and corticosteroid axis abnormalities is essential even if neonatal testing was normal. Sudden death may occur if these abnormalities are not identified and promptly treated (see text box below [p.257]).

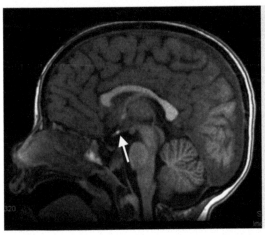

Fig. 30.2 Brain magnetic resonance imaging in a patient with septo-optic dysplasia, revealing ectopic pituitary "bright spot" (*arrow*).

Systemic Syndromes Associated with Optic Nerve Hypoplasia (ONH) (OMIM)*

- Aarskog syndrome (305400).
- Aicardi syndrome (304050).
- Albinism.
- Blepharophimosis syndrome (110100).
- CHARGE (Coloboma of the eye, Heart defects, Atresia of the nasal choanae, Retardation of growth and/or development, Genital and/or urinary abnormalities, and Ear abnormalities with or without deafness) syndrome (214800).
- Duane syndrome (126800).
- Goltz syndrome (109400).
- Goldenhar syndrome (164210).
- Neonatal central diabetes insipidus.
- Nevus sebaceous of Jadassohn (163200).
- Noonan syndrome (163950).
- Proteus syndrome (176920).
- Smith–Lemli–Optiz syndrome (270400).
- STAR syndrome (300707; toe syndactyly, telecanthus, anogenital, and renal malformations).
- SUNCT (Short-lasting Unilateral Neuralgiform headache attacks with Conjunctival injection and Tearing) syndrome.
- Trisomy 18.
- Vici syndrome (242840).
- Walker–Warburg syndrome (236670).

*Most relevant syndromes included

30.2 Molecular Genetics

Most patients with ONH will not have an identifiable molecular cause. Rarely, homozygous or heterozygous pathogenic variations in *HESX1* have been seen in patients with SOD. *SOX2*, *SOX3*, *PAX6*, and *OTX2* have also been implicated in ONH. Compound heterozygosity for two pathogenic variants in *SLC25A1*, which encodes the mitochondrial citrate transporter, has also been reported. *FGFR1*, *FGF8*, and *PROKR2* mutations have been associated with ONH. Although *ATOH7* polymorphisms have been associated with ONH, sequencing in these patients has not shown pathogenic variants.

30.3 Differential Diagnosis

30.3.1 Optic Nerve Atrophy

Pallor of the optic nerve is the hallmark sign of optic nerve atrophy. Optic atrophy can result in abnormal visual acuity, visual fields, and color vision. Causes include tumor, trauma, ischemia, papilledema, toxins, dietary deficiencies, inflammation, infiltration, primary genetic etiologies, and infection. It is distinguished from ONH in that the size of the optic nerve is normal in optic atrophy.

30.3.2 Tilted Disc Syndrome

This congenital anomaly occurs in up to 2% of the general population. Although it is mostly sporadic, there are reports of AD inheritance. It is defined by tilting of the optic disc, but can also have inferonasal crescent (peripapillary atrophy), situs inversus, and/or inferior staphyloma. It is usually bilateral. It can be associated with high myopia. Visual field can show bitemporal superior visual field defects.

30.3.3 Glaucoma

A small optic nerve and double ring can be confused with the cup and the rim, respectively.

30.3.4 Optic Nerve Coloboma

Optic nerve coloboma may be rarely confused with ONH (▶ Fig. 30.3).

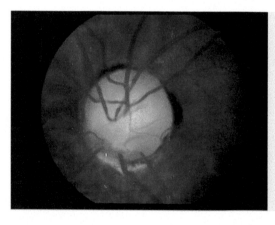

Fig. 30.3 Coloboma involving the optic nerve.

30.4 Uncommon Manifestations

Although rare, sudden death has been reported in ONH largely due to abnormalities in the corticosteroid hormonal axis.

Optic nerve aplasia, a rare developmental anomaly characterized by congenital absence of the optic nerve, retinal blood vessels, and retinal ganglion cells, can be a severe presentation of the ONH spectrum.

30.5 Clinical Testing

30.5.1 Optical Coherence Tomography

Particularly useful to identify thin nerve fiber and ganglion cell layers. Some patients may also have mild foveal hypoplasia.

30.5.2 Electroretinogram

Electroretinogram is typically normal in ONH.

30.5.3 Visual Evoked Potential

Waveforms may be delayed in amplitude and implicit times.

30.5.4 Magnetic Resonance Imaging

High-resolution orbital MRI, with emphasis on the pituitary axis, is warranted in most cases.

30.5.5 Endocrine Workup

Endocrine workup, including levels of cortisol, prolactin, adrenocorticotropic hormone (ACTH), insulin-like growth factor-1 (IGF1), insulin-like factor binding protein-3 (IGFBP3), thyroid stimulating hormone (TSH), and free T4, is recommended.

30.6 Genetic Testing

Genetic testing is currently not effective to identify a molecular cause of isolated ONH, pending new gene discovery. Testing for mutations in HEX1 is clinically available in multiple labs for those suspected of having SOD. Genomic testing, including chromosomal microarray (CMA) or exome sequencing in individuals with syndromic presentation that does not fit a known phenotype may be considered and should be ordered by a genetics professional. Research combining natural history studies and genomic testing to identify candidate molecular causes may one day improve availability of commercial testing.

30.7 Problems

30.7.1 Case 1

A 6-month-old boy comes for ophthalmic evaluation. His parents note that his vision is "not so good." Past medical history shows a normal delivery, no medical problems, and normal growth and development. Neonatal thyroid screening was normal. On examination, he has nystagmus and subnormal visual responses. Pupillary reflexes are normal. Anterior segment is normal, but fundus examination reveals bilateral ONH with a double-ring sign. MRI reveals a thin corpus callosum and absent septum pellucidum. Which from the following seems the most appropriate next step?

a) Sequence HESX1.
b) Request levels of cortisol, TSH, and T4.
c) Request serum vitamin B_{12}.
d) Refer to pediatric neurosurgeon for further evaluation.

Correct answer is b.

Although physical examination and previous thyroid screening tests were normal, approximately 50% of patients with bilateral ONH and dysgenesis of corpus callosum have hypothalamic–pituitary dysfunction in patients with ONH. Thyroid testing may be abnormal even if neonatal screening was normal.

a) **Less appropriate.** HESX1 gene mutations in ONH are infrequent.
b) **Correct.**
c) **Incorrect.** Vitamin B_{12} deficiency may result in optic atrophy but not ONH.
d) **Incorrect.** Although hydrocephalus is rarely observed in SOD, the anomalies seen in this patient do not require surgery consultation.

30.7.2 Case 2

A 9-year-old girl is referred to you for a second opinion. Her ophthalmologist found "small optic discs." Pregnancy and delivery were unremarkable. Physical examination is normal. On ophthalmic evaluation, best corrected vision is 20/25 OD (oculus dextrus) and 20/30 OS (oculus sinister) with –19.00 sph OU (oculus uterque). Axial length is 29.5-mm OD and 28.97-mm OS. Color vision is normal. Pupillary reflexes are normal. Anterior segment is normal. The optic discs are vertically elongated with temporal peripapillary alterations. There is no double-ring sign. Which from the following seems the most appropriate next step?

a) Examination under anesthesia.
b) Orbital MRI.
c) Optic nerve optical coherence tomography (OCT) and optic nerve imaging.
d) None of the above.

Correct answer is d.

This patient has tilted discs, which can mimic ONH. Vision is good, axial length long, and there is no double-ring sign. No workup is needed.

a) **Incorrect.** Clinical presentation is compatible with tilted discs. No further information likely to be gained from EUA (exam under anesthesia).
b) **Incorrect.** Tilted discs are not associated with intracranial abnormalities.
c) **Incorrect.** Although OCT may be helpful in confirming diagnosis, and in particular an expected normal nerve fiber layer, the diagnosis of tilted disc can be made clinically in most cases.
d) **Correct.**

30.7.3 Case 3

A 3-year-old boy comes for ONH evaluation. Past medical history is unrevealing and there are no other known affected family members. Physical examination is normal. He has nystagmus and subnormal vision. Pupillary reflexes are mildly sluggish. Anterior segment is normal, but fundus examination shows severe ONH with double-ring sign. MRI confirms ONH, but reveals no brain anomalies. Endocrine workup is normal. Which of the following tests would you recommend?

a) Microarray.
b) *PAX6*.
c) *SOX2*.
d) None of the above.

Correct answer is d.

Genetic testing is currently not effective in identifying a molecular cause of isolated ONH. Although mutations in *HESX1* have been reported, the chance of this test being positive on a sporadic case of ONH is so low as to make this test largely ineffective.

a) **Incorrect.** There is no indication for chromosomal microarray in an otherwise well child with ONH.

b) **Incorrect.** Although mutations in *PAX6* can cause aniridia with associated ONH, mutations in this gene have not been known to cause isolated ONH.

c) **Incorrect.** Although mutations in *SOX2* can cause microphthalmia with associated ONH, mutations in this gene have not been known to cause isolated ONH.

d) **Correct.**

Suggested Reading

[1] Borchert M, McCulloch D, Rother C, Stout AU. Clinical assessment, optic disk measurements, and visual-evoked potential in optic nerve hypoplasia. Am J Ophthalmol. 1995; 120(5):605–612

[2] Acers TE. Optic nerve hypoplasia: septo-optic-pituitary dysplasia syndrome. Trans Am Ophthalmol Soc. 1981; 79:425–457

[3] Cohen RN, Cohen LE, Botero D, et al. Enhanced repression by HESX1 as a cause of hypopituitarism and septooptic dysplasia. J Clin Endocrinol Metab. 2003; 88(10):4832–4839

[4] Benner JD, Preslan MW, Gratz E, Joslyn J, Schwartz M, Kelman S. Septo-optic dysplasia in two siblings. Am J Ophthalmol. 1990; 109(6):632–637

[5] Kelberman D, Dattani MT. Septo-optic dysplasia - novel insights into the aetiology. Horm Res. 2008; 69(5):257–265

[6] McCabe MJ, Alatzoglou KS, Dattani MT. Septo-optic dysplasia and other midline defects: the role of transcription factors: HESX1 and beyond. Best Pract Res Clin Endocrinol Metab. 2011; 25(1):115–124

[7] Taban M, Cohen BH, David Rothner A, Traboulsi EI. Association of optic nerve hypoplasia with mitochondrial cytopathies. J Child Neurol. 2006; 21(11):956–960

[8] Phillips PH, Spear C, Brodsky MC. Magnetic resonance diagnosis of congenital hypopituitarism in children with optic nerve hypoplasia. J AAPOS. 2001; 5(5):275–280

[9] Dutton GN. Congenital disorders of the optic nerve: excavations and hypoplasia. Eye (Lond). 2004; 18(11):1038–1048

[10] Lambert SR, Hoyt CS, Narahara MH. Optic nerve hypoplasia. Surv Ophthalmol. 1987; 32(1):1–9

[11] Kim RY, Hoyt WF, Lessell S, Narahara MH. Superior segmental optic hypoplasia. A sign of maternal diabetes. Arch Ophthalmol. 1989; 107(9):1312–1315

[12] Petersen RA, Holmes LB. Optic nerve hypoplasia in infants of diabetic mothers. Arch Ophthalmol. 1986; 104(11):1587

[13] Garcia-Filion P, Borchert M. Prenatal determinants of optic nerve hypoplasia: review of suggested correlates and future focus. Surv Ophthalmol. 2013; 58(6):610–619

[14] Hellström A, Wiklund LM, Svensson E. Diagnostic value of magnetic resonance imaging and planimetric measurement of optic disc size in confirming optic nerve hypoplasia. J AAPOS. 1999; 3(2):104–108

[15] Wakakura M, Alvarez E. A simple clinical method of assessing patients with optic nerve hypoplasia. The disc-macula distance to disc diameter ratio (DM/DD). Acta Ophthalmol (Copenh). 1987; 65(5):612–617

[16] Zeki SM, Dudgeon J, Dutton GN. Reappraisal of the ratio of disc to macula/disc diameter in optic nerve hypoplasia. Br J Ophthalmol. 1991; 75(9):538–541

[17] Pilat A, Sibley D, McLean RJ, Proudlock FA, Gottlob I. High-resolution imaging of the optic nerve and retina in optic nerve hypoplasia. Ophthalmology. 2015; 122(7):1330–1339

31 Leber Hereditary Optic Neuropathy

Pablo Romero

Abstract

Leber hereditary optic neuropathy (LHON) is caused by mutations in the mitochondrial genome. It is usually bilateral although often sequential. Vision loss is acute or subacute and painless. Patients usually have a large central or cecocentral scotoma. LHON is expressed predominantly in males with approximately 80 to 90% of affected patients being male, but it can affect either gender at almost any age. All mitochondrial deoxyribonucleic acid (mtDNA) pathogenic mutations associated with LHON have incomplete clinical penetrance, so symptoms are not always present in individuals who have the mutation. Depending on the underlying mtDNA point mutation and haplotype, up to 60% of patients may have some degree of spontaneous improvement. A younger age at the time of initial visual loss is associated with a better visual outcome.

Keywords: Leber hereditary optic neuropathy, optic nerve hyperemia, mitochondrial mutation, optic atrophy

Key Points

- Leber hereditary optic neuropathy is a disorder of the mitochondrial genome characterized by bilateral, acute or subacute, and painless vision loss.
- It is most frequently seen in previously healthy young males, but can affect any gender at any age.
- Three primary mitochondrial deoxyribonucleic acid (mtDNA) point mutations are found in more than 95% of affected patients.

31.1 Overview

Leber hereditary optic neuropathy (LHON) is due to mutations in the mitochondrial genome. The worldwide prevalence of LHON is estimated to be between 1:30,000 and 1:50,000. This prevalence varies in different populations and in most populations is unknown. It is usually bilateral although often sequential. Vision loss is acute or subacute and painless. Patients usually have a large central or cecocentral scotoma. LHON is expressed predominantly in males with approximately 80 to 90% of affected patients being male, but it can affect either gender at almost any age. The reason for male predominance is not well understood.

All mitochondrial deoxyribonucleic acid (mtDNA) pathogenic mutations associated with LHON have incomplete clinical penetrance, so symptoms are not always present in individuals who have the mutation. This variable penetrance may reflect the action of unlinked modifier genes, epigenetic changes, or environmental factors. For example, alcohol intake or smoking seem to raise the chance of vision loss, and may negatively affect the chance of spontaneous recovery in those who experience loss of vision. The phenotypic expression of LHON may also be affected by the type of mtDNA mutation and mitochondrial haplotype.

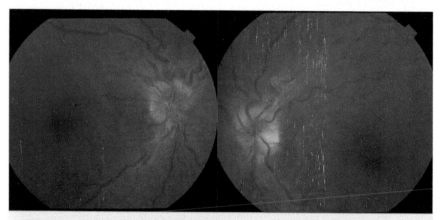

Fig. 31.1 Bilateral acute Leber hereditary optic neuropathy. Examination reveals hyperemic, "pseudo-edematous" optic nerves with peripapillary telangiectasias, and tortuosity of retinal arterioles.

Most patients deteriorate to acuities of 20/200 or worse. Color vision is affected early and severely, and visual fields typically show central or cecocentral defects. Depending on the underlying mtDNA point mutation and haplotype, up to 60% of patients may have some degree of spontaneous improvement. A younger age at the time of initial visual loss is associated with a better visual outcome. It has been suggested that the pupillary function is relatively preserved in the affected eyes of LHON patients. Some cases have been reported of partial spontaneous recovery of visual acuity, especially in children and with m.14484T > C mutation. The eyes can be affected simultaneously or sequentially, with an average interval between eyes being affected of approximately 2 months.

Funduscopic abnormalities may be seen, particularly during the acute phase of visual loss, when there may be hyperemia of the optic nerve head, dilatation and tortuosity of vessels, hemorrhages, circumpapillary telangiectatic microangiopathy, or circumpapillary nerve fiber layer swelling (► Fig. 31.1). Over time, the optic nerves become pale without distinguishing clinical features. There may also be nonglaucomatous cupping of the disc and arterial attenuation.

31.2 Molecular Genetics

The precise pathogenesis of LHON has not yet been fully determined. Three primary mtDNA point mutations are found in more than 95% of patients: m.11778G > A (ND4), m.3460G > A (ND1), and m.14484T > C (ND6). More than 30 other infrequent mitochondrial mutations have also been associated with LHON. mtDNA mutations associated with LHON may be heteroplasmic or homoplasmic based on blood testing. Although there may be some correlation between clinical expression and degree of heteroplasmy, it must be remembered that mutation load can vary greatly from one tissue to another. Therefore, blood testing may not directly reflect the mutation load at the level of the optic nerve. Symptomatic individuals are typically homoplasmic for an mtDNA mutation in their blood, but there are exceptions and affected individuals with varying degrees of heteroplasmy for the family mtDNA mutation have been reported. This limitation to test interpretation is one of the many challenges in counseling at-risk family members.

31.3 Differential Diagnosis

31.3.1 Autosomal Dominant Optic Atrophy (OMIM 165500)

Autosomal dominant (AD) optic atrophy, also known as Kjer's optic atrophy, is the most common form of hereditary optic neuropathy. It is caused by mutations in *OPA1* (3q29). The incidence is approximately 1 in 10,000 to 50,000 live births. It is a childhood-onset disorder typically characterized by a bilateral slow and progressive loss in central vision, dyschromatopsia, and paracentral scotomas. The optic disc pallor is typically sectorial and temporal, sometimes referred to as "pie in the sky" atrophy, but may be more severe and complete. The expression displays both inter- and intrafamilial variability with incomplete penetrance. Symptoms typically start during the first or second decade of life. Some patients with mutations in *OPA1* may also develop extraocular neurologic features, such as deafness, progressive external ophthalmoplegia, muscle cramps, hyperreflexia, and/or ataxia ("optic atrophy plus syndrome").

In addition, there are other known loci for optic atrophy, which are included in
▶ Table 31.1.

31.3.2 3-Methylglutaconic Aciduria Type III (OMIM 258501)

This autosomal recessive (AR) condition is also known as recessive optic atrophy type 3 (OPA3) or optic atrophy plus syndrome. It is an allelic disorder of OPA3, and is caused by mutation in the *OPA3* gene. It presents as a neurophthalmologic syndrome, which

Table 31.1 Other known loci for optic atrophy

Clinical condition	Gene/locus	Additional information
OPA2 (OMIM 311050)	Xp11.4-p11.21	X-linked. Early childhood onset and slow progression
OPA3 (OMIM 165300)	*OPA3*; 19q13.32	AD. Optic atrophy, cataract, with or without extrapyramidal findings and ataxia
OPA4 (OMIM 605293)	*OPA4*; 18q12	AD
OPA5 (OMIM 610708)	*OPA5*; 22q12.1-q13.1	AD
OPA6 (OMIM 258500)	*OPA6*; 8q21-q22	AR
OPA7 (OMIM 612989)	*TMEM126A*; 11q14.1	AR. With or without auditory neuropathy. Usually presents with early onset
OPA8 (OMIM 616648)	*OPA8*; 16q21–22	AD. Progressive visual loss during the first or second decade of life. Some individuals may present late-onset sensorineural hearing loss or, rarely, mitral valve prolapse or insufficiency
OPA9 (OMIM 616289)	*ACO2*; 22q13	AR
OPA10 (OMIM 616732)	*RTN4IP1*; 6q21	AR. Can present with or without ataxia, mental retardation, and seizures

Abbreviations: AD, autosomal dominant; AR, autosomal recessive; OPA, optic atrophy.

consists of early-onset bilateral optic atrophy and later-onset spasticity, extrapyramidal dysfunction, and cognitive deficit. It can be confused with Behr syndrome. Diagnostic testing includes urinary excretion of 3-methylglutaconic acid and 3-methylglutaric acid.

31.3.3 Behr Syndrome (OMIM 210000)

This AR condition is caused by homozygous or compound heterozygous mutations in *OPA1*. It is characterized by early-onset optic atrophy accompanied by neurologic findings, such as ataxia, pyramidal signs, spasticity, and mental retardation.

31.3.4 Wolfram Syndrome (OMIM 222300)

This condition is a rare and severe AR neurodegenerative disease defined by diabetes mellitus, diabetes insipidus, optic atrophy, and deafness (DIDMOAD syndrome). More mild AD forms are also known. Other clinical findings may include renal abnormalities, ataxia, premature dementia or developmental delay, and diverse psychiatric illnesses. It is caused by mutations in *WFS1* (4p16.3).

31.3.5 Bosch–Boonstra–Schaaf Optic Atrophy Syndrome (OMIM 615722)

Bosch–Boonstra–Schaaf optic atrophy syndrome (OMIM 615722) is an AD disorder characterized by delayed development, moderate intellectual disability, and optic atrophy. Most of the affected individuals also have cortical visual impairment. Dysmorphic findings include protruding ears, high nasal bridge, upturned nose, epicanthal folds, upslanting palpebral fissures, and tapering fingers. Other features include hypotonia, obsessive compulsive disorder, and autistic features. It is caused by heterozygous mutation in *NR2F1* (5q15).

31.3.6 Lamb–Shaffer Syndrome (OMIM 616803)

This AD disorder is caused by heterozygous mutation in *SOX5* (12p12). A contiguous deletion syndrome has also been reported. Individuals with larger deletions tend to present more dysmorphic and musculoskeletal findings compared to those with smaller deletions. Lamb–Shaffer syndrome is a neurodevelopmental disease defined by global developmental delay, intellectual disability, speech disorder, and facial dysmorphism (frontal bossing, ear abnormalities, and low nasal bridge). Other findings include strabismus, behavioral problems, seizures, hypotonia, clumsiness, poor balance, articulation difficulties, and scoliosis.

31.3.7 Mohr–Tranebjaerg Syndrome (OMIM 304700)

Mohr–Tranebjaerg syndrome (OMIM 304700) is an X-linked recessive (XLr) disorder caused by mutation in *TIMM8A* (Xq22). It is characterized by progressive deafness and optic atrophy. Patients have normal speech development until hearing deteriorates. Ocular features include myopia, decreased visual acuity, constricted visual fields, and "abnormal electroretinogram." Cortical blindness, dystonia, fractures, and mental deficiency have also been reported. The combination of deafness, optic atrophy, and dementia caused by *TIMM8A* mutations has been called Jensen syndrome.

31.3.8 Mitochondrial DNA Depletion Syndrome 4A (OMIM 203700)

Also known as Alpers syndrome, this disorder is associated with biallelic mutations in the nuclear gene encoding mtDNA polymerase gamma (*POLG*; 15q26). This disorder is characterized by psychomotor retardation, intractable epilepsy, and liver failure in infants and young children. The condition is progressive and often leads to death from hepatic failure or status epilepticus before the age of 3 years. Optic atrophy is a variable feature.

31.3.9 Charcot–Marie–Tooth Disease Type 1B (OMIM 118200)

Charcot–Marie–Tooth disease type 1B (OMIM 118200) is caused by heterozygous mutation in *MPZ* (1q23.3). Pathogenic variants in this gene can produce several sensorineural neuropathies, including Dejerine–Sottas disease, congenital hypomyelinating neuropathy, and other forms of axonal Charcot–Marie–Tooth disease.

Charcot–Marie–Tooth disease is a sensorineural peripheral polyneuropathy. It is the most frequent inherited disorder of the peripheral nervous system. It can be AD, AR, and XLr. In general, this disorder is characterized by an insidious onset and slowly progressive weakness and atrophy of the distal limb muscles, usually starting in the legs and feet. Both motor and sensory nerve functions are affected. The onset is typically in the first or second decade of life. There is a wide clinical presentation, ranging from severe distal atrophy and marked hand and foot deformity to affected individuals whose only feature is pes cavus and subtle distal muscle weakness. Argyll–Robertson pupils and severe optic atrophy have been rarely described.

31.3.10 Spinocerebellar Ataxia 1 (OMIM 164400)

Spinocerebellar ataxia 1 (SCA1; OMIM 164400) is caused by an expanded (CAG)n trinucleotide repeat in *ATXN1* (6p22). This AD cerebellar degenerative disorder presents with variable involvement of the brainstem and spinal cord. Clinical features include ataxia, hypotonia, and spastic paraplegia. Optic atrophy can also be observed.

31.3.11 Nongenetic Differential Diagnosis

Nongenetic differential diagnosis includes idiopathic optic atrophy, toxic optic neuropathy, infiltrative disease, status post papillitis or papilledema, abusive head trauma, and end stage of optic neuritis.

31.4 Uncommon Manifestations

Early and late onsets of the disease are uncommon. The onset of visual loss typically occurs between the ages of 15 and 35 years, but otherwise classic LHON has been noted in patients ranging in age from 1 to 90 years. Age of onset variability is seen even among members of the same family. Subjects with the A2 haplogroup on average had later onset of disease.

Pedigrees of LHON due to the 11,778 mutation have been reported in which females are predominantly affected.

Other infrequent findings include white matter changes, headaches, Wolff–Parkinson–White and Lown–Ganong–Levine (paroxysms of tachycardia and electrocardiogram findings of a short PR interval and normal QRS duration) syndromes.

31.5 Clinical Testing

31.5.1 Intravenous Fluorescein Angiography

Although not commonly needed to make the diagnosis, unlike true disc edema, the LHON disc does not leak on fluorescein angiography.

31.5.2 Optical Coherence Tomography

Patients with LHON show thickened RNFL (retinal nerve fiber layer) when the time of onset is shorter than 6 months and severely thinned in atrophic LHON, when the duration is longer than 6 months. The temporal fibers (papillomacular bundle) are the first and most severely affected; the nasal fibers seem to be partially spared even in the late stage of the disease.

31.6 Genetic Testing

As the mitochondrial mutations 11778G > A, 14484T > C, and 3460G > A account for approximately 95% of LHON mutations, most laboratories will offer testing for these three mutations as a panel. The 11778G > A mutations account for approximately 70% of LHON mutations. The 3460G > A and 14484T > C mutations each account for approximately 13 to 14% of LHON mutations. If these tests are normal, then further searching for other mtDNA mutations can be carried out by sequencing of the mitochondrial genome.

31.7 Problems

31.7.1 Case 1

A 21-year-old man complains of bilateral decreased visual acuity over the last 5 days. He was previously healthy. He has one maternal cousin who had similar symptoms a few years ago. Brain MRI (magnetic resonance imaging) is normal. The optic nerves appear mildly edematous with some tiny telangiectatic vessels and peripapillary hemorrhages. Visual field shows a central scotoma in one eye and a cecocentral scotoma in the other eye. Which of the following tests would be most appropriate?

a) Nuclear DNA testing for *CEP290*.
b) Testing for *MT-TL1*, *MT-ND1*, *MT-ND5*, *MT-TH*, and *MT-TV*.
c) mtDNA testing for m.11778G > A, m.3460G > A, and m.14484T > C.
d) mtDNA testing for *MT-ATP6* (or ATP6).

Correct answer is c.

This is a typical presentation of LHON although one might not see the optic nerve changes. LHON produces a bilateral or sequential, subacute, and painless vision loss most commonly in previously healthy young males. Family history is compatible with a mitochondrial pattern of inheritance. Three primary mtDNA point mutations (m.11778G > A, m.3460G > A, and m.14484T > C) are found in more than 95% of patients with LHON.

a) **Incorrect.** *CEP290* is associated with Leber congenital amaurosis.

b) **Incorrect.** *MT-TL1*, *MT-ND1*, *MT-ND5*, *MT-TH*, and *MT-TV* are most associated with an unlikely phenotype, more than 80% of all cases of mitochondrial encephalomyopathy, lactic acidosis, and strokelike episodes (MELAS).

c) **Correct.**

d) **Incorrect.** Mutations in *MT-ATP6* are associated with neuropathy, ataxia, and retinitis pigmentosa (NARP syndrome).

31.7.2 Case 2

In a family with a known LHON mutation, four siblings aged between 25 and 35 years have the mutation (two males and two females), but just one male has the clinical disease. This is best explained by:

a) Heteroplasmy.

b) Mosaicism.

c) Anticipation.

d) Lyonization.

Correct answer is a.

Higher levels of heteroplasmy are associated with a greater chance of manifesting clinical LHON. In addition, males are more likely to be clinically affected than females.

a) **Correct.**

b) **Incorrect.** Mosaicism denotes the presence of two or more populations of cells with different nuclear genotypes in one individual who has developed from a single fertilized egg. LHON is a mitochondrial disorder.

c) **Incorrect.** Anticipation is a phenomenon in which the symptoms and signs of the genetic disorder become apparent at an earlier age and/or with more severity with each successive generation. Some examples are Huntington's disease and myotonic dystrophy. This is a phenomena seen with trinucleotide repeat expansion in nuclear genes and therefore not applicable to mitochondrial disorders.

d) **Incorrect.** Lyonization refers to inactivation of one copy of a female's two X chromosomes in every cell. It does not apply to the mitochondrial genome.

31.7.3 Case 3

An entirely well, nonsmoking, 21-year-old male student who enjoys a normal diet and takes no medications, alcohol, or recreational drugs is referred for evaluation of decreased visual acuity. On physical examination, his vision is 20/200 in both eyes. Pupils are equal, round, and reactive to light and accommodation. His father and his paternal grandfather have an "optic nerve condition." Fundus examination show bilateral optic atrophy. Assuming the affected family members have the same condition as the proband, the clinical findings are suggestive of:

a) LHON.

b) AD optic atrophy.

c) Wolfram syndrome.

d) Toxic optic atrophy.

Correct answer is b.

AD inheritance is characterized in particular by male-to-male transmission, which rules out both X-linked and maternal mitochondrial inheritance.

a) **Incorrect.** There is male-to-male transmission, thus ruling out mitochondrial genome mutation.

b) **Correct.**

c) **Incorrect.** Otherwise known as DIDMOAD syndrome, Wolfram syndrome is associated with diabetes insipidus, diabetes mellitus, and deafness in addition to optic atrophy.

d) **Incorrect.** There are no risk factors in the history.

Suggested Reading

[1] Spruijt L, Kolbach DN, de Coo RF, et al. Influence of mutation type on clinical expression of Leber hereditary optic neuropathy. Am J Ophthalmol. 2006; 141(4):676–682

[2] Harding AE, Sweeney MG, Govan GG, Riordan-Eva P. Pedigree analysis in Leber hereditary optic neuropathy families with a pathogenic mtDNA mutation. Am J Hum Genet. 1995; 57(1):77–86

[3] Yu-Wai-Man P, Griffiths PG, Hudson G, Chinnery PF. Inherited mitochondrial optic neuropathies. J Med Genet. 2009; 46(3):145–158

[4] Carelli V, Ross-Cisneros FN, Sadun AA. Mitochondrial dysfunction as a cause of optic neuropathies. Prog Retin Eye Res. 2004; 23(1):53–89

[5] Yu-Wai-Man P, Turnbull DM, Chinnery PF. Leber hereditary optic neuropathy. J Med Genet. 2002; 39(3):162–169

[6] Wong LJ. Pathogenic mitochondrial DNA mutations in protein-coding genes. Muscle Nerve. 2007; 36(3):279–293

[7] Torroni A, Petrozzi M, D'Urbano L, et al. Haplotype and phylogenetic analyses suggest that one European-specific mtDNA background plays a role in the expression of Leber hereditary optic neuropathy by increasing the penetrance of the primary mutations 11778 and 14484. Am J Hum Genet. 1997; 60(5):1107–1121

[8] Hudson G, Carelli V, Spruijt L, et al. Clinical expression of Leber hereditary optic neuropathy is affected by the mitochondrial DNA-haplogroup background. Am J Hum Genet. 2007; 81(2):228–233

[9] Hudson G, Keers S, Yu-Wai-Man P, et al. Identification of an X-chromosomal locus and haplotype modulating the phenotype of a mitochondrial DNA disorder. Am J Hum Genet. 2005; 77(6):1086–1091

[10] Kerrison JB, Newman NJ. Clinical spectrum of Leber hereditary optic neuropathy. Clin Neurosci. 1997; 4(5):295–301

[11] Nikoskelainen EK, Huoponen K, Juvonen V, Lamminen T, Nummelin K, Savontaus ML. Ophthalmologic findings in Leber hereditary optic neuropathy, with special reference to mtDNA mutations. Ophthalmology. 1996; 103(3):504–514

[12] Newman NJ, Lott MT, Wallace DC. The clinical characteristics of pedigrees of Leber hereditary optic neuropathy with the 11778 mutation. Am J Ophthalmol. 1991; 111(6):750–762

[13] Stone EM, Newman NJ, Miller NR, Johns DR, Lott MT, Wallace DC. Visual recovery in patients with Leber hereditary optic neuropathy and the 11778 mutation. J Clin Neuroophthalmol. 1992; 12(1):10–14

[14] Wakakura M, Yokoe J. Evidence for preserved direct pupillary light response in Leber hereditary optic neuropathy. Br J Ophthalmol. 1995; 79(5):442–446

32 Complex Ocular Disorders

with contributions by Christian R. Diaz

Abstract

Primary open angle glaucoma, keratoconus, age-related macular degeneration, and strabismus are examples of complex ocular genetic disorders. These disorders are likely associated with the effects of multiple genes in combination with environmental factors and lifestyle. Although multifactorial disorders often cluster in families, they do not have a well-defined pattern of inheritance. This makes it difficult to determine an individual's specific risk of inheriting these disorders. Complex disorders are also difficult to study because the specific factors that cause them have not yet been identified and some may be environmental.

Keywords: complex disorders, multifactorial disorders, primary open angle glaucoma, keratoconus, age-related macular degeneration, strabismus

Key Points

- Complex multifactorial disorders are likely associated with the effects of multiple genes in combination with environmental factors.
- Primary open angle glaucoma, keratoconus, age-related macular degeneration, and strabismus are examples of complex ocular genetic disorders.
- Currently, the costs and risks of routine genetic testing, combined with the need for greater understanding, outweigh the benefits for patients with these conditions.

Common medical conditions such as heart disease, diabetes, and obesity do not have a single gene as an identifiable cause. These disorders are likely associated with the effects of multiple genes in combination with environmental factors and lifestyle. These conditions are called complex or multifactorial disorders. Although multifactorial disorders often cluster in families, they do not have a well-defined pattern of inheritance. This makes it difficult to determine an individual's specific risk of inheriting these disorders. Complex disorders are also difficult to study because the specific factors that cause them have not yet been identified and some may be environmental.

Primary open angle glaucoma, keratoconus, age-related macular degeneration (ARMD), and strabismus are examples of complex ocular genetic disorders. ► Table 32.1, ► Table 32.2, ► Table 32.3, and ► Table 32.4 elucidate genes in which polymorphisms, and in some cases mutations, predispose to the development of the disorder but in isolation are insufficient to cause the disease. It may be that the combination of certain polymorphisms (haplotype) is required to confer sufficient risk to get the disorder. Different genes may confer risk via different pathophysiologic pathways. For example, genes involved with disc size, corneal thickness, or aqueous humor production may play a role. For strabismus, individual genes may affect refraction, accommodation, or fusion, which then contribute in unique ways to various forms of strabismus. There are also single gene strabismus disorders (► Table 32.1). All other CFEOM (congenital fibrosis of the extraocular muscles) refers to at least eight genetically defined strabismus syndromes: CFEOM1A, CFEOM1B, CFEOM2, CFEOM3A, CFEOM3B, CFEOM3C, Tukel

Table 32.1 Genes and Loci associated with strabismus

Locus	Identified gene	Note
7p22.1	None	STBMS1 (OMIM 185100). Susceptibility to strabismus
12q12	KIF21A	CFEOM1 (OMIM 135700) AD
11q13.4	PHOX2A	CFEOM2 (OMIM 602078) AR
16q24.3	TUBB3	CFEOM3A (OMIM 600638) AD
12q12	KIF21A	CFEOM3B (OMIM 135700) AD
13q12.11	None	CFEOM3C (OMIM 609384) AD
21q22	None	CFEOM4 (OMIM 609428) AR Tukel syndrome: nonprogressive restrictive ophthalmoplegia with ptosis and postaxial hand oligodactyly/oligosyndactyly
4q25	COL25A1	CFEOM5 (OMIM 616219) AR
20q13.2	SALL4	Duane-radial ray syndrome (607323) AD Also known as Okihiro syndrome, characterized by upper limb anomalies, ocular anomalies, and, in some cases, renal anomalies
7p15.2	HOXA1	Bosley–Salih–Alorainy syndrome (OMIM 601536) AR. Duane syndrome associated with profound sensorineural deafness and, in some cases, external ear defects and/or delayed motor milestones
8q13	None	DURS1 (OMIM 126800) AD
2q31.1	CHN1	DURS2 (OMIM 604356)
20q12	MAFB	DURS3 (OMIM 617041) AD
13q12.2-q13	None	Moebius syndrome, a congenital, nonprogressive facial weakness with limited abduction of one or both eyes. Other findings: hearing loss and other cranial nerve dysfunction, as well as motor, orofacial, musculoskeletal, neurodevelopmental, and social problems (OMIM 157900). There are also reports of hereditary congenital facial palsy and comitant esotropia with homozygous mutation in HOXB1 (17q21)
19q13.1	RYR1	Congenital ophthalmoplegia, facial weakness, predisposition to malignant hyperthermia, skeletal myopathy, scoliosis, ptosis
18p11.22	PIEZO2	Ptosis, ophthalmoplegia, and/or strabismus, in addition to contractures of the skeletal muscles. Pulmonary hypertension has also been reported (OMIM 108145)
2q37.1	ECEL1	AR distal arthrogryposis type 5D. Ptosis, hyperopic astigmatic refractive error, and exotropia (OMIM 615065)
11q24.2	ROBO3	Horizontal gaze palsy with progressive scoliosis with or without brainstem hypoplasia (OMIM 607313).
Xq26.3	SLC9A6	Christianson syndrome: microcephaly, impaired ocular movements, severe global developmental delay, developmental regression, hypotonia, abnormal movements, and early-onset seizures (OMIM 300243)

Abbreviations: AD, autosomal dominant; AR, autosomal recessive; OMIM, Online Mendelian Inheritance in Man.
Note: Duane retraction syndrome (DURS) is a congenital eye movement disorder that presents with a failure of the abducens nerve to develop normally. This results in restriction or absence of abduction, adduction, or both, and narrowing of the palpebral fissure in adduction. Retraction of the globe on attempted adduction may be seen as well.

Table 32.2 Genes and Loci associated with primary open angle glaucoma (POAG)

Locus	Identified gene	Additional information
1q24.3	MYOC	GLC1A (OMIM 137750) AD. JOAG Heterozygous mutations in the CYP1B1 gene can also be associated with digenic inheritance
2cen-q13	None	GLC1B (OMIM 606689)
3q21-q24	None	GLC1C (OMIM 601682) AD
8q23	None	GLC1D (OMIM 602429) AD
10p13	OPTN	GLC1E (OMIM 137760) AD Normal tension glaucoma
7q36.1	ASB10	GLC1F (OMIM 603383)
5q22.1	WDR36	GLC1G (OMIM 609887)
2p16-p15	None	GLC1H (OMIM 611276)
15q11-q13	None	GLC1I (OMIM 609745)
9q22	None	GLC1J (OMIM 608695). JOAG
20p12	None	GLC1K (OMIM 608696) AD. JOAG 8% is associated with MYOC mutations
3p21-p22	None	GLC1L (OMIM 137750)
5q22.1-q32	None	GLC1M (OMIM 610535) AD. JOAG
15q22-q24	None	GLC1N (OMIM 611274) AD. JOAG.
19q13.33	NTF4	GLC1O (OMIM 613100)
12q14	TBK1	GLC1P (OMIM 177700) AD.
9q33.3	LMX1B	Nail–patella syndrome (OMIM 161200) Glaucoma and dysplasia of the nails and absent or hypoplastic patellae. Other findings are iliac horns, abnormality of the elbows, and rarely nephropathy
3q29 10p13	OPA1 OPTN	Normal tension glaucoma (OMIM 606657)
11p15.5	IGF-II	Insulin growth factor is a recognized optic nerve trophic factor, which is associated with apoptosis
1p13.3	GSTM1	Oxidative stress pathway
22q11.23	GSTT1	Oxidative stress pathway
19q13.32	APOE	Neuronal degeneration may occur with APOE mutations
3q24	AGTR1	The renin–angiotensin–aldosterone system is involved in the regulation of aqueous humor dynamics. Polymorphisms in AGTR1 may be risk factors for glaucoma, in particular in the Japanese population
4q31.23	EDNRA	Endothelin is a potent vasoconstrictor
10q25.3	ADRB1	β-adrenergic receptor is significantly expressed in the ciliary body and trabecular meshwork
17p13.1	P53	Apoptosis mechanism
6p21.31	P21	Apoptosis mechanism
6p21.33	TNFα	Optic nerve degeneration through overexpression of tumor necrosis factor
17q11.1	NOS2A	Apoptosis regulation through nitric oxide pathway
1p36.22	MTHFR	Homocysteine overproduction induces apoptosis in retinal ganglion cells

Table 32.2 (continued)

Locus	Identified gene	Additional information
1q32.1	OPTC	OPTC gene is expressed in iris, trabecular meshwork, ciliary body, retina, vitreous, and optic nerve
6p21.33	HSP70	Association study in Japanese population
2q13	IL-1	Association study in Chinese population
6p21.32	TAP1	Association study in Chinese population
16q22.1	CDH-1	Association study in Chinese population
10p12.31	None	Susceptibility loci for POAG
12q21.31	None	Susceptibility loci for POAG
2p16	None	Susceptibility loci for POAG
2q31-q34	None	Susceptibility loci for POAG
13q14	None	JOAG

Abbreviations: AD, autosomal dominant; JOAG, juvenile open angle glaucoma; OMIM, Online Mendelian Inheritance in Man.

Table 32.3 Genes and Loci associated with keratoconus

Locus	Identified gene	Note
20p11.2	VSX1	KTCN1 (OMIM 605020) Visual system homeobox 1, transcription factor
16q22.3-q23.1	None	KTCN2 (OMIM 608932)
3p14-q13	None	KTCN3 (OMIM 608586)
2p24	None	KTCN4 (OMIM 609271)
5q14.1-q21.3	None	KTCN5 (OMIM 614622)
9q34	None	KTCN6 (OMIM 614623)
13q32	None	KTCN7 (OMIM 614629)
14q24.3	None	KTCN8 (OMIM 614628)
15q22-q25	miR-184	Micro-RNA involved in regulation of transcriptional activity of key genes in corneal development and maintenance
5q23.2	LOX	Lysyl oxidase (OMIM 153455), participates in collagen and elastin cross-linking
9q34.2-q34.3	COL5A1	Collagen type V, α-1 chain (OMIM 120215), part of fibril-forming corneal collagen
5q15	CAST	Calpain/calpastatin (OMIM 114090), proteolytic degradation
2q21.3	RAB3GAP1	1 Rab GTPase activating protein (OMIM 602536), regulates exocytosis
7q21.1	HGF	Hepatocyte growth factor (OMIM 142409), involved in corneal wound healing
3q26.31	FNDC3B	Fibronectin (OMIM 135600), extracellular matrix protein
13q14.1	FOXO1	(OMIM 136533) Transcription factor
5q31.1	TGFBI	Transforming growth factor β induced (OMIM 601692)
16q24.2	ZNF469	Transcription factor (OMIM 612078), regulates corneal collagen structure and synthesis, brittle cornea syndrome

Table 32.3 (*continued*)

Locus	Identified gene	Note
13q32.3	DOCK9	Dedicator of cytokinesis 9 (OMIM 607325), guanine nucleotide exchange factor
9p23	MPDZ	(OMIM 603785)
2q35	WNT10A	(OMIM 606268) member of WNT gene family of secreted signaling proteins
10p11.22	ZEB1	Zinc finger E box transcription factor homeobox 1 (OMIM 189909)
21q22.11	SOD1	Superoxide dismutase 1 (OMIM 147450) cytoplasmic antioxidant enzyme
2q13	IL1A	Interleukin-1α, cytokine (OMIM 147760)
2q13	IL1B	Interleukin-1β, cytokine (OMIM 147720)
2q36.3	COL4A3	Collagen type IV, α-3 chain (OMIM 120070), structural part of corneal membranes
2q36.3	COL4A4	Collagen type IV, α-4 chain (OMIM 120131), structural part of corneal membranes
5q31.3-g32	SPARC	(OMIM 182120)

Abbreviations: OMIM, Online Mendelian Inheritance in Man.
Source: Published with permission from Christian R. Díaz, MD.

Table 32.4 Genes and Loci associated with age related macular degeneration

Locus	Identified gene	Note
1q25.3-q31.1	HMCN1	ARMD1 (OMIM 603075) AD
1q31.3	CFHR3	ARMD1 (OMIM 603075) AD
1q31.3	CFHR1	ARMD1 (OMIM 603075) AD
19q13.32	APOE	ARMD1 (OMIM 603075) AD
1p22.1	ABCA4	ARMD2 (OMIM 153800) AD
14q32.12	FBLN5	ARMD3 (OMIM 608895) AD Can also present as neuropathy with or without age-related macular degeneration
1q31.3	CFH	ARMD4 (OMIM 610698)
10q11.23	ERCC6	ARMD5 (OMIM 613761)
19p13.3	RAX2	ARMD6 (OMIM 613757)
10q26.13	HTRA1	ARMD7 (OMIM 610149) Susceptibility to neovascular ("wet") ARMD
10q26.13	LOC387715	ARMD8 (OMIM 613778)
19p13.3	C3	ARMD9 (OMIM 611378)
9q32-q33	None	ARMD10 (OMIM 611488)
20p1121	CST3	ARMD11 (OMIM 611953)
3p22.2	CX3CR1	ARMD12 (OMIM 613784)
4q25	CFI	ARMD13 (OMIM 615439) AD
6p21.33	C2 CFB	ARMD14 (OMIM 615489). Reduced risk of ARMD
5p13.1	C9	ARMD15 (OMIM 615591)

Abbreviations: AD, autosomal dominant; AR, autosomal recessive; ARMD, age-related macular degeneration; OMIM, Online Mendelian Inheritance in Man.

syndrome, and CFEOM3 with polymicrogyria. It is defined by congenital nonprogressive ophthalmoplegia with or without ptosis, due to fibrosis and muscle dysfunction, which result from abnormalities of development of the cranial nerve nuclei serving the extraocular muscles and the nerves that arise from those nuclei.

Each of these disorders may also be seen as part of another genetic syndrome for which a genetic cause is known but via which the isolated condition does not occur: glaucoma in nail–patella syndrome, keratoconus in trisomy 21, and strabismus in a variety of genetic syndromes. Finally, the role of environmental factors is particularly difficult to unravel. For example, diet in ARMD or smoking in glaucoma.

Knowledge of an individual's genotype may confer useful information with regard to risk of being affected, prognosis, and perhaps even therapeutic options. The latter have been termed "personalized medicine" whereby a genotype identifies optimal choices for treatment. Much information remains to be elucidated for these disorders. There are risks to testing as well. For example, one may falsely underestimate risk based on genotype and needlessly abandon screening in an individual who has environmental risk factors. Currently, the costs and risks of routine genetic testing, combined with the need for greater understanding, outweigh the benefits for patients with these conditions, in particular ARMD, for which genetic testing is commercially available.

32.1 Problems

32.1.1 Case 1

A 30-year-old woman comes for genetic consultation with her 60-year-old father and 85-year-old paternal grandmother, both of whom were diagnosed in their 50s with primary open angle glaucoma. Her paternal uncle, a 68-year-old man, is also affected. She wants to know if she will also be affected. Which from the following seems the best genetic test to answer her question?
a) *MYOC*.
b) *OPA1*.
c) Whole exome sequencing (WES).
d) None.

Correct answer is d.
Primary open angle glaucoma is a complex disease, associated with the effects of multiple genes likely in combination with environmental factors. Single gene testing is not likely to be helpful.
a) **Incorrect.** Mutations in *MYOC* are associated with juvenile open angle glaucoma.
b) **Incorrect.** *OPA1* mutations play a role in normal tension glaucoma.
c) **Incorrect.** Although WES may detect mutations or polymorphisms in genes known to be associated with glaucoma or the anterior segment, it is unable at this time to provide a truly diagnostic profile.
d) **Correct.**

32.1.2 Case 2

A 55-year-old, smoking woman comes for genetic consultation. Her deceased father had wet ARMD and was treated more than 15 times with intravitreal injections. She has two paternal aunts with dry ARMD. She wants to be treated "as soon as possible" to avoid "what her father suffered." She read on the internet that this disease is genetic and she wants to learn her risk. Based on the clinical information, which is her probable risk of inheriting the condition?

a) 50%.
b) 25%.
c) 8%.
d) None of the above.

Correct answer is d.

It is impossible to predict recurrence risks for complex disorders even with the use of multiple gene sequencing.

a) **Incorrect.**
b) **Incorrect.**
c) **Incorrect.**
d) **Correct.**

33 Albinism

Abstract

Albinism is a group of disorders characterized by ocular hypopigmentation with or without hypopigmentation of the skin and hair. Most common findings include iris transillumination, nystagmus, and macular hypoplasia. Visual acuity ranges from 20/40 to 20/400, depending primarily on the level of foveal hypoplasia which is in turn related to genotype. Although phenotype may help guide molecular testing strategies, genotype is difficult to predict clinically.

Keywords: albinism, iris transillumination, nystagmus, macular hypoplasia, tyrosinase

Key Points

- Albinism is a group of disorders characterized by ocular hypopigmentation with or without hypopigmentation of the skin and hair.
- Iris transillumination, nystagmus, and macular hypoplasia are the most common features. Visual acuity is between 20/40 and 20/400, depending primarily on the level of foveal hypoplasia.
- Although phenotype may help guide molecular testing strategies, genotype is difficult to predict clinically.

33.1 Overview

Albinism is a group of disorders characterized by reduced pigmentation resulting in ocular abnormalities with or without hypopigmentation of the skin and hair. The latter circumstance is referred to as oculocutaneous albinism (OCA). If only the eyes are affected, the patient has ocular albinism (OA).

Ocular manifestations of albinism include infantile nystagmus, iris transillumination (► Fig. 33.1), fundus hypopigmentation, macular hypoplasia (► Fig. 33.2), and gray optic nerves with or without optic nerve hypoplasia. Iris transillumination is perhaps the most constant feature although it rarely can be absent and sometimes is difficult to detect, especially in the presence of nystagmus. Visual acuity ranges between 20/40 and 20/400, depending primarily on the level of foveal hypoplasia. There is also a higher incidence of strabismus and refractive errors.

Differentiating OA, which is usually an X-linked recessive (XLr) disorder, from autosomal recessive (AR) and the uncommon autosomal dominant (AD) forms of OCA can be aided by examination of the parents. Carriers of all forms of albinism may show subtle, or even more frank, iris transillumination, most often in the inferior iris. Lyonization in female carriers of XLr OA (OA1) may result in irregular retinal pigmentation known as the "mud-splattered fundus," with patches of retinal pigment epithelium (RPE) cells expressing the normal X chromosome, which are pigmented, interspersed with hypopigmented patches of RPE cells expressing the abnormal chromosome X (► Fig. 33.3). A careful search of the skin may reveal hypopigmented patches also due to lyonization.

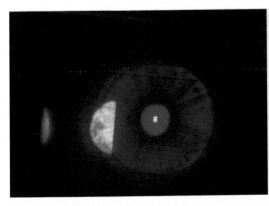

Fig. 33.1 Marked iris transillumination in albinism allowing visualization of the ciliary processes and lens behind the iris.

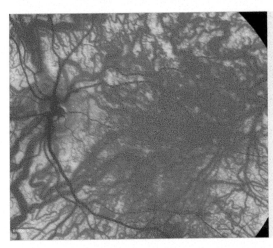

Fig. 33.2 Macular hypoplasia in albinism. Note prominence of choroidal vessels due to hypopigmentation and absence of foveal reflex. One retinal vessel aberrantly enters area where fovea should be.

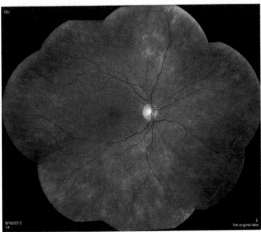

Fig. 33.3 Retina of female carrier of X-linked recessive ocular albinism showing "mud-splattered fundus" due to lyonization. Note patchy retinal pigmentation due to patches of retinal pigmented epithelial cells expressing a normal *GPR143* gene interspersed with hypopigmented patches of cells expressing the abnormal X chromosome copy of this gene.

33.2 Molecular Genetics

Tyrosinase, encoded by the *TYR* gene, is the key enzyme involved in melanin synthesis, through the hydroxylation of tyrosine to L-DOPA (L-3,4-dihydroxyphenylalanine) and the oxidation of L-DOPA to DOPAquinone. There are two types of melanin: eumelanin, which is a darker pigment commonly associated with tanning, and pheomelanin, which is responsible for yellow, orange, and reddish coloration. When eumelanin production is reduced, the pathway is shunted toward pheomelanin production.

Melanin is located in intracellular vesicles called melanosomes, most often found in melanocyte cells. In the eye, melanin is found in the iris-pigmented posterior epithelium, phagocytic clump cells in the iris stroma, retinal pigmented epithelium, and choroidal melanocytes.

Albinism has a gene-based nomenclature (▶ Table 33.1).

33.3 Differential Diagnosis

The presence of iris transillumination is usually abnormal even in lightly pigmented ethnic groups but can occur in other conditions, such as trauma, secondary atrophy (e.g., herpetic uveitis), and prematurity. Albinism should be considered in any child with nystagmus, but in the absence of other cardinal signs, such as iris transillumination or macular hypoplasia, nystagmus is not due to albinism. Macular hypoplasia can be due to isolated *PAX6* mutation or with aniridia, both not associated with iris transillumination. Prematurity can be a cause of iris transillumination. The three-lead visual evoked potential (VEP) may show asymmetric decussations in any condition that leads to signal asymmetry, such as unilateral anophthalmia, severe microphthalmia, or severe amblyopia.

33.3.1 Åland Island Eye Disease (OMIM 300600)

This XLr condition is characterized by fundus hypopigmentation, decreased visual acuity, nystagmus, astigmatism, protan color vision defect, progressive myopia, and

Table 33.1 Albinism gene-based nomenclature

Name	Gene	Inheritance
Tyrosine negative (OCA1)	*Tyr*	AR
Yellow variant (OCA1B)	*Tyr*	AR
Minimal pigment (OCA1MP)	*Tyr*	AR
Temperature sensitive (OCA1TS)	*Tyr*	AR
Type 2 OCA (OCA2)	*OCA2*	AR
Type 3 OCA (OCA3)	*TYRP1*	AR
Type 4 OCA (OCA4)	*SLC45A2*	AR
Type 6 OCA (OCA6)	*SLC24A5*	AR
Type 7 OCA (OCA7)	*C10orf11*	AR
Hermansky–Pudlak syndrome	Nine types	AR
Chediak–Higashi syndrome	*LYST*	AR
X-linked ocular albinism (OA1)	*GPR143*	XLr

Abbreviations: OCA, oculocutaneous albinism; AR, autosomal recessive; XLr, X-linked recessive.

defective dark adaptation. Because of fundus hypopigmentation, it has been labeled as a form of albinism, but there is no misrouting of the optic nerves in the three-lead VEP. Iris transillumination may be seen. This condition is caused by mutation in the *CACNA1F* gene, which also causes XLr incomplete congenital stationary night blindness (CSNB2A; OMIM 300071).

33.3.2 BADS (Behavioral Assessment of the Dysexecutive) Syndrome (OMIM 227010)

This phenotype, also known as ermine phenotype, includes OA, black lock, and deafness. Molecular cause is unknown.

33.3.3 Griscelli Syndrome Type 1 (OMIM 214450)

This rare AR disorder is characterized by hypomelanosis with a primary neurologic deficit but without immunologic impairment or manifestations of hemophagocytic syndrome. It is caused by mutations in the gene encoding myosin VA (*MYO5A*; 15q21.2). Griscelli syndrome with immune impairment is known as Griscelli syndrome type 2 (*RAB27A* gene). Griscelli syndrome type 3 is characterized by hypomelanosis with no immunologic or neurologic manifestations (*MLPH* or *MYO5A* genes).

33.3.4 Elejalde Syndrome (OMIM 256710)

Also known as neuroectodermal melanolysosomal disease, this entity is characterized by profound psychomotor retardation, seizures, hypotonia, involuntary movements, generalized hypopigmentation, and silver-colored hair from early in life. It has been proposed that Elejalde disease and Griscelli syndrome type 1 (*MYO5A* gene) are allelic.

33.3.5 Waardenburg Syndrome

This AD condition is caused by heterozygous mutation in *PAX3* (2q36). It is an auditory–pigmentary syndrome characterized by pigmentary anomalies of the hair (white forelock and premature graying), skin, and eyes (heterochromia irides and brilliant blue eyes), congenital sensorineural hearing loss, and dystopia canthorum. Waardenburg syndrome has been classified into four main phenotypes. Type 1 is distinguished by the presence of dystopia canthorum. Type 2 is characterized by the absence of dystopia canthorum. Type 3 has dystopia canthorum and upper limb abnormalities. Type 4 is also known as Waardenburg–Shah syndrome, and has the additional finding of Hirschsprung's disease.

33.3.6 Prader–Willi/Angelman Syndrome (OMIM 176270/105830)

Prader–Willi syndrome is characterized by diminished fetal activity, obesity, muscular hypotonia, mental retardation, short stature, hypogonadotropic hypogonadism, and small hands and feet. Between 70 and 80% of cases are caused by a contiguous gene deletion of the paternal copy of the imprinted *SNRPN* gene, *NDN* gene, and other genes within the region 15q11-q13. Uniparental disomy of the maternal copy of 15q11-q13 region and de novo unbalanced chromosome translocation have been reported in rare cases. Angelman syndrome is a neurodevelopmental disorder characterized by mental retardation, movement or balance disorder, typical abnormal behaviors, and severe limitations in speech and language. Angelman syndrome can be caused by de novo maternal deletions involving chromosome 15q11.2-q13, paternal uniparental disomy of 15q11.2-q13, imprinting defects, or mutations in the *UBE3A* gene. Both Prader–Willi and Angelman syndromes can present with retinal and skin hypopigmentation as well as pale irides and iris transillumination when caused by a contiguous gene deletion involving the p gene.

33.3.7 Brachymetapody–Anodontia–Hypotrichosis– Albinoidism (OMIM 211370)

There is a Finnish family with three siblings who have congenital anodontia, short stature, shortening of the metacarpals and metatarsals, hypotrichosis, albinoidism, and other ocular anomalies (strabismus, nystagmus, distichiasis, lenticular opacities, and high-grade myopia).

33.3.8 Albinoidism

This AD form of oculocutaneous hypopigmentation differs from albinism because of the absence of hypoplastic foveae, nystagmus, and photophobia. Visual acuity is usually normal, but iris transillumination is present. The patients otherwise appear to be affected with OCA, often with white hair and fair skin complexion.

33.3.9 Albinism Deafness Syndrome (OMIM 300700)

This rare XLr condition (Xq24-q26) describes the combination of profound deafness and OCA. Molecular cause is unknown.

33.3.10 Microcephaly, Oculocutaneous Albinism, and Digital Anomalies Syndrome (OMIM 203340)

There is a report of two siblings with microcephaly, OCA, and hypoplasia of the distal phalanx of several fingers and agenesis of the distal part of the first toe.

33.3.11 Cross Syndrome (OMIM 257800)

This condition includes oculocutaneous hypopigmentation, microphthalmia, spasticity, mental and physical retardation, and athetoid movements. Molecular cause is unknown.

33.3.12 Preus Syndrome (OMIM 257790)

This condition is characterized by growth retardation, dolichocephaly, cataracts, highly arched palate, small and widely spaced teeth, generalized hypopigmentation, psycho-motor retardation, and hypochromic anemia. Molecular cause is unknown.

33.4 Uncommon Manifestations

Albinism may also be associated with systemic findings. Hermansky–Pudlak syndrome is a group of disorders characterized by OCA with widely variable intra- and interfamilial expression; symptoms include a bleeding disorder (platelet storage pool deficiency) and sometimes pulmonary fibrosis or granulomatous colitis. Chediak–Higashi syndrome is associated with cellular immunodeficiency due to abnormalities of white cell chemotaxis. Diagnosis is based on identification of abnormal white blood cell granules on blood smear. Other systemic findings that may be seen in albinism include hearing loss and humoral immunodeficiency.

33.5 Clinical Testing

Patients usually have abnormal visual pathway decussations, with over-decussation of the nerve fibers from each eye to the contralateral cerebral hemisphere. This can be detected by three-lead VEP testing.

33.6 Genetic Testing

Although phenotype may offer some help to approach molecular diagnosis, genotype is often difficult to predict clinically. Most patients with OCA are compound heterozygotes which greatly affects the phenotype. For example, when both copies of *TYR* have null mutations (OCA1A), a severe phenotype is observed, with visual acuity ranging between 20/200 and 20/400. If tyrosinase activity is only partially reduced (e.g., OCA1B), patients will have a milder phenotype, with more pigmentation and better vision acuity. Compound heterozygosity for null and other mutations that variably alter tyrosinase activity will yield a spectrum of phenotypes. Several other genes involved with the pigmentation pathway have been associated with different forms of albinism (see ▶ Table 33.1). Many commercial labs offer multigene test panels to assist in determining an individual's type of albinism.

33.7 Additional Resources

www.albinism.org

33.8 Problems

33.8.1 Case 1

A 6-year-old male patient was referred for nystagmus. Careful examination in a dark room reveals iris transillumination in each eye and mild macular hypoplasia with small gray optic nerves. The child has light-brown hair and a fair complexion. Both parents have light-brown hair and fair complexions. Each parent is examined, and the mother is found to have subtle iris transillumination. Which of the following is true?
a) The child most likely has OCA.
b) Gray optic nerves indicate pigmentation, so the child does not have albinism.
c) The phenotype is diagnostic of OCA1.
d) The child's three-lead VEP will likely be normal.

Correct answer is a.

The diagnosis of albinism, in most cases, is clinical. The presence of nystagmus, iris transillumination, macular hypoplasia, and mild optic nerve hypoplasia with a grayish appearance confirms the diagnosis of albinism.

a) **Correct.**

b) **Incorrect.** Although gray optic nerves are an ocular finding in albinism, the color is not due to melanin.

c) **Incorrect.** OCA phenotypes are a poor predictor of genotype.

d) **Incorrect.** Most patients with OCA show pattern reversal on three-lead VEP as a result of asymmetric visual pathway decussation.

33.8.2 Case 2

A 1-year-old male patient is referred for evaluation of nystagmus. Examination reveals light-colored hair, visual acuity of 20/200 in each eye, iris transillumination, and macular hypoplasia. Further testing reveals asymmetric decussations by three-lead VEP. Both parents are blonde and can tan. Their ocular examinations are normal. What type of OCA does the patient have?

a) OCA1A.

b) OCA1B.

c) OA1.

d) Cannot be determined.

Correct answer is d.

Although history and complete examination can provide important clues, especially when signs of lyonization are found in female carriers, clinical information usually does not correlate well with molecular genetic results, particularly in the first year of life when phenotypes can be similar despite different genotypes.

a) **Incorrect.** *TYR* sequence analysis is the only way to differentiate OCA1A and OCA1B.

b) **Incorrect.** Same as a.

c) **Incorrect.** The question arises as to whether a child is blonde due to family pigmentation and happens to have OA or is blonde because of OCA. If the mother of a male child shows no signs of lyonization, then it is unlikely that the child has OA1.

d) **Correct.**

33.8.3 Case 3

A 5-year-old male with albinism was referred by the pediatrician for "shaky eyes." Examination reveals blonde hair, horizontal symmetric nystagmus, iris transillumination, and hypopigmented fundi with macular hypoplasia in both eyes. You also note that the child has multiple bruises and his mother reveals some occasional bleeding when she brushes his teeth. Further testing reveals normal complete blood count (CBC), platelets, PT (prothrombin time), PTT (partial thromboplastin time), INR (international normalized ratio), and skeletal survey. What is your diagnosis?

a) Chediak–Higashi syndrome.

b) Leukemia.

c) Hermansky–Pudlak syndrome.

d) Child abuse.

Correct answer is c.

This child has a clinical diagnosis of OCA in association with bleeding manifestations but in the absence of an obvious coagulopathy on routine blood testing. The most likely diagnosis is Hermansky–Pudlak syndrome. Screening for pulmonary and gastrointestinal involvement may also be indicated. Confirmation of the diagnosis can be obtained via platelet electron microscopy showing abnormal or absent dense bodies, platelet aggregation/function studies, and/or DNA (deoxyribonucleic acid) analysis of genes known to cause this disorder when mutated.

a) **Incorrect.** Chediak–Higashi syndrome should be suspected in children with OCA and recurrent infection, but bleeding may also be a manifestation when bone marrow involvement occurs.

b) **Incorrect.** Normal blood count should be enough to rule out leukemia in this setting. There is no association between leukemia and albinism.

c) **Correct.**

d) **Incorrect.** Although child abuse should always be considered in a child with multiple unexplained bruises, especially when the child is not ambulatory or the bruises occur on surfaces not commonly injured (e.g., back, trunk, proximal extremities), the history, clinical findings, and normal skeletal survey decrease the chance of abuse.

33.8.4 Case 4

An 8-month-old male patient comes for nystagmus evaluation. The parents are very anxious as they were told that the child would be blind. Hair and skin pigmentation is normal and consistent with the family members. Ocular examination reveals that each eye can fix and follow equally with pendular horizontal symmetric moderate-frequency and large-amplitude nystagmus. There is also iris transillumination, macular hypoplasia, and gray optic nerves. Three-lead VEP reveals pattern reversal. Maternal examination shows a large hypopigmented skin patch on her lower back, mild inferior bilateral iris transillumination, and a "mud-splattered fundus." What is the chance for the next pregnancy of this mother to result in an affected child?

a) 8%.

b) 50%.

c) 25%.

d) 100%.

Correct answer is c.

This child has XLr OA. The large-amplitude nystagmus is common in childhood and often gives the false impression of nonfixation. The mother demonstrates typical features of lyonization. As a heterozygote, there is a 50% chance that any pregnancy will be conceived using an egg that carries the mutated copy of her OA1 gene (*GPR143*). If that egg is fertilized by a sperm carrying an X chromosome, the resulting child will be a female carrier. If the sperm has a Y chromosome, the son will be affected. Therefore, there is a 25% chance of having a carrier daughter, 25% of having an unaffected daughter, 25% chance of having an unaffected son, and a 25% chance of having an affected son.

a) **Incorrect.**

b) **Incorrect.**

c) **Correct.**

d) **Incorrect**

33.8.5 Case 5

A 7-year-old male patient with OCA has been followed by you over the past 4 years without any significant clinical change other than the usual reduction in nystagmus amplitude and the onset of a small face turn-in while fixating straight ahead. The child has marked iris transillumination, white hair, and very fair complexion. The child has no systemic signs or malformations. Parents were interested in molecular genetic testing for pregnancy planning. Which from the following list is most appropriate to begin genetic testing?

a) Albinism multigene panel.
b) *TYR* deletion/duplication analysis.
c) Chromosome microarray.
d) Whole exome sequencing.

Correct answer is a.

In North America, the most common causes of OCA are mutations in either *TYR* or the p gene. As phenotype is a poor predictor of genotype, the use of commercially available multigene panels is a more cost-effective way of optimizing the yield of genetic testing by searching for mutations in several genes in one test, as opposed to testing individual genes one at a time. For example, one laboratory offers testing for OCA1, OCA2, OCA3, and OCA4 while simultaneously screening genes that when mutated cause Hermansky–Pudlak and Chediak–Higashi syndromes. Excellent resources for identifying laboratories that provide such panels (as well as single gene tests where indicated) include Gene Tests (http://www.genetests.org/tests/) and Genetic Testing Registry (https://www.ncbi.nlm.nih.gov/gtr/).

a) **Correct.**
b) **Incorrect.** A *TYR* deletion/duplication is present in less than 1% of albinism. If a multigene panel did not uncover a mutation that explains the patient phenotype, then deletion analysis could be considered.
c) **Incorrect.** Chromosome microarray does not identify intragenic mutations. This test is useful to find copy number variation (e.g., duplications or deletions) that usually affect more than one gene, resulting in findings in addition to the primary disorder. An example would be del15q leading to albinism (p gene deletion) along with Prader–Willi syndrome.
d) **Incorrect.** WES (whole exome sequencing) is only indicated when there is no available or identifiable single gene disorder that can be tested and would explain the patient's condition or such tests return with negative results. It is costly. In addition, as it screens all coding genes it may reveal mutations in genes unrelated to the condition that prompted testing (e.g., Alzheimer's disease, cancer genes), which may raise uncertainty and ethical dilemmas with regard to disclosure.

Suggested Reading

[1] Chiang PW, Spector E, Tsai AC. Oculocutaneous albinism spectrum. Am J Med Genet A. 2009; 149A(7):1590–1591

[2] Hutton SM, Spritz RA. Comprehensive analysis of oculocutaneous albinism among non-Hispanic Caucasians shows that OCA1 is the most prevalent OCA type. J Invest Dermatol. 2008; 128(10):2442–2450

[3] Pott JW, Jansonius NM, Kooijman AC. Chiasmal coefficient of flash and pattern visual evoked potentials for detection of chiasmal misrouting in albinism. Doc Ophthalmol. 2003; 106(2):137–143

[4] Schmitz B, Schaefer T, Krick CM, Reith W, Backens M, Käsmann-Kellner B. Configuration of the optic chiasm in humans with albinism as revealed by magnetic resonance imaging. Invest Ophthalmol Vis Sci. 2003; 44 (1):16–21

[5] Simeonov DR, Wang X, Wang C, et al. DNA variations in oculocutaneous albinism: an updated mutation list and current outstanding issues in molecular diagnostics. Hum Mutat. 2013; 34(6):827–835

[6] Levin AV, Stroh E. Albinism for the busy clinician. J AAPOS. 2011; 15(1):59–66

Index

Note: Page numbers set **bold** or *italic* indicate headings or figures, respectively.

Index